Social Marketing for Public Health

Global Trends and Success Stories

EDITED BY

Hong Cheng, PhD
Associate Professor of Advertising
E. W. Scripps School of Journalism
Ohio University

Philip Kotler, PhD
S. C. Johnson Distinguished Professor of International Marketing
Kellogg School of Management
Northwestern University

Nancy R. Lee, MBA
President
Social Marketing Services Inc.
Adjunct Faculty
Evans School of Public Affairs
University of Washington
College of Public Health
University of South Florida

JONES AND BARTLETT PUBLISHERS
Sudbury, Massachusetts
BOSTON   TORONTO   LONDON   SINGAPORE

World Headquarters

Jones and Bartlett Publishers
40 Tall Pine Drive
Sudbury, MA 01776
978-443-5000
info@jbpub.com
www.jbpub.com

Jones and Bartlett Publishers
Canada
6339 Ormindale Way
Mississauga, Ontario L5V 1J2
Canada

Jones and Bartlett Publishers
International
Barb House, Barb Mews
London W6 7PA
United Kingdom

Jones and Bartlett's books and products are available through most bookstores and online booksellers. To contact Jones and Bartlett Publishers directly, call 800-832-0034, fax 978-443-8000, or visit our website, www.jbpub.com.

Substantial discounts on bulk quantities of Jones and Bartlett's publications are available to corporations, professional associations, and other qualified organizations. For details and specific discount information, contact the special sales department at Jones and Bartlett via the above contact information or send an email to specialsales@jbpub.com.

This publication is designed to provide accurate and authoritative information in regard to the Subject Matter covered. It is sold with the understanding that the publisher is not engaged in rendering legal, accounting, or other professional service. If legal advice or other expert assistance is required, the service of a competent professional person should be sought.

Production Credits
Publisher: Michael Brown
Editorial Assistant: Catie Heverling
Editorial Assistant: Teresa Reilly
Senior Production Editor: Tracey Chapman
Senior Marketing Manager: Sophie Fleck
Manufacturing and Inventory Control Supervisor: Amy Bacus
Composition: Cape Cod Compositors, Inc.
Cover Design: Scott Moden
Photo Research and Permissions Manager: Kimberly Potvin
Associate Photo Researcher: Jessica Elias
Cover Image: © Kay1979/Dreamstime.com (world map); © Dennis Richardson/Dreamstime.com (African woman with bread); © Andersen Ross/age fotostock (vending machine); © Konstantin Sutyagin/ShutterStock, Inc. (runners); © Kristy Tillotson/Dreamstime.com (water pump); © Science Photo Library/age fotostock (patch); © Anette Romanenko/Dreamstime.com (doctor taking blood)
Chapter Openers: Courtesy of the U.S. Central Intelligence Agency/University of Texas Libraries
Printing and Binding: Malloy, Inc.
Cover Printing: Malloy, Inc.

Library of Congress Cataloging-in-Publication Data
Social marketing for public health : global trends and success stories / Edited By Hong Cheng, Philip Kotler, Nancy R. Lee.
     p.   cm.
  Includes bibliographical references and index.
  ISBN-13: 978-0-7637-5797-7 (pbk.)
  ISBN-10: 0-7637-5797-7 (pbk.)
  1. Health promotion. 2. Social marketing. 3. Public health. I. Cheng, Hong. II. Kotler, Philip.
III. Lee, Nancy, 1932–
  RA427.8.S625 2009
  362.1068'8—dc22

                                              2009022876

6048

Printed in the United States of America
13 12 11 10 09   10 9 8 7 6 5 4 3 2 1

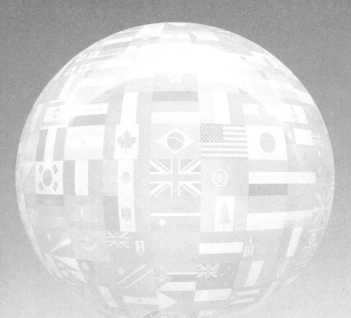

Contents

CHAPTER 2

Reducing Tobacco Use in the United States: A Public Health Success Story . . . So Far   31

Nancy R. Lee

CHAPTER 15

**Social Marketing Practices: Government and Private Partnerships in
Controlling Diseases and Promoting a Healthy Lifestyle in Singapore   357**

Kavita Karan

CHAPTER 16

**Reducing Drink Driving Road Deaths: Integrating Communication and
Social Policy Enforcement in Australia   383**

Samantha Snitow and Linda Brennan

Preface

Of the United Nations' eight Millennium Development Goals, four are related to public health: to eradicate extreme poverty and hunger; to reduce child mortality; to improve maternal health; and to combat HIV/AIDS, malaria, and other diseases (Haider & Rogers, 2005). With the commitment of 189 U.N. member nations to achieving these goals in the years to come (Millennium project, 2006), improving public health has never become so significant, intensive, and time-bound in a global sense.

Identified as an "adaptation [of marketing] to public health imperatives" (Manoff, 1985, p. 35) and one of the "key health communications tools" (Merrick 2005, p. xxv), social marketing has been playing a pivotal role in the improvement of public health since its launch about four decades ago (e.g., Coreil, Bryant, & Henderson, 2001; Kotler & Lee, 2008; Kotler & Zaltman, 1971; Ling, Franklin, Lindsteadt, & Gearon, 1992; Manoff, 1985). This role is continuing and expanding today in achieving the U.N.'s Millennium Development Goals in general and in reaching individual nations' public health-related goals in particular.

Unfortunately, little has been done to synthesize and showcase the practice and success of social marketing in helping to improve public health in the world. This book is the first substantial effort to present in-depth stories of public health campaigns successfully conducted in different parts of the world using the social marketing model.

Featuring success stories from 15 countries spread out across five continents, the book examines how social marketing is used as a strategy for influencing positive health behaviors in the world today. Our book highlights successful and measurable health behavior–changing campaigns launched by governments, citizens, and (in one case) corporations. Each chapter focuses on a unique public health challenge and social marketing solution.

This book is positioned as a supplementary textbook for upper-level undergraduate and graduate courses in social marketing, public health, health communication, international marketing, international advertising, consumer behavior, social change, and public communication. The book's central theme is that knowledge, techniques, and technologies now exist to organize and implement effective health programs globally. To facilitate the book's use in the classroom, discussion questions are provided at the end of each chapter, and a PowerPoint presentation has been created for each chapter as well.

We would like to thank all the chapter authors earnestly. They come from a broad spectrum of intellectual, professional, and cultural backgrounds. Without their valuable contributions, this volume would not be as rich in breadth and depth.

We wish to express our heartfelt thanks to Jones and Bartlett, the book's publisher. In particular, we want to thank Mr. Robert W. Holland Jr., Jones and Bartlett President and Publisher, and Mr. Michael Brown, Publisher for Jones and Bartlett's public health books, for their keen interest and strong support of this book. We especially appreciate the excellent assistance of Jones and Bartlett's Ms. Katey Birtcher, a former Associate Editor and current Acquisitions Editor of the Clinical Nutrition list, Ms. Tracey Chapman, a Senior Production Editor, and Ms. Catie Heverling and Ms. Teresa Reilly, two Editorial Assistants.

REFERENCES

Coreil, J., Bryant, C. A., & Henderson, J. N. (with contributions from M. S. Forthofer & G. P. Quinn). (2001). *Social and behavioral foundations of public health.* Thousand Oaks, CA: Sage Publications.

Haider, M., & Rogers, E. M. (2005). Public health communication: Utility, value, and challenges. In M. Haider (Ed.), *Global public health communication: Challenges, perspectives, and strategies* (pp. xxvii–xxxvii). Sudbury, MA: Jones and Bartlett Publishers.

Kotler, P., & Lee, N. R. (2008). *Social marketing: Influencing behaviors for good* (3rd ed.). Thousand Oaks, CA: Sage Publications.

Kotler, P., & Zaltman, G. (1971). Social marketing: An approach to planned social change. *Journal of Marketing, 35*(3), 3–12.

Ling, J. C., Franklin, B. A. K., Lindsteadt, J. F., & Gearon, S. A. N. (1992). Social marketing: Its place in public health. *Annual Review of Public Health, 13,* 341–362.

Manoff, R. K. (1985). *Social marketing: New imperative for public health.* New York: Praeger Publishers.

Merrick, T. W. (2005). Foreword. In M. Haider (Ed.), *Global public health communication: Challenges, perspectives, and strategies* (p. xxv). Sudbury, MA: Jones and Bartlett Publishers.

Millennium Project. (2006). Core MDG documents. United Nations. Retrieved July 28, 2009, from http://www.unmillenniumproject.org/goals/core_mdgs.htm

Hong Cheng
E. W. Scripps School of Journalism
Ohio University

Philip Kotler
Kellogg School of Management
Northwestern University

Nancy R. Lee
Social Marketing Services Inc.
Adjunct Faculty
Evans School of Public Affairs
University of Washington
College of Public Health
University of South Florida

About the Editors

Hong Cheng (PhD, Pennsylvania State University) is an associate professor of advertising in the E. W. Scripps School of Journalism at Ohio University. His research interests center on social marketing, international and cross-cultural advertising, and global branding. His work has appeared as dozens of journal articles, book chapters, and conference papers. He co-authored (with Guofang Wan) *The Media-Savvy Student* (Chicago: Zephyr Press, 2004) and co-edited (with Kara Chan) *Advertising and Chinese Society: Impacts and Issues* (Copenhagen Business School Press, 2009). He was head of the Advertising Division (2008–2009) and the International Communication Division (2002–2003) of the Association for Education in Journalism and Mass Communication (AEJMC) and was secretary (2005) of the American Academy of Advertising (AAA). He is an associate editor of the *Asian Journal of Communication*, a member of the Editorial Advisory Board of *Journalism and Mass Communication Quarterly*, and a member of the National Academic Committee of the American Advertising Federation (AAF).

Philip Kotler (MA, University of Chicago; PhD, Massachusetts Institute of Technology) is the S. C. Johnson Distinguished Professor of International Marketing at the Kellogg School of Management, Northwestern University. In 2009, he published the Kotler/Keller 13th edition of *Marketing Management*, the world's leading textbook in teaching marketing to MBAs. He also published or co-published *Principles of Marketing, Strategic Marketing for Nonprofit Organizations, Marketing Places, Kotler on Marketing, Marketing Insights A to Z, Lateral Marketing, Social Marketing, Museum Strategies and Marketing, Standing Room Only, Corporate Social Responsibility*, and 30 other books. His research covers strategic marketing, innovation, consumer marketing, business marketing, services marketing, healthcare marketing, and social marketing. He has been a consultant to IBM, Bank of America, Merck, General Electric, Honeywell, and many other companies. He has received honorary doctorate degrees from 11 major universities in the United States and abroad.

Philip Kotler is credited, along with Gerald Zaltman, as having invented the field of social marketing in their article "Social Marketing: An Approach to Planned Social Change" (*Journal of Marketing*, July 1971, pp. 3–12). He wrote the first book discussing this new field, *Social Marketing* (The Free Press, 1989), along with Ned Roberto. Since then, he has been working with Nancy Lee on new editions of *Social Marketing* and social marketing projects. He is also the co-author of *Strategic Marketing for Health Care Organizations: Building a Customer-Driven Health Care System* (Jossey-Bass, 2008).

Nancy R. Lee (BS, University of Illinois; MBA, University of Puget Sound) has more than 25 years of professional marketing experience, with special expertise in social marketing, nonprofit marketing, marketing in the public sector, marketing research, and marketing communications. She is an adjunct faculty member, teaching social marketing, marketing for nonprofit organizations, and strategic marketing for public sector agencies at the University of Washington, the University of South Florida, and Seattle University. She has held numerous corporate marketing positions including vice president and director of marketing for Rainier Bank and director of marketing for Children's Hospital and Regional Medical Center in Seattle. As president of Social Marketing Services Inc. in Seattle since 1993, Nancy Lee has participated in the development of more than 100 social marketing campaign strategies for public sector and nonprofit agencies. She has co-authored five books with Philip Kotler: *Social Marketing: Improving the Quality of Life* (Sage, 2002), *Corporate Social Responsibility: Doing the Most Good for Your Company and Your Cause* (Wiley, 2005), *Marketing in the Public Sector: A Roadmap for Improved Performance* (Wharton School Publishing, 2006), *Social Marketing: Influencing Behaviors for Good* (Sage, 2008), and *UP and OUT of Poverty: The Social Marketing Solution* (Wharton School Publishing, 2009).

About the Contributors

Paola Artoni is a physician specializing in hygiene and preventive medicine. Since 2005, she has been working in the Communication and Social Marketing Department of the Local Health Unit of Modena (Italy). She is part of the scientific secretarial staff of the Health Marketing national competition and co-author of articles related to health promotion and social marketing in Italian magazines.

Jaidev Balakrishnan has more than 15 years of experience working with reputed advertising agencies such as Chaitra Leo Burnett and Percept Advertising. A postgraduate student in marketing at Lucknow University, he is currently working as a senior communication manager with Population Services International, managing social marketing projects. He has been instrumental in the design of three multimedia communication campaigns in the field of maternal and child health in the states of Uttar Pradesh, Uttaranchal, and Rajasthan.

Anurudra Bhanot's 20-year career in advertising and marketing has seen him work for dairy cooperatives, pharmaceuticals, and market research agencies across Asia and Africa. He currently heads the Research and Learning division for South Asia at BBC World Service Trust office in New Delhi. His work includes formative, pretesting, and summative research support for BBC WST's Development Communication projects in the region. A postgraduate student of the Institute of Rural Management, Anand, Anurudra completed advanced training in Market Research Analysis from the Indian Institute of Management, Ahmedabad.

Linda Brennan holds a PhD from the University of Melbourne and a Bachelor of Business (Honours) from Monash University in Australia. She is Deputy Dean in the Faculty of Business & Enterprise at Swinburne University of Technology in Melbourne. In the lead-up to becoming a full-time academic associate professor, she had an active consulting practice in marketing and strategic research. Her clients have included government, not-for-profit, and educational marketers. Her research interests are social and government marketing and, especially, the influence of marketing communications and advertising on behavior.

Sameer Deshpande moved to North America and earned his PhD from the University of Wisconsin–Madison, after spending his early years in India. Currently, he is an associate professor in marketing in the Faculty of Management and faculty member of the Centre for Socially Responsible Marketing at the University of Lethbridge, Canada. His research interests include applying social marketing thought to a variety of public health issues. In 2007, thanks to a faculty fellowship from the Shastri Indo-Canadian Institute, he investigated how social marketing organizations manage their stakeholders to promote contraceptives in India.

Sanjeev Dham has worked on large-scale operations through various positions, translating strategic thinking into action for more than 15 years in Population Services International. He planned and executed innovative behavioral change communication strategies for four birth spacing programs and one HIV/AIDS program. He conceptualized and implemented a unique and cost-effective rural sales distribution model that provided a new approach to the family planning programs. He also promoted the use of modern contraceptive methods in the rural population using the unique child health route as a hook. He is presently working as a state director.

Karin M. Ekström is a professor of marketing at University of Borås and former director and initiator of Center for Consumer Science, Sweden. Her research concerns family consumption, consumer socialization, collecting, and brands. She has edited several books, including *Children, Media and Consumption, on the Front Edge* (2007), *Little Monster, (De)Coupling Assemblages of Consumption* (2007), and *Elusive Consumption* (2004). Her academic works have appeared in the *Journal of Consumer*

Behaviour, Research in Consumer Behavior, Advances in Consumer Research, Academy of Marketing Science Review, and *Journal of Consumer Research.* She is a member of the editorial review board for *Consumption, Markets and Culture, Journal of Consumer Behaviour, Journal of Macromarketing, Young Consumers,* and *Academy of Marketing Science Review* and a member of the Royal Society of Arts and Sciences in Göteborg.

Giuseppe Fattori is a physician with vast experience in the management of healthcare services. Since 2000, he has been the director of the Communication and Social Marketing Department at the Local Health Unit of Modena (Italy), where he develops and leads health communication and prevention activities. In this field, he studies and tests social marketing strategies for health promotion. In reference to these topics, he has published several articles in Italian magazines. He is head of the research area relevant to Social Marketing and Health Communication and the National Social Marketing Work Group, activated by the Italian Association of Public and Institutional Communication. He is also the president of the Health Marketing national competition panel and collaborates with the University of Bologna on a specialist degree course in Public, Social, and Political Communication Science, where he teaches in the Social Marketing Educational Lab.

Lena Hansson is a researcher at the Center for Consumer Science (CFK) at School of Business, Economics and Law, University of Gothenburg, Sweden. She holds a PhD in business administration and conducts research on consumption and design, universal design and social sustainability, and gender issues related to design. A recent project concerns market communication and older consumers (55+ consumers). Her thesis "Universal Design—A Marketable or Utopian Concept?" was published in 2006. Other publications include "The Impact of Design. Allies Fighting Design Exclusion" in *Little Monsters, (De)Coupling Assemblages of Consumption* (2007, edited by Brembeck, Ekström, & Mörck), and "Designing for Inclusion Rather than Exclusion" in *European Advances in Consumer Research* (vol. 7, 2006). Before pursuing her academic career, she was a consultant and project leader with information technology and software development projects.

Emma Heesom joined the National Social Marketing Centre (in London) in 2005. She has a diverse public sector and not-for-profit sector communications background, having worked for several agencies, including the National Blood Service and the Salvation Army. Emma worked on secondment to the NSM Centre in 2005/2006 and became a freelancer in 2006, when she took up a post as media and campaign manager for the School Food Trust. She has a tested and comprehensive range of communications and public relations skills, having been actively involved in campaigning for smoke-free legislation; developing a highly successful advertising and public affairs campaign; and, more recently, managing a busy press office.

Morikazu Hirose is an associate professor of marketing and advertising in the Faculty of Business Administration, Tokyo Fuji University, Japan. His research interests center on corporate communications, advertising media, and sales promotion. He has published in the *International Journal of Advertising*, *Tourism Management*, and the proceedings of the American Academy of Advertising, the Global Marketing Conference, the European Marketing Academy, and the International Conference on Research in Advertising.

Steven W. Honeyman is the director of global capacity building at Population Services International and is based in Bangkok, Thailand. He leads a team that strengthens PSI-affiliated social marketing organizations in more than 60 countries and assists in the professional development of PSI's 8,000 employees worldwide. Prior to his current position, he led 47 international social marketing and social franchising projects and launched 28 products and services in Burma/Myanmar, the Central African Republic, and Nepal over the past 15 years. He has been the executive producer of several award-winning social marketing media projects and won the Population Institute's Global Media Award for "Best Television Documentary" in 2004. He has been on expert panels and given papers or presentations at some two dozen international public health and social marketing conferences. He has contributed to Philip Kotler and Nancy Lee's *Social Marketing: Influencing Behaviors for Good* (Sage, 2008) and *Marketing in the Public Sector: A Roadmap for Improved Performance* (Wharton School Publishing, 2006).

Kavita Karan teaches in the School of Journalism, College of Mass Communication and Media Arts at Southern Illinois University Carbondale. She received her PhD from the London School of Economics and Political Science. She has extensively investigated issues related to the representation of women and men in advertising, health communication, Internet and rural communities in Asia, Indian cinema, and political communication. She teaches courses in research methods, marketing, and advertising. She has presented papers at various international conferences and contributed several papers for journals and chapters for books. Her edited and co-edited books include *Cyber Communities in Rural Asia: A Study of Seven Asian Countries* and *Commercializing Women: Images of Asian Women in the Media*.

Cathie Kryzanowski is the manager of *Saskatchewan in Motion*. For the past 30 years, she has promoted physical activity and active living in her various positions with local, provincial, and national organizations, such as the YMCA, Boys and Girls Clubs, City of Regina, Tourism Regina, and ParticipACTION. She was elected to the Active Living Canada Board of Stewards in 1995 and became the founding chair of the national Coalition for Active Living in 1999. As a frequent public speaker, she has shared her many experiences at conferences and seminars across North America and elsewhere in the world.

François Lagarde is a Canadian social marketing and communications consultant and trainer for numerous organizations in the health, philanthropy, development aid, and housing fields in Canada and in nine countries abroad. From 1984 to 1991, he worked for ParticipACTION, a national fitness promotion agency, where he served as vice president and manager of national media campaigns. He is an adjunct professor in the Faculty of Medicine at the University of Montreal, where he teaches social marketing in the health administration and public health programs. He has published numerous reports, book chapters, cases, guides, and articles. He is a member of the *Social Marketing Quarterly* editorial review board. He is also a member of the steering committee for the "Innovations in Social Marketing" conference. As part of his consultancy, he acts as a senior advisor to *Saskatchewan in Motion*.

Ruth Massingill has more than 20 years experience in journalism, public relations, and advertising as a professional communicator as well as an administrator and faculty member at Sam Houston State University in Huntsville, Texas. Recent awards she has received include the 2008 Excellence in Teaching Award and the 2007 Achievement in Mass Communication Award for Outstanding Research and Scholarship (SHSU College of Humanities and Social Science), Outstanding Educator (American Advertising Federation, 2002), and Outstanding Faculty (University of Phoenix-Houston, 2003). She is lead author for a book on prison communications, *Prison City: Life with the Death Penalty in Huntsville, Texas* (Peter Lang, 2007), and regularly presents communication research papers at national and international conferences. She holds an MA in journalism from the University of Wyoming and is currently working toward a PhD in social marketing from the University of Teesside in Middlesbrough, England.

Rowena Merritt is program manager at the National Social Marketing Centre (in London), leading development of the local practitioner development and support program. She has helped develop training, skills, and related resources and has overseen the establishment of a number of collaborative demonstration initiatives with local organizations. She is also the convenor for the National Social Marketing Academic Advisory Group, which is helping expand academic sector capacity in social marketing. She graduated in 2001 from Imperial College with a first in business studies. She spent the third year of the course working with Depression Alliance, a mental health charity, coordinating its marketing and publications. This experience awoke an interest in applying marketing techniques to the alleviation of depression. She commenced a DPhil with the University of Oxford in 2002. Her doctoral thesis, completed in 2006, explores the use of social marketing techniques to improve clinical outcomes for depressed patients.

James H. Mintz is the director of the Centre of Excellence for Public Sector Marketing. He is also the program director of the Public Sector and Non-Profit Marketing Certificate and Executive Certificate at Carleton University's Sport School of Business. He lectures at the University of South Florida College of Public Health (Tampa). He was formerly the director of marketing and corporate communications at Health Canada. For more than 20 years, his responsibilities included directing major social marketing and communications campaigns. He was also an adjunct professor of marketing at the University of Ottawa School of Management. He is a member of the steering committee for the "Innovations in Social Marketing" conference and serves on the planning committee for MARCOM. He has also provided social marketing advice and consultation to a number of government departments and nonprofit organizations.

Jun Qiao (PhD, Nanjing Normal University) is the dean and a professor of the School of Marketing and Logistics at Nanjing University of Finance and Economics, China. He was a visiting scholar at Ohio University in 2007. His research interests center on branding theory and service marketing. He has published more than 150 articles, including articles in the *World of Management*, *China Industrial Economics*, and *China Advertising*. He is the author of five books, including *Principles of Marketing* (Nanjing: Dongnan University Press, 2006) and *Brand Value Theories* (Beijing: China Finance and Economics Press, 2007). He is the deputy secretary of the Academic Committee of the China Advertising Association, the chair of the editorial board for *Marketing Weekly*, and an associate editor of *Marketing Guide* in China.

Lucy Reynolds joined the National Social Marketing Centre (in London) in 2007, after working as a regeneration consultant based at London Bridge. She has broad project management experience and has worked with public and private sector clients, including NDCs, Business Enterprise Centres, Voluntary Service deliverers, and community practitioners. Her move to the NSM Centre resulted from a growing interest in health interventions and issues of sustainability and was prompted by project work undertaken for SureStart. She completed her DPhil at Oxford University, where she wrote on 19th-century poetry and philology. She brings with her strong research and communication skills, combined with a commitment to achieving social good. She is currently working across the programs, with a particular interest in childhood diet and obesity interventions, as well as environmental change.

Donald Ruschman is a marketing/marketing communications and management specialist concentrating in the areas of market development and reform and social marketing. He has more than 25 years of both domestic (U.S.) and international client service experience in the Former Soviet Union, Near East, Asia, and the Caribbean. He holds an MBA in marketing and international business. From 1994 to 1999, he served as the regional director for the USAID-funded SOMARC (Futures Group—Social Marketing for Change) Central Asian Project, based in Almaty, Kazakhstan, and covering the Former Soviet Republics of Kazakhstan, Uzbekistan, Kyrgyzstan, Turkmenistan, and Tajikistan. He has also worked as the Futures Group's Manager for the Near-East, Asia, and Caribbean under USAID's first worldwide social marketing effort, SOMARC I, from 1984 to 1986, and as a consultant to the predecessor to SOMARC, USAID's ICSMP (International Contraceptive Social Marketing Project) in Sri Lanka and the Caribbean.

Willard D. Shaw is an international development professional with extensive experience in the design and implementation of programs in malaria prevention, public–private partnerships, child survival, behavior change communication, and adult education. He has worked on long-term field assignments in Asia and Africa and overseen technical assistance to dozens of other countries. From 2000 to 2005, he served as NetMark's Africa-based field manager, setting up programs in seven countries aimed at establishing sustainable commercial markets for insecticide-treated nets, working with nine multinational companies and 41 African distributors. He has published articles on public health and educational issues. He holds a BA from Princeton University, an MA from the University of Hawaii, and an MEd and EdD from the Center for International Education of the University of Massachusetts Amherst. He is a vice president in the Global Health, Population, and Nutrition Group of the AED (U.S.).

Samantha Snitow holds a BA from Tufts University and an MA from the Royal Melbourne Institute of Technology. She conducted research on the subject of drink driving and communications as a Fulbright Scholar to Australia and has worked in the fields of road safety and communications at the Transport Accident Commission of Victoria and the Walsh Group of Bethesda, Maryland.

Tatiana Stafford has 15 years of international experience in project management, marketing, and communications. Fluent in Russian, English, and Spanish, she has worked in Russia, the United States, Central Asia, and Latin America. She holds a master's degree in computerized design systems. From 1997 to 1999, she acted as the project manager for the USAID-funded SOMARC (Futures Group—Social Marketing for Change) Project in Almaty, Kazakhstan. She also served as country coordinator for the Central Asian follow-on program to SOMARC, the USAID-funded PSI (Population Services International) and CMS (Commercial Market Strategies) project for the final two years of USAID support during the project's transition to the commercial sector and local NGO management.

Marcello Tedeschi is a professor of marketing. He teaches graduate and postgraduate courses (at both the master's and PhD levels) in marketing, consumer behavior, and psychology of decisions. He developed his research activities with particular focuses on consumer attitude, heuristics, and biases in decision-making processes. He is a member of the ACR (Association for Consumer Research) and IAREP (International Association for Research in Economic Psychology). Since 2006, he has been the director of the Marketing Research and Lab in the Department of Cognitive, Quantitative, and Social Sciences at the University of Modena and Reggio Emilia (Italy).

Randi Thompson is a marketing communication specialist with 30 years of experience in developing outcome-based marketing and communications projects designed to effect social change, including 15 years in Russia, Eurasia, the Caribbean, and South America. Currently, she is chief executive officer/executive director of Kidsave International, a social change organization she co-founded in 1997, which is dedicated to transforming child welfare systems worldwide so that every child has the opportunity to grow up in a family. She also spent 15 years with the public relations and social marketing firm, Porter Novelli, as its executive vice president. She holds an MA in communications from the University of Maryland. From 1994 to 1998, she headed marketing/communications for the USAID-funded SOMARC, Central Asian Project in Kazakhstan and Uzbekistan. She also served as a communications and marketing consultant under USAID's pre-SOMARC project, the IC-SMP (International Contraceptive Social Marketing Project) from 1979 to 1981 in Haiti; in SOMARC II in the Philippines; and in SOMARC III in Senegal, Morocco, Niger, and Ghana.

Aiden Truss joined the National Social Marketing Centre (in London) in 2006. He has a background in information technology, with nearly 10 years of experience in systems administration and project management as well as Web design and implementation. He has worked in both the public and private sectors. Prior to joining the Centre, he managed the information technology systems for the National Consumer Council. Within the team, he is responsible for marketing and new media. This includes managing the Centre's Web site, producing regular bulletins for its e-network, production of new marketing materials, and writing articles for publication. He is currently studying part-time for an MA in cultural and critical studies.

Huixin Zhang (MA, Shanghai Normal University) is the editor-in-chief and president of *China Advertising* and an adjunct professor with the Department of Advertising at Shanghai University. His research is focused on advertising strategies and advertising creativity. He did research in these areas at the Dentsu Group in Japan in 2003 and published dozens of articles over the years. He is the author of several books, including *Brand Positing Strategies in China* (Shanghai University of Finance and Economics Press, 2006) and *Advertising Creativity and Design* (Shanghai Periodical Publishing House, 2006). He is a member of the Academic Committee of the China Advertising Association, the Advertising Committee of the China Enterprise United Association, and the International Advertising Institute (IAI) in China.

CHAPTER 1

Social Marketing for Public Health

An Introduction

Hong Cheng, Philip Kotler, and Nancy R. Lee

SOCIAL MARKETING: A BRIEF OVERVIEW

Evolution and Definition

When this book was completed in 2009, it had been exactly 40 years since the publication of Kotler and Levy's (1969) pioneering article, "Broadening the Concept of Marketing." It was in this article that the idea of social marketing was first introduced and discussed. Kotler and Levy clearly proposed that as "a pervasive societal activity," marketing "goes considerably beyond the selling of toothpaste, soap, and steel," urging marketing researchers and practitioners to consider "whether traditional marketing principles are transferable to the marketing of organizations, persons, and ideas" (p. 10).

Subsequently, the term *social marketing* was formally introduced in 1971 (e.g., Basil, 2007; Kotler & Lee, 2008), when Kotler and Zaltman (1971) coined the term.

In their article, they provided a clear definition for social marketing, discussed the requisite conditions for effective social marketing, elaborated on the social marketing approach, outlined the social marketing planning process, and deliberated on the social implications of social marketing.

Kotler and Zaltman (1971) defined *social marketing* as:

> the design, implementation, and control of programs calculated to influence the acceptability of social ideas and involving considerations of product planning, pricing, communication, distribution, and marketing research. (p. 5)

Over the years, modifications have been made to the definition of social marketing (e.g., Andreasen, 1995; French & Blair-Stevens, 2005; Kotler & Roberto, 1989). Although wording in the definitions of social marketing varies, the essence of social marketing remains unchanged. In this book, we adopt the following definition:

> Social marketing is a process that applies marketing principles and techniques to create, communicate, and deliver value in order to influence target audience behaviors that benefit society as well as the target audience. (P. Kotler, N. R. Lee, & M. Rothschild, personal communication, September 19, 2006)

As indicated in this definition, several features are essential to social marketing:

- It is a distinct discipline within the field of marketing.
- It is for the good of society as well as the target audience.
- It relies on the principles and techniques developed by commercial marketing, especially the marketing mix strategies, conventionally called the 4Ps—product, price, place, and promotion.

Here, two points deserve more of our attention—one is the integration of the 4Ps; the other is the focus on behavior change in any social marketing campaign. As Bill Smith of the Academy for Educational Development, a Washington, DC–based nonprofit organization "working globally to improve education, health, civil society, and economic development" (AED, 2009), aptly observed:

> the genius of modern marketing is not the 4Ps, or audience research, or even exchange, but rather the management paradigm that studies, selects, balances, and manipulates the 4Ps to achieve behavior change. We keep shortening "The Marketing Mix" to the 4Ps. . . . [I]t is the "mix" that matters most. This is exactly what all the message campaigns miss—they never ask about the other 3Ps and that is why so many of them fail. (Kotler & Lee, 2008, p. 3)

As Kotler and Lee (2008) emphasized, "social marketing is about influencing behaviors"; "[s]imilar to commercial sector marketers who sell goods and services, social marketers are selling behaviors" (p. 8). As they elaborated, social marketers typically try to influence their target audience toward four behavioral changes:

> (1) *accept* a new behavior (e.g., composting food waste), (2) *reject* a potential undesirable behavior (e.g., starting smoking), (3) *modify* a current behavior (e.g., increasing physical activity from 3 to 5 days of the week), or (4) *abandon* an old undesirable one (e.g., talking on a cell phone while driving). (p. 8)

Applications

Social marketing principles and techniques can be used to benefit society in general and the target audience in particular in several ways. There are four major arenas that social marketing efforts have focused on over the years: health promotion, injury prevention, environmental protection, and community mobilization (Kotler & Lee, 2008).

Health promotion–related behavioral issues that could benefit from social marketing include tobacco use, heavy/binge drinking, obesity, teen pregnancy, HIV/AIDS, fruit and vegetable intake, high cholesterol, breastfeeding, cancers, birth defects, immunizations, oral health, diabetes, blood pressure, and eating disorders.

Injury prevention–related behavioral issues that could benefit from social marketing include drinking and driving, seatbelts, head injuries, proper safety restraints for children in cars, suicide, drowning, domestic violence, gun storage, school violence, fires, injuries or deaths of senior citizens caused by falls, and household poisons.

Environmental protection–related behavioral issues that could benefit from social marketing include waste reduction, wildlife habitat protection, forest destruction, toxic fertilizers and pesticides, water conservation, air pollution from automobiles and other sources, composting garbage and yard waste, unintentional fires, energy conservation, litter (such as cigarette butts), and watershed protection.

Community mobilization–related behavioral issues that could benefit from social marketing include organ donation, blood donation, voting, literacy, identity theft, and animal adoption (Kotler & Lee, 2008).

For a more detailed review of these applications of social marketing, please see Kotler and Lee's 2008 text, *Social Marketing: Influencing Behaviors for Good*, pages 18–21. In this book, we focus on the successful applications of social marketing principles and techniques on public health–related issues.

SOCIAL MARKETING AND PUBLIC HEALTH

Defining Public Health

Throughout human history, the major health problems that individuals have faced have been occurring at the levels of their communities, their countries, or even the entire world (such as the control of transmittable diseases, the improvement of the physical environment, the quality and supply of water and food, the provision of medical care, and the relief of disability and destitution). Although emphasis placed on each of these problems has varied from time to time and from country to country, "they are all closely related, and from them has come public health as we know it today" (Rosen, 1993, p. 1).

In this book, a widely cited quotation by C.-E. A. Winslow, "the founder of modern public health in the United States" (Merson, Black, & Mills, 2006, p. xiii), is borrowed to define *public health* as:

> the science and art of preventing disease, prolonging life, and promoting physical health and efficiency through organized community efforts for the sanitation of the environment, the control of communicable infections, the education of the individual in personal hygiene, the organization of medical and nursing services for the early diagnosis and preventive treatment of disease, and the development of the social machinery which will ensure to every individual a standard of living adequate for the maintenance of health; organizing these benefits in such a fashion as to enable every citizen to realize his birthright of health and longevity. (Winslow, 1920, as cited in Merson et al., 2006, p. xiii)

Public health has several distinguishing features:

- *It uses prevention as a prime intervention strategy* (such as the prevention of illness, deaths, hospital admissions, days lost from school or work, or consumption of unnecessary human or fiscal resources).
- *It is grounded in a broad array of sciences* (including epidemiology, biological sciences, biostatistics, economics, psychology, anthropology, and sociology).
- *It has the philosophy of social justice as its central pillar* (so the knowledge obtained about how to ensure a healthy population must be extended equally to all groups in any society).
- *It is linked with government and public policy* (which have strong impacts on many public health activities carried out by nonprofit organizations and/or the private sector; Merson et al., 2006).

Social Marketing for Public Health

Social marketing has been widely used in solving public health problems, has fast become "part of the health domain" (Ling, Franklin, Lindsteadt, & Gearon, 1992,

p. 360), and will "play a bigger role in public health" (p. 358). For example, it has been used to:

- Reduce AIDS risk behaviors.
- Prevent teen smoking.
- Fight child abuse.
- Increase utilization of public health services.
- Combat various chronic diseases.
- Promote family planning, breastfeeding, good nutrition, physical exercise, contraceptive use, infant weaning foods, childhood immunizations, and oral rehydration therapy. (Coreil, Bryant, & Henderson, 2001)

Today, social marketing has been applied to an even broader array of public health activities and programs—from the safe drinking water campaign in Madagascar, to the promotion of mosquito nets in Nigeria, and then to the anti–drink driving program in Australia (yes, *drink* driving!), to mention but a few of the cases covered in this book.

Social marketing has offered public health professionals "an effective approach for developing programs to promote healthy behaviors" (Coreil et al., 2001, p. 231). It has also provided public health with "a new institutional mindset," in which "solutions to problems are solicited from consumers" (p. 231), mainly through *formative research* that obtains insights into target audience's needs and wants. An organization that has adopted the social marketing mindset "continually evaluates and remakes itself so as to increase the likelihood that it is meeting the needs of its ever-changing constituency" (p. 231).

USING SOCIAL MARKETING FOR PUBLIC HEALTH: GLOBAL TRENDS

A major purpose of this book is to identify some global trends in using social marketing for public health. Due to limited space, we could only cover cases from 15 countries, carefully selected. These cases speak volumes for what is going on in today's world regarding how social marketing is being applied in public health. At least 10 trends are noteworthy in our view.

Trend 1: Going Global for Public Health

Social marketing can be seen as an "American invention" in the 20th century, because the concept was initially formulated in the United States (see Kotler & Levy, 1969), and the term was then coined by U.S. scholars (see Kotler & Zaltman, 1971).

Today, social marketing practice and successful social marketing campaigns can be found all over the world. Countries active in applying social marketing techniques to public health vary at the levels of economic and technological developments and differ in social, cultural, and regulatory environments.

The case studies presented in this book are just a small sample of the success stories. Here are a few "indicators" of the global scope of social marketing:

- In 1996, Alan Andreasen of Georgetown University in Washington, DC, launched the Social Marketing Listserv, listproc@listproc.georgetown.edu, a worldwide e-mail list for social marketers. Currently, the listserv has about 2,100 subscribers from more than 40 countries, who constantly share information and discuss questions about social marketing research and practice via this server. A large part of their discussions involve public health (A. R. Andreasen, personal communication, August 12, 2009).

- On September 29 and 30, 2008, a World Social Marketing Conference was held in Brighton, England. More than 700 delegates from all over the world came together "to network, learn, and share knowledge and experience" at this first global conference of its kind (World Social Marketing Conference, 2008). During this two-day conference, many success stories on social marketing for public health, among others, were told.

- In the same year, the *International Journal of Nonprofit and Voluntary Sector Marketing* ran a special issue on social marketing. Most of the articles published in this special issue were about public health (Wymer, 2008).

- Also in 2008, a survey conducted by the U.S.–based Advertising Council, in partnership with the International Advertising Association (IAA), revealed that IAA members are "dedicated to promoting social causes and advocate for increased participation across the globe" (Survey finds, 2008, p. 1). According to the survey, 66% of respondents have been actively involved in social marketing efforts. In addition, 84% of respondents say the media outlets in their countries support social marketing efforts through donated media space or time. The research also indicates that most respondents think "social marketing efforts in other countries could be useful learning tools" and believe "working together on issues of common interest could bring about positive social change" (Survey finds, 2008, p. 1). More than half of the respondents expressed interest in collaborating on social marketing campaigns internationally (Survey finds, 2008).

Trend 2: Integration of Downstream, Midstream, and Upstream Efforts

Social marketing was once called "an administrative theory" because it was perceived as "essentially source-dominated" (Baran & Davis, 2009, p. 259). The critics held that social marketing "assumes the existence of a benign information provider seeking to bring about useful, beneficial social change" (Baran & Davis, 2009, p. 259). These critics failed to see the complete picture of today's social marketing theory and practice. In 2006, Andreasen described the expanded roles for social marketing in his book, *Social Marketing in the 21st Century*, seeing social marketing as "about making the world a better place for everyone—not just for investors or foundation executives" (p. 11). As he elaborated,

> the same basic principles [of marketing] that can induce a 12-year-old in Bangkok or Leningrad to get a Big Mac and a caregiver in Indonesia to start using oral rehydration solutions for diarrhea can also be used to influence politicians, media figures, community activities, law officers and judges, foundation officials, and other individuals whose actions are needed to bring about widespread, long-lasting, positive social change. (p. 11)

"[T]o take social marketing to the 'next level' of influence and impact" (p. 11), Andreasen (2006) outlined a vertical perspective, in addition to the "traditional" horizontal perspective. As he put it,

> [w]e need *vertical perspectives* to understand where social problems come from, how they arise on various social agendas, and how they are addressed. A *horizontal perspective* then is needed to consider the range of players who need to act and the kinds of changes that have to happen for the social change process to move forward. (p. 12)

Andreasen's (2006) thought has actually been put into practice in many social marketing campaigns. In this book, Chapters 3 and 5 illustrate social marketing successes for public health in both horizontal and vertical perspectives. The only difference lies in the different terms used in these chapters. While the horizontal perspective is called *downstream* efforts in the chapters, the vertical perspective is described as *upstream* efforts. Between these two types of efforts, a third dimension of social marketing—midstream efforts—is also introduced in Chapter 5. *Midstream* efforts are made to reach "those with the ability to influence others in the target markets' community," including family members, neighbors, co-workers, and friends. Midstream efforts could be as critical as downstream and upstream efforts for the success of a social marketing campaign. Chapter 3 describes how a mass media campaign (to reach the main segment of the target audience) and an advocacy campaign (to reach key stakeholders and decision makers) were integrated in the "Saskatchewan in motion" campaign in Canada.

Trend 3: Building Partnerships

Public health issues are often so complex that no single agency is able to "make a dent by itself." No wonder some social marketers even deem partnership as one of the "additional social marketing Ps" (Weinreich, 2006, p. 1).

Partners for social marketers can be nonprofit organizations (at local, national, or international levels), private sectors, governments, media organizations, local communities (or online communities), and even individuals (like volunteers).

This book reviews some creative and effective short-term and long-term partnerships. In Chapter 9, social marketers for mosquito nets in Nigeria partnered with international net and insecticide manufacturers as well as Nigerian distributors. In Chapter 10, social marketers of the safe drinking water program in Madagascar had more than 12,000 government volunteer community healthcare workers as partners; they also partnered with the government and nongovernmental organizations (NGOs) in the training of those volunteers for the program. In Chapter 12, the Chinese government, public health organizations, a global pharmaceutical company, marketing professionals, media outlets, and voluntary individuals (such as popular singing and movie stars) partnered in a nationwide anti–hepatitis B campaign. In Chapter 15, the National Environment Agency (NEA) in Singapore partnered with other government agencies, private organizations (such as construction companies), schools, and town councils in an anti–dengue fever campaign.

Trend 4: Corporate Social Initiatives to Support Social Marketing Efforts

Research has documented that "[i]n response to pressures to be more socially responsible, corporations are becoming more active in global communities through direct involvement in social initiatives" (Hess & Warren, 2008, p. 163). Defined as "a commitment to improving community well-being through discretionary business practices and contributions of corporate resources" (Kotler & Lee, 2005, p. 3), *corporate social initiatives* include six major options for doing social good:

- *Corporate cause promotions* to increase awareness and concern for social causes.
- *Cause-related marketing* to make contributions to social causes based on product sales.
- *Corporate social marketing* to support behavior-changing campaigns.

- *Corporate philanthropy* to make direct contributions to social causes.
- *Community volunteering* to have employees donate their time and talents.
- *Socially responsible business practices*, which involve discretionary business practices and investments to support social causes. (Kotler & Lee, 2005)

The case reviewed in Chapter 13 illustrates a successful example of how corporate social initiatives are practiced by Terumo Corporation, a Tokyo-headquartered global medical products and equipment manufacturer. In that case, many of the aforementioned options were implemented.

Successful corporate social initiatives often create a win–win situation for both the social marketing program and the corporation. Such initiatives have "the potential to achieve sustainability" (Agha, Do, & Armand, 2006, p. 28). For example, when a donor-funded project partners with a manufacturer and/or distributor willing to market a contraceptive at a price lower than those of other commercial brands, this partnership may make it profitable for the commercial partner(s) because the brand awareness and loyalty created through the social marketing program could continue to benefit the manufacturer and/or distributor after the donor support is over (Agha et al., 2006).

Successful corporate social initiatives are also believed to be an effective way to break through clutter, a major challenge all commercial marketers and advertisers are facing today. No wonder some say, "if there is nothing more distinctive about your brand of cell phone, then surely there is a cause you can identify with, which will raise your brand way above those of your competitors" (Sparg, 2008, p. 1). Nowadays, in many smart companies, corporate social initiatives have been shifted "from obligation to strategy" (Kotler & Lee, 2005, p. 7).

As more and more private companies are engaged in corporate social initiatives, social marketing, as a subfield of marketing, originally "derived" from commercial marketing, will "reblend" with commercial sectors. This "reblend" is created through reaching shared objectives—to do a social good and to create a win–win situation for both social causes and private companies involved.

Trend 5: Integration of the 4Ps

The 4Ps in social marketing mix strategies cannot be developed in isolation—it is the "mix," or "synergy," of the 4Ps that makes a truly successful social marketing campaign possible. Social marketing for public health is more than health communication. The other 15 chapters in this book illustrate the need for social marketers to develop products, or at least include them in campaign efforts, and the benefit of integrating the 4Ps to achieve campaign success.

Trend 6: Integration of Various Communication Formats and Media

The success of a social marketing campaign utilizes various communication formats and media. The *communication formats* consist mainly of advertising (including public service advertising, simply called PSA), public relations, special events (like public meetings and national exhibitions), sponsorships, and personal communication (including word of mouth, such as clinic counseling and family visits).

Communication media include *traditional media* (such as newspapers, magazines, radio, television, cinemas, billboards, and transits), *nontraditional media* (e.g., computer desktop kits, desktop wallpaper, plastic cups, posters, T-shirts, bike lights, and point-of-purchase materials), *addressable media* (like direct mail, flyers, postcards, pamphlets, and booklets), and *digital* and/or *interactive* media (such as the Internet, video games, DVDs, and mobile phones).

What really represents a current trend in social marketing for public health is not only the increasing number of communication formats and media, it is also the *integration* of those different channels to achieve a "one-sight, one-sound" effect (Schultz & Schultz, 2004, p. 23) in all those communication efforts. The rationale and goals for integrating various communication efforts are twofold:

1. To more effectively orchestrate the delivery of messages into the marketplace.
2. To apply the strengths of each communication discipline or technique so that the whole is greater than the sum of the parts and the optimal message impact is achieved. (Schultz & Schultz, 2004, p. 23)

In some social marketing campaigns covered in this book, emerging media were actively adopted. As "the evolution of utilizing technology to share information in new and innovative ways" (EM, 2009), *emerging media* involve:

> an explosion in digital media with the development and expansion of social networks, blogs, forums, instant messaging, mobile marketing, e-mail marketing, rich media and paid and organic search all the way to offline trends in discovering the power of word of mouth marketing (WOM) techniques and strategies that become a part of media and marketing campaigns. (EM, 2009, p. 1)

Due to the disparity in economic and technological development and in media access to target audiences among those countries covered in the book, the adoption of new and emerging media for social marketing has been uneven in some of those countries.

As a sea of change is surging over the traditional media landscape globally, social marketers have begun to venture into *social media* (e.g., YouTube, MySpace, and Twitter) to connect with the target audience, especially the "digital natives," who were "born into the digital age (after 1980), with access to networked digital technologies and strong computer skills and knowledge" (Palfrey & Gasser, 2008, p. 346).

While "social marketing is one of the fastest-growing areas of marketing and communications, it is also frequently one of the most misunderstood" (Houghton, 2008, p. 1). The most severe and widely spread misunderstanding about social marketing is that many people seem to have confused it with social media nowadays. In a brief Google search, we found the following misuses of social marketing as social media or social networking:

Misuse 1: What people are saying about a product in chat rooms, on blogs, on review sites, and in social networks is mistakenly regarded as "social marketing."

Misuse 2: Web 2.0 technology, "a phase in Web development where users, and not just professional content creators, write Web-based, Google-searched content," is regarded as a practice of "social marketing."

Misuse 3: Two European countries held the "first international social advertising and marketing competition . . . to recognize online marketing and advertising ideas that incorporate the importance of social networks."

Misuse 4: A Fortune 500 company, which wants to sell more pads and tampons to young girls, has found "social marketing" more effective than traditional advertising—not because of its initiative for any social good, but "as a result of the company's proven ability to listen to customers and respond effectively" through social networking.

Misuse 5: A new university course in the United States on "the benefits of social networking" and the techniques on how to use "online networking sites such as Facebook, MySpace, and LinkedIn" to increase "membership or patronage, and potential improvement of revenues" for companies is called "Social Marketing in the 21st Century."

Although definitions of social media vary in focus and format (Definitions, 2009), social media are *not* social marketing. Social media can be communication tools and channels for social marketing, but merely social networking—typical of social media—is not the social marketing that has been defined and practiced since this term was born in 1971 (Kotler & Zaltman, 1971). The confusion between *social marketing* and *social media* has given rise to a serious challenge to the identity of social marketing as a field of practice, research, and education. To clean this "muddy water" is a battle that all social marketers have to fight right now—and in the years to come.

Trend 7: Edutainment

Edutainment, a term coined from educational entertainment, is a type of entertainment designed to be educational (Merriam-Webster, 2009). "Lessons" embedded in edutainment tend to be delivered to the target audience through entertainment formats familiar to the audience, such as entertainment shows, radio and TV programs, computer and video games, films, and Web sites.

"The entertainment-education approach to social change rests on this notion of fluid boundaries between learning and enjoying" (Cooper-Chen, 2005, p. 5). It is for this reason that edutainment, if used appropriately, could be an effective way to convey social marketing messages, including those focused on public health, to the target audience.

As demonstrated in this book, edutainment was successfully used in some social marketing campaigns. As shown in Chapter 12 on the anti–hepatitis B campaign in China, for example, MTV and a campaign theme song, starring singers popular among the public, helped catch the attention of target audiences, increase their awareness, and reinforce their memory of the campaign messages.

A word of caution is in place here, however: Edutainment has to be used appropriately in social marketing campaigns. It was reported in a study on the fundraising effect of situating the social marketing of organ donation against a broader backdrop of entertainment and news media coverage that the storylines for organ donations heavily featured on broadcast television in medical and legal dramas and soap operas actually did not work because they were highly sensational. As a result, "the marketing of organ donation for entertainment essentially create[d] a counter-campaign to organ donation, with greater resources and reach than social marketers [had] access to" (Harrison, Morgan, & Chewning, 2008, p. 33).

Trend 8: Paying Attention to Social, Cultural, and Regulatory Environments

Social marketing campaigns for public health are often affected by the social, cultural, and regulatory environments in the countries or regions in which they are carried out. The cases presented in this book all have one thing in common: They were designed and carried out in a way that best fit their social, cultural, and regulatory contexts in order to maximize their effectiveness.

Take the anti–hepatitis B campaign in China reviewed in Chapter 12, again, for example. For more than two decades, public service advertising (PSA) has been enthusiastically embraced by the Chinese government and Chinese media. The first PSA spot was aired by a Chinese TV station in 1986, and since 1996, the Chinese government and media have been jointly hosting annual national PSA campaigns and presenting awards to outstanding pieces (Cheng & Chan, 2009). Given this unique social environment in China, the Chinese government played a major role in this nationwide anti–hepatitis B campaign, which was, in fact, co-sponsored by the China Foundation for Hepatitis Prevention and Control and the Information Office of the Ministry of Health, with donations of expertise from McCann Healthcare China and airtime and space from many media outlets.

Cultural influences on social marketing campaigns for public health are abundant in this book. In the anti–HIV/AIDS case study in Mexico in Chapter 4, the campaign focused on "redefin[ing] gender norms among Mexican youth," because the traditional inequitable gender roles between young men and young women in Mexico was identified as a root cause of risky sexual behaviors among them. In Singapore's anti–dengue fever campaign examined in Chapter 15, all communication materials were produced in four languages—English, Chinese, Malay, and Tamil—because they are all official languages in this multiethnic nation.

As Willard Shaw, author of the case study on insecticide-treated mosquito nets in Nigeria, concluded in Chapter 9, "Keeping an eye on both . . . regular monitoring and adapting to changing circumstances is the only way to achieve success." An example he gave in the chapter in terms of campaign agility to deal with unpredictable government regulations was that tariff increases in the country could jump from 5% to 75% overnight during the campaign.

Trend 9: Valuing Marketing Research

A commonality among all the case studies in this book is that research played a pivotal role in all these success stories of social marketing for public health. As "the systematic design, collection, analysis, and reporting of data and findings relevant to a specific marketing situation facing the organization" (Kotler & Lee, 2008, p. 74), *marketing research* can be divided as formative, pretest, monitoring, and evaluation. While *formative research* helps "form strategies, especially to select and understand target audiences and develop draft marketing strategies" (Kotler & Lee, 2008, p. 75), *pretest research*, *monitoring research*, and *evaluation research* are conducted before, during, and after a marketing campaign is launched, respectively.

The success stories of social marketing for public health all resorted to some types of marketing research. One of the major lessons provided in these success stories is that "properly focused marketing research can make the difference between a brilliant plan and a mediocre one" (Kotler & Lee, 2008, p. 44).

Because the social, cultural, economic, and technological conditions in those countries are quite different, you will find that marketing researchers paid great attention to not only the *appropriateness* of a research method for a target market, but also the *feasibility* of research in a target market. That is why, while relatively large-scale surveys (either online or offline) were conducted in some countries, observation and personal interviews were done in others.

The strong emphasis on marketing research in these success stories has also demonstrated how social marketing "focuses clearly on the audience," how "[i]t has gone so far as to describe [itself] as 'being obsessed with the audience,'" and how "[i]t starts and ends with the target audience" (Sparg, 2008, p. 1).

Trend 10: Focusing on Behavior Changes

The last, but by no means the least, trend you will observe in the public health campaigns reviewed in this book is their clear, strong, and consistent focus on behavior change, the hallmark of social marketing. Each campaign yielded some measurable behavior changes in the target audience, from quitting smoking to beginning to do more physical exercise and from increased adoption of mosquito nets, contraceptives, or new needles (for diabetic patients) to the reduced rate of drink driving (yes, again, *drink* driving, as in Chapter 16).

SOCIAL MARKETING FOR PUBLIC HEALTH: CHAPTER HIGHLIGHTS

This volume has several major features: broad geographic coverage, variety in public health campaigns examined, currency of campaigns reviewed, consistency in presentation format, and, most important of all, measurable outcomes in each case.

Geographically, this book covers 15 countries spread across five continents. These selected countries include highly developed nations, emerging new economic powerhouses, and countries where the economy has not yet significantly developed. Starting from the United States, where the concept of social marketing originated, the 15 countries covered in the book are presented in a roughly clockwise order on a "U.S.–made" world map (which has the United States as the central focus point).

For each country, one—occasionally, two—successful social marketing campaign(s) dealing with a public health issue especially important or unique to that country was (were) presented. These successful campaigns varied from anti-smoking campaigns to HIV/AIDS prevention, from promotions for healthy lifestyles to battles against obesity, and from public educational campaigns on hepatitis B to contraceptive social marketing.

Each success story in this book is told in two parts: The first part is a brief country overview, including some essential background information about the country, the major public health challenges the country is facing, and its government policies and regulations on public health. The major part of each chapter goes to an in-depth case study, including campaign background and environment; campaign target audiences; campaign objectives and goals; campaign target audience barriers, motivations, and competition; and campaign strategies, implementation, and evaluation. At the end of each chapter, a concise summary is provided, with a focus on the "lessons learned," followed by a few questions for discussion.

All case studies represent recent social marketing campaigns for public health. Some of them are even still ongoing.

As mentioned earlier in this chapter, the hallmark for a successful social marketing campaign is always behavior change. The most important criterion for selecting cases for this book has been measurable and documented changes in target audience behavior. Each chapter devotes considerable space to the report of such changes.

In Chapter 2, Nancy Lee reviews the tobacco problem in the United States and major milestones and strategies in the reduction of tobacco use in the country. She presents two case studies. The first one is about the **truth**® Campaign, "the largest national youth smoking prevention campaign" in U.S. history and "the only national prevention campaign not directed by the tobacco industry." The next case study is about a local campaign, focusing on the Tobacco Quit Line Campaign in Washington State. Both cases document the success of the two anti-smoking social marketing campaigns.

Chapter 3, by François Lagarde, Cathie Kryzanowski, and James Mintz, describes a community-based, provincewide social marketing campaign in Canada. Called "Saskatchewan in motion," this campaign promotes physical activity among the people of a Western province in the country. The authors give a thorough examination of the campaign, after a review of the healthcare system, major public health issues, and the current status of social marketing as used to address those issues in Canada.

In Chapter 4, Ruth Massingill reviews how social marketing is used in Mexico to achieve HIV/AIDS prevention through redefining gender norms among youth. In the early part of the chapter, Massingill takes a look at how HIV/AIDS entered the picture of public health issues in the country and how social marketing was determined to be an appropriate tool to deal with this public health issue. After an analysis of two successful companion campaigns—Programas Hombres and Mujeres, the author concludes that it is critical in HIV prevention targeting young men and women to address unequal gender norms, especially machismo attitudes.

In Chapter 5, Nancy Lee examines how social marketing is used successfully in Peru's prevention and treatment of tuberculosis (TB). She first highlights the TB problems in the world and in Peru. In her in-depth case study, she discusses how downstream efforts (focused on reaching high-risk TB groups), midstream efforts (aimed at those who could influence high-risk TB groups, such as family members, neighbors, co-workers, and healthcare providers), and upstream efforts (geared toward policy makers, the media, and the commercial sector) were integrated in the national anti-TB campaign in Peru.

In Chapter 6, Rowena Merritt, Aiden Truss, Lucy Reynolds, and Emma Heesom demonstrate how social marketing is used to increase school meal uptake in "a deprived region" in northeast England. Given the complex nature of school meal uptake, the campaign has adopted "a multipronged approach" that involves head teachers, parents, and schoolchildren. Details on the setup of a steering committee for the campaign are also provided in the early part of the chapter.

In Chapter 7, Giuseppe Fattori, Paola Artoni, and Marcello Tedeschi direct our attention to food vending machines in Italy. After an overview of public health issues and the application of social marketing in dealing with those issues in Italy, the authors focus on the Choose Health campaign. Designed for obesity prevention and healthy lifestyle promotion, this campaign is an experiment, as the authors call it, on how to transform vending machines into a tool to achieve these purposes. Although the creation of a healthy food portfolio, a reasonable pricing strategy, and an easily recognizable healthy product identity are pivotal to the campaign success, a good definition of good purchasing behaviors and habits at vending machines is essential, according to the authors.

Karin Ekström and Lena Hansson's Chapter 8 focuses on Systembolaget, the alcohol retail monopoly in Sweden. The authors first review Swedish alcohol policy and give necessary background information on Systembolaget. Then they provide a detailed examination of two recent pro-alcohol monopoly campaigns, showing how the Swedish public's understanding and positive attitude toward Systembolaget were successfully increased through store atmosphere, quality assortment, and customer service, as well as advertising.

In Chapter 9, Willard Shaw tells the story of how a commercial market for insecticide-treated mosquito nets has been created in Nigeria. He first reviews how severe malaria, largely carried by night-biting anopheles mosquitoes in Africa, is as a public health issue. Then he discusses how public–private partnerships helped achieve sustainable malaria prevention in Nigeria. He particularly emphasizes the importance of having a catalyst for this partnership to bring the two sectors together and help them create a win–win situation for both sides. The Nigeria case also indicates the need for a close implementer–client relationship. As Shaw elaborates in his chapter, the best scenario is when the implementer and the client function as a team, both focusing on their overall goals and constantly and frankly discussing the steps ahead in the campaign.

Also focusing on Africa, Steven Honeyman has a different focus in Chapter 10, describing how social marketing has been used in Madagascar to promote clean drinking water for reducing diarrhea-related mortality. The author first reviews how unsafe water-related diarrheal disease threatens millions of people's health and lives and some global trends in household water treatment. Through a detailed examination of the "Safe Water Saves Lives" campaign, he draws a number of valuable lessons, from project design to the production of safe water product components, from regulatory environment to marketing and communication, and from creating partnerships to pricing and cost recovery.

In Chapter 11, Donald Ruschman, Randi Thompson, and Tatiana Stafford examine how a social marketing campaign called Red Apple in the Republic of Kazakhstan was able to make contraceptives widely available commercially. They analyze how this "comprehensive, multipronged, and short-term" campaign convinced Kazakhstani women to adopt contraceptives as an alternative to abortion, and then how the commercial contraceptive market in this former Soviet republic became largely self-sufficient by transferring principal responsibility for maintaining these newly found gains to the private, commercial sector. The chapter describes a challenging social marketing problem: changing consumer beliefs and setting up a new distribution system.

In Chapter 12, Hong Cheng, Jun Qiao, and Huixin Zhang review a nationwide campaign for hepatitis B prevention and education in China. First, they describe major public health issues in the country, including hepatitis B, and the Chinese government's strategies and policies in dealing with these issues. Then they focus their attention on a recent "Love Your Liver, Improve Your Health" campaign. To evaluate the campaign effectiveness, they conducted a survey in five selected cities in China and reported the survey results in the chapter. Based on the survey, the campaign was found to have been highly effective.

In Chapter 13, Morikazu Hirose examines how a Japanese company integrated its corporate social initiatives. After reviewing emerging public health issues and the health policy in Japan, the author focuses on Terumo, a Tokyo-headquartered global manufacturer of healthcare products and equipment. He narrates how Terumo's corporate philosophy of "contributing to society through health care" has driven the company in its development of painless syringe needles for diabetic patients and its enhancement of the public's understanding of diabetes, through communication strategies, advertising campaigns, and educational TV programs.

In Chapter 14, Sameer Deshpande, Jaidev Balakrishnan, Anurudra Bhanot, and Sanjeev Dham document successful social marketing campaigns for contraceptive products in India. After a review of major public health issues and trends in using social marketing and health communication in the country, they present two cases in the chapter. The first one is an emergency contraception campaign conducted by the Washington, DC–based Population Services International (PSI); the other is BBC World Service Trust's anti–HIV/AIDS campaign. Among the lessons to be learned from the successful PSI campaign are the importance of interpersonal communication in the behavior-change process and the value of mass media in providing credibility to ground-level campaign activities. The edutainment approach and the appropriate media selection for campaign messages are two valuable lessons from the successful BBC campaign.

In Chapter 15, Kavita Karan discusses how the Singapore government, private companies, schools, and communities partner in disease control and healthy lifestyle promotion. These partnerships are demonstrated through an anti–dengue fever campaign and a national healthy lifestyle program. Important lessons learned from these two successful campaigns include effective strategies and tactics that the Singapore government has used in preventing the spread of dengue fever in the country, the importance of using new media techniques in health communication, and the impact of cultural factors on campaign success.

In Chapter 16, the last but by no means the least chapter, Samantha Snitow and Linda Brennan take us to Australia. They first review the drink driving (yes, *drink driving*, as Australians say; not merely *drunk driving*) problem in Australia and provide prior anti–drink driving efforts and major milestones in the country. Then they demonstrate how the integration of legislation, law enforcement, and social marketing (especially public service advertising) has significantly reduced drink driving road deaths.

Through the following 15 chapters, you will be exposed to the breadth and depth of social marketing as successfully practiced in various countries to change target audience public health–related behaviors. These campaigns differ in their specific objectives due to different public health issues, and they vary in specific campaign designs and implementations due to different campaign environments—social, cultural, economic, regulatory, and media, to mention a few. They all have one thing in common: namely, they all share the key elements of social marketing campaigns, which are highlighted in the next section of this chapter.

DEVELOPING A SOCIAL MARKETING CAMPAIGN: STEP BY STEP[1]

In *Social Marketing: Influencing Behaviors for Good*, Kotler and Lee (2008) divided the development of a typical social marketing campaign into 10 steps and illustrated

[1]This section is adapted from Kotler & Lee (2008) with permission from SAGE Publications.

each in great detail. Here, we adopt these steps and present them concisely. In the next 15 chapters of this book, you will notice that all the cases examined by our contributors contain many, if not all, of these steps.

Step 1: Define the Problem, Purpose, and Focus

Any social marketing campaign for public health needs a clearly determined public health *problem*, which might be a severe epidemic (like SARS), an evolving issue (like the increases in teen smoking), or a justifiable need (like public education on the prevention of hepatitis B). The problem could be precipitated by an unusual happening such as tsunami or may be simply triggered by an organization's mandate or mission such as "contributing to society through health care." Adequate background information is provided at this step to put the public health problem in perspective. When defining the public health problem, it is critical to identify the campaign's sponsor(s) and summarize the factors that led to the rationale and decision for developing such a campaign. The rationale and decision are based on sufficient research data, epidemiological or scientific, in order to substantiate and quantify the problem defined.

Once the public health problem is defined, a *purpose statement* is needed to make it clear what impact and benefits that the social marketing campaign, when successful, would generate.

A *focus* is determined to narrow down the scope of the social marketing campaign to best use the resources available, maximize the campaign impact, and ensure the campaign feasibility. The campaign focus is selected from a number of options that have some potential to help achieve the campaign purpose.

Step 2: Conduct a Situation Analysis

Typically, a SWOT (strengths, weaknesses, opportunities, and threats) analysis is conducted at this step to provide a quick audit of *organizational* strengths and weaknesses and *environmental* opportunities and threats. Strengths to maximize and weaknesses to minimize include internal factors such as levels of funding, management support, current partners, delivery system capabilities, and the sponsor's reputation. Opportunities to take advantage of and threats to prepare for include major trends and events outside your influence—those often associated with demographic, psychographic, geographic, economic, cultural, political, legal, and technological forces. At this step, you will also conduct a literature review and environmental scan of current and prior campaigns, especially those with similar efforts, and summarize their major activities conducted, major effects achieved, and major lessons learned.

Step 3: Select Target Audiences

A *target audience* is quite like the bull's-eye; it is selected through *segmentation*, a process to divide a broad audience (population) into homogeneous subaudiences (groups), called *audience segments*. An audience segment is identified and aggregated by the shared characteristics and needs of the people in a broad audience, including similar demographics, psychographics, geographics, behaviors, social networks, community assets, and stage of change.

It is ideal that a social marketing campaign focuses on one primary target audience, but secondary audiences are often identified, based on the marketing problem, purpose, and focus of the campaign defined earlier. An estimated size and informative description of the target audience(s) is needed at this step. An ideal description of the target audience will make you believe that if a member of the audience walked into the room, you would "recognize" her or him.

Step 4: Set Marketing Objectives and Goals

A social marketing campaign needs clear marketing objectives and goals. Specifying desired behaviors and changes in knowledge, attitudes, and/or beliefs, *marketing objectives* always includes a *behavior objective*—something you want the target audience to do as a result of the campaign (e.g., to choose healthy foods and/or beverages available at vending machines). Marketing objectives also often include a *knowledge objective*, which makes clear the information or facts that the target audience needs to be aware of through the campaign (e.g., to know what a healthy lifestyle is and what advantages it has), and a *belief objective*, which relates to the things the target audience needs to believe in order to "change its mind" (e.g., to believe that a healthy lifestyle can be achieved through simple everyday actions).

A social marketing campaign also needs to establish quantifiable measures, called *marketing goals*, relevant to the marketing objectives. Marketing goals, responding to behavior objectives, knowledge objectives, and belief objectives should be ideally SMART—specific, measurable, achievable, relevant, and time-bound (Haughey, n.d.) in terms of knowledge, attitudes, and behavior changes. What is determined here will have strong implications for budgets, will guide marketing mix strategies, and will direct evaluation measures in the later planning process in a social marketing campaign.

Step 5: Identify Factors Influencing Behavior Adoption

Before positioning your social marketing campaign and establishing the marketing mix strategies for the campaign, the social marketer needs to take the time, effort, and resources needed to understand what the target audience is doing or prefers to do and what is affecting its behaviors and preferences. Specifically, barriers, benefits, competitors, and the influencers need to be identified at this step.

Barriers refer to reasons, real or perceived, the target audience may not want the behavior to be promoted, or may not think it can be adopted. *Benefits* are the "gains" that the target audience could see through adopting the targeted behavior, or that the social marketing program may promise the target market. *Competitors* refer to any related behaviors (or organizations promoting them) that the target audience is currently engaged in, or prefers to have, rather than the ones to be promoted. *Influencers* include any "important others" who could have some bearing on the target audience, such as family members, social networks, the entertainment industry, and religious leaders.

Step 6: Craft a Positioning Statement

A *positioning statement* describes what the target audience is supposed to feel and think about the targeted behavior and its related benefits. A positioning statement, together with brand identity, is inspired by the description of the target audience and its barriers, competitors, and influencers. It differentiates the targeted behavior from alternative or preferred ones. Effective positioning will guide the development of the marketing mix strategies in the next step, helping ensure that the offer in a social marketing campaign will land on and occupy a distinctive place in the minds of the target audience.

Step 7: Develop Marketing Mix Strategies: The 4Ps

The traditional marketing toolbox contains four major devices: product, price, place, and promotion. Like their counterparts in commercial sectors, social marketers resort to these tools to create, communicate, and deliver values for their targeted behaviors. The 4Ps can be thought of as independent, though not isolated, variables used as determinants to influence the dependent variables—the behaviors of the target market.

The 4Ps should be developed and presented in the following order, with the product strategy at the beginning of the sequence and the promotion strategy at the end. Promotion is at the end because it ensures that the target markets become aware of the targeted product, its price, and its accessibility, which need to be developed prior to the promotion strategy. Great attention is called for the "mix" of the 4Ps, which should not be developed in isolation—it is the synergy of the 4Ps that makes a truly successful social marketing campaign possible.

Product Strategy

It is essential to have a clear description of the product in a social marketing campaign, at core, actual, and augmented levels. A *core product* comprises the benefits that the target audience will experience or expect in exchange for performing the targeted behavior, or that will be highlighted in a social marketing campaign (e.g., a healthier life and the reduction in the risk of becoming obese or overweight). An *actual product* is the desired behavior, often embodied by its major features and described in specific terms (such as healthy foods or beverages available at vending machines). An *augmented product* refers to any additional tangible objects and/or services that will be included in the offer and promoted to the target market. An augmented product helps perform the targeted behavior or increase its appeal (e.g., information on healthy products available in vending machines).

Price Strategy

A price strategy sums up the costs that the target audience will "pay" for adopting the desired behavior that leads to the promised benefits. These costs could be monetary in the real sense, such as those for tangible goods and services. Most of the time, however, social marketers sell behaviors that require something else in exchange: time, effort, energy, psychological costs, and/or physical discomfort. A sensible price strategy is aimed at minimizing these costs by maximizing incentives (monetary and nonmonetary alike) to reward desired behaviors (again, monetary or nonmonetary) or to discourage competing, undesirable behaviors. (The other three Ps are also needed in the effort to reduce these costs.)

Place Strategy

Place is largely where and when the target audience will be encouraged to perform the desired behavior and/or to obtain tangible products or services associated with the campaign. As in commercial marketing, place can be regarded as the delivery system or a distribution channel for a social marketing campaign. Strategies related to the system or channel management need to be provided here to ensure that they will be as convenient and pleasant as possible for the customer to engage in the targeted behavior and access related products and services.

Promotion Strategy

Information on product benefits and features, fair price, and easy accessibility needs effective and efficient communications to bring to the target audience and inspire action. Promotion strategy is needed to maximize the success of the communications. The development of these communications is a process that begins with the determination of key messages, continues with the selection of messengers and communication formats and channels, moves on to the creation of communication elements, and ends up with the implementation of those communications.

The determination of key *messages* needs to be aligned with marketing objectives, because they determine what a social marketing campaign wants its target audience to know, to believe, and to do. Information on barriers, benefits, competitors, and influencers will help shape message choices. *Messengers* are those who deliver the messages. Credibility, expertise, and likability are some key considerations for selecting messengers.

Messages are delivered through various *communication channels* (including media channels), such as advertising (including PSA), public relations, events, sponsorships, and personal selling and word of mouth. As far as media channels are concerned, they can be online or offline, or both. Online media range from e-mail, Web sites, and "smart" mobile phones to blogs, podcasts, and tweets, but by no means are limited to these options. Offline media include newspapers, magazines, radio, and television, as well as direct mail, billboards, transit (e.g., buses, taxes, and subways), and kiosks.

As we all know, thanks to the ongoing technology revolution, the line between online and offline media has become increasingly blurred. For example, radio and television can be both online and offline, while more and more newspapers and magazines are going online. The fast-changing media landscape is both a blessing and a "curse" for marketers; social marketers are no exception. As a blessing, social marketers have more and more media choices to target their audiences more precisely and effectively. As a "curse," the increasingly perplexing media landscape requires social marketers to think "out of the box"—not only considering those traditional media or the media they are familiar with, but also thinking about those nontraditional and emerging media that their target audiences often tend to use or be exposed to. At the same time, in the media selection and planning, social marketers need to make sure the selected media will complement each other; communications via various media must be consistent over time. Social marketers should also consider making their communications with their target audiences more interactive.

Because different communication channels have different characteristics, it could be more effective and efficient to have a good idea of the media budget and media options that a social marketing campaign could have before communication elements are created. *Creative elements* translate the content of intended, desired messages into specific communication elements, which include copy, graphic images, and typeface for traditional print media, and interactive features and audio and/or video streams for online media.

Step 8: Outline a Plan for Monitoring and Evaluation

A plan for monitoring and evaluating a social marketing campaign is needed before final budget and implementation plans are made. It needs to be referred back to the goals established for the campaign. *Monitoring* is a measurement conducted sometime after the launch of a new campaign, but before its completion. Monitoring is executed to determine if midcourse corrections are needed to ensure that marketing goals of the program will be reached. An *evaluation* refers to a measurement and a final report on what happened through the campaign. It needs to address questions like: Were the marketing goals reached? What components of the campaign can be linked with outcomes? Was the program on time and within budget? What worked well and what did not? What should be done differently next time?

Measures fall into three categories—*output* measures for program activities; *outcome* measures for target audience responses and changes in knowledge, beliefs, and behavior; and *impact* measures for contributions to the plan purposes (e.g., reductions in obesity as a result of many more people buying healthy foods and/or beverages due to a social marketing campaign).

In the development of a monitoring and evaluation plan, five basic questions need to be taken into account:

- Why will this measurement be conducted? For whom?
- What inputs, processes, and outcomes/impacts will be measured?
- What methods (such as interview, focus group, survey, and/or online tracking) will be used for these measurements?
- When will these measurements be conducted?
- How much will these measurements cost?

Step 9: Establish Budgets and Find Funding Sources

The budgets for a social marketing campaign reflect the costs for developing and implementing it, which include those associated with marketing mix strategies (the 4Ps) and additional costs anticipated for monitoring and evaluation. In ideal objective-and-task budgeting, these anticipated costs become a preliminary budget, based on what is needed to achieve the established marketing goals. When the preliminary budget exceeds available funds, however, options for additional funding and the potential for adjusting campaign phases (such as spreading out costs over a longer period of time), revising strategies, and/or reducing behavior change goals need to be considered. Additional funding sources may include government grants and appropriations, nonprofit organization and foundation supports, advertising and media partnerships and coalitions, and corporation donations. Only a final budget is presented in this section, which delineates secured funding sources and reflects contributions from partners.

Step 10: Complete the Plan for Campaign Implementation and Management

At this last step, the planning for a social marketing campaign is wrapped up with specifics on *who* will do *what*, with *how much*, and *when*. In a nutshell, an implementation and management plan is aimed at transforming marketing strategies into specific actions for those who are involved in the campaign. It functions like a concise working document to share and track planned efforts. So, to some, this section of the planning is the "real" social marketing plan or even a "stand-alone" piece that they will share internally. More often than not, a social marketing plan is for a minimum of one year of activities; ideally, it can be designed for a two- or three-year time span. (For a quick summary of the 10 steps, please see Box 1-1.)

BOX 1-1   Social Marketing Planning: A Summary Outline

Executive Summary
Brief summary highlighting campaign stakeholders, background, purpose, target audience, marketing objectives and goals, desired positioning, marketing mix strategies (4Ps), and evaluation plans, budgets, and implementation plans.

1.0 Background, Purpose, and Focus
   Who are sponsors? Why are they doing this? What social issue and population will the plan focus on, and why?

2.0 Situation Analysis
2.1 SWOT: organizational strengths and weaknesses and environmental opportunities and threats
2.2 Literature review and environmental scan of programs focusing on similar efforts: activities and lessons learned

3.0 Target Audience Profile (see Note 1 regarding alternative terminology)
3.1 Demographics, psychographics, geographics, relevant behaviors, social networks, community assets, and stage of change
3.2 Size of target audience

(continues)

BOX 1-1   Social Marketing Planning (continued)

4.0   Marketing Objectives and Goals

Campaign objectives: targeted behaviors and attitudes (knowledge and beliefs)

SMART goals: specific, measurable, achievable, relevant, time-bound changes in behaviors and attitudes

5.0   Factors Influencing Adoption of the Behavior (see Note 2 regarding the *iterative process*)

Perceived barriers to targeted behavior

Potential benefits for targeted behavior

Competing behaviors/forces

Influence of important others

6.0   Positioning Statement

How do we want the target audience to see the targeted behavior and its benefits relative to alternative/preferred ones?

7.0   Marketing Mix Strategies (using the 4Ps to create, communicate, and deliver value for the behavior)

7.1   *Product: benefits from performing behaviors and any objects or services offered to assist adoption*

Core product: desired audience benefits promised in exchange for performing the targeted behavior

Actual product: features of basic product (e.g., HIV/AIDS test, physical exercise, daily intake of fruits and vegetables)

Augmented product: additional objects and services to help perform the behavior or increase appeal

7.2   *Price: costs that will be associated with adopting the behavior*

Costs: money, time, physical effort, and/or psychological discomfort

Price-related tactics to reduce costs: monetary and/or nonmonetary; incentives and/or disincentives

7.3   *Place: making access convenient*

Creating convenient opportunities to engage in the targeted behaviors and/or access products and services

BOX 1-1   **Social Marketing Planning (continued)**

7.4   *Promotion: persuasive communications highlighting product benefits and features, fair price, and ease of access*

Messages

Messengers

Creative/executional strategy

Media channels and promotional items

8.0   Plan for Monitoring and Evaluation

Purpose and audience for monitoring and evaluation

What will be measured: inputs, outputs, outcomes (from Steps 4 and 6) and impact

How and when measures will be taken

9.0   Budget

9.1   Costs for implementing marketing plan, including additional research and monitoring/evaluation plan

9.2   Any anticipated incremental revenues, cost savings, and/or partner contributions

10.0 Plan for Campaign Implementation and Management

Who will do what, when—including partners and their roles

Special Notes:

1. Alternative terms include *target market* (a traditional term), *priority market*, and *priority audience*.
2. The process is an iterative one. For example, you may need to revise objectives and goals after hearing of barriers and benefits in Step 5, or promotional ideas based on final budget realities in Step 9.
3. A separate plan will be needed for each target audience, even though it is part of one campaign.
4. Research will be needed to develop most steps, especially formative research for Steps 2–6 and pretesting for finalizing Step 7.

Source: Developed 2008 by Philip Kotler and Nancy Lee, with input and review by Alan Andreasen, Carol Bryant, Craig Lefebvre, Bob Marshall, Mike Newton-Ward, Michael Rothschild, and Bill Smith.

QUESTIONS FOR DISCUSSION

1. What are the major contributions that social marketing—as a theory, a practice, and/or a movement—has made to society in general and to marketing in particular? What are some of the most important advances in social marketing over the past 40 years?

2. Why is social marketing regarded as a "natural fit" for public health? In your opinion and/or based on your experience, what are the most valuable contributions that social marketing has made to public health globally or in your country? What area(s) in public health still need(s) more help from social marketers nowadays?

3. In your view, what are the three most noteworthy global trends in social marketing for public health? What other trend(s) have you noticed besides the 10 highlighted in this chapter?

4. What has given rise to the widespread confusion between *social marketing* and *social media*? What do you think should and can be done to clean up the "muddy water" and protect the identity of social marketing?

REFERENCES

Academy for Educational Development (AED). (2009). *AED helps build a better future.* Retrieved July 28, 2009, from http://www.aed.org/About/index.cfm

Agha, S., Do., M., & Armand, F. (2006). When donor support ends: The fate of social marketing products and the markets they help create. *Social Marketing Quarterly* 12(2), 28–42.

Andreasen, A. R. (1995). *Marketing social change: Changing behavior to promote health, social development, and the environment.* San Francisco: Jossey-Bass.

Andreasen, A. R. (2006). *Social marketing in the 21st century.* Thousand Oaks, CA: Sage Publications.

Baran, S. J., & Davis, D. K. (2009). *Mass communication theory: Foundations, ferment, and future* (5th ed.). Boston: Wadsworth Cengage Learning.

Basil, D. Z. (2007). Foreword. In D. Z. Basil & W. Wymer (Eds.), *Social marketing: Advances in research and theory* (pp. xvii–xxi). Binghamton, NY: Haworth Press.

Cheng, H., & Chan, K. (2009). Public service advertising in China: A semiotic analysis. In H. Cheng & K. Chan (Eds.), *Advertising and Chinese Society: Impacts and Issues* (pp. 203–221). Copenhagen, Denmark: Copenhagen Business School Press.

Cooper-Chen, A. (2005). The world of television. In A. Cooper-Chen (Ed.), *Global entertainment media: Content, audiences, and issues* (pp. 1–15). Mahwah, NJ: Lawrence Erlbaum Associates.

Coreil, J., Bryant, C. A., & Henderson, J. N. (with contributions from M. S. Forthofer & G. P. Quinn). (2001). *Social and behavioral foundations of public health.* Thousand Oaks, CA: Sage Publications.

Definitions of social media on the Web. (2009). Retrieved July 28, 2009, from http://www
.google.com/search?hl=en&defl=en&q=define:Social+media&ei=ij_OSefRB9DflQfo4ZzICQ
&sa=X&oi=glossary_definition&ct=title

Emerging Media (EM). (2009). Retrieved July 28, 2009, from http://emergingmedia.org/

French, J., & Blair-Stevens, C. (2005). *Social marketing pocket guide.* London: National Social
Marketing Centre of Excellence.

Harrison, T. R., Morgan, S. E., & Chewning, L. V. (2008). The challenge of social marketing of
organ donation: News and entertainment coverage of donation and transplantation.
Health Marketing Quarterly 12(1/2), 33–65.

Haughey, D. (n.d.). Smart goals. Retrieved July 28, 2009, from http://www.projectsmart.co.uk/
smart-goals.html

Hess, D., & Warren, D. E. (2008). The meaning and meaningfulness of corporate social initiatives. *Business and Society Review* 113(2), 163–197.

Houghton, A. (2008, July 31). *Social marketing set to make a big difference to business.* Retrieved
July 28, 2009, from http://www.ldpbusiness.co.uk/liverpool-news/liverpool-business-news/
2008/07/31/opinion-social-marketing-set-to-make-a-big-difference-to-businesses-96026-
21438250/

Kotler, P., & Lee, N. (2005). *Corporate social responsibility: Doing the most good for your company
and your cause.* Hoboken, NJ: John Wiley & Sons.

Kotler, P., & Lee, N. R. (2008). *Social marketing: Influencing behaviors for good* (3rd ed.).
Thousand Oaks, CA: Sage Publications.

Kotler, P., & Levy, S. J. (1969). Broadening the concept of marketing. *Journal of Marketing*
33(1), 10–15.

Kotler, P., & Roberto, E. L. (1989). *Social marketing: Strategies for changing public behavior.* New
York: Free Press.

Kotler, P., & Zaltman, G. (1971). Social marketing: An approach to planned social change.
Journal of Marketing 35(3), 3–12.

Ling, J. C., Franklin, B. A. K., Lindsteadt, J. F., & Gearon, S. A. N. (1992). Social marketing: Its
place in public health. *Annual Review of Public Health,* 13, 341–362.

Merriam-Webster Online. (2009). Edutainment. Retrieved July 28, 2009, from http://www
.merriam-webster.com/dictionary/edutainment

Merson, M. H., Black, R. E., & Mills, A. J. (Eds.). (2006). *International public health: Diseases,
programs, systems, and policies* (2nd ed.). Sudbury, MA: Jones and Bartlett Publishers.

Palfrey, J., & Gasser, U. (2008). *Born digital: Understanding the first generation of digital natives.*
New York: Basic Books.

Rosen, G. (1993). *A history of public health* (expanded ed.). Baltimore: Johns Hopkins University
Press.

Schultz, D., & Schultz, H. (2004). *IMC—The next generation: Five steps for delivering value and
measuring returns using marketing communication.* New York: McGraw-Hill.

Sparg, M. (2008, January 21). *Social marketing—The next big thing in 2008.* Retrieved July 28,
2009, from http://www.bizcommunity.com/Article/196/11/21177.html

*Survey finds great involvement in social marketing campaigns among international advertising
community.* (2008, April 8). Retrieved July 28, 2009, from http://www.library.ohiou.edu
:2256/us/lnacademic/results/docview/docview.do?docLinkInd=true&risb=21_T70300619

10&format=GNBFI&sort=RELEVANCE&startDocNo=1&resultsUrlKey=29_T70300619
13&cisb=22_T7030061912&treeMax=true&treeWidth=0&csi=299219&docNo=1

Weinreich, N. K. (2006). *What is social marketing?* Retrieved July 28, 2009, from http://www
.social-marketing.com/Whatis.html

World Social Marketing Conference. (2008). Retrieved July 28, 2009, from http://www
.tcp-events.co.uk/wsmc/index.html

Wymer, W. (2008). Editorial: Special issue on social marketing. *International Journal of Nonprofit
and Voluntary Sector Marketing* 13, 191.

CHAPTER 2

Reducing Tobacco Use in the United States

A Public Health Success Story ... So Far

Nancy R. Lee

Knowing is not enough; we must apply.
Willing is not enough; we must do.
                    —Goethe

In 1964, almost half (42%) of the adults in the United States smoked cigarettes. By 2007, that number had declined to 20% (CDC, 2007; IOM, 2007). And among youth, the prevalence of daily smoking among 12th-graders decreased from 23% in 1999 to 12% in 2006 (IOM, 2007). These near 50% declines have been characterized as one of the 10 greatest achievements for the United States in public health in the 20th century (IOM, 2007). The stories, strategies, and unfinished business for this public health hazard are covered in this chapter, with a focus on inspirational youth smoking prevention and adult cessation efforts.

UNITED STATES: A COUNTRY OVERVIEW

The United States of America is situated mostly in central North America and is comprised of 50 states plus Washington, DC, the capital district. The United States also possesses several territories in the Caribbean and Pacific. At 3.8 million square miles (9.83 million square kilometers) and with more than 300 million people (*BBC News*, 2008), the United States is the third largest country in the world, by land area and by population. The major religion is Christianity, and it is one of the world's most ethnically diverse nations, the product of large-scale immigration from many countries. In terms of gross national product (GNP), it is the largest national economy in the world (*BBC News*, 2008).

The United States is fundamentally structured as a representative democracy, and the federal government is composed of three branches: legislative, executive, and judiciary. Politics in the United States have operated under a two-party system (currently, the Democratic and Republican parties) for virtually all of the country's history. The greatest challenges facing the country (judging by the 2008 presidential debates) include the war in Iraq, the economy, illegal immigration, health care, education, and the environment.

Life expectancy in the United States is 76 years for men and 81 years for women (*BBC News*, 2008). The following 10 current leading health indicators reflect the major public health concerns in the United States, chosen based on their ability to motivate action, the availability of data to measure their progress, and their relevance as broad public health issues: *physical activity*; *overweight and obesity*; *tobacco use*; *substance abuse*; *responsible sexual behavior*; *mental health*; *injury and violence*; *environmental quality*; *immunization*; and *access to health care*. Goals for each of these indicators have been established for 2010 and are used to help measure the health of the nation (Healthy People 2010, 2005).

The Tobacco Problem in the United States

Tobacco use is the single most preventable cause of death and disease in the United States. An estimated 21% of adults (45.3 million; CDC, 2007), 20% of high school students, and 6% of middle school students smoke cigarettes (CDC, 2009). Annually, cigarette smoking causes approximately 440,000 deaths, and for every person who dies from tobacco use, another 20 suffer with at least one serious tobacco-related illness (CDC, 2008). Astoundingly, approximately one in every five deaths in the United States is smoking related, accounting for more deaths than those from AIDS, alcohol use, cocaine use, heroin use, homicides, suicides, motor vehicle crashes, and fires combined (IOM, 2007).

And then there are economic costs. Estimates are that this addiction costs the nation more than $96 billion per year in direct medical expenses as well as more than $97 billion annually in lost productivity. Furthermore, there are the effects of exposure to secondhand smoke, costing the United States an additional $10 billion per year (CDC, 2008).

In terms of demographics, smoking among this nation's adults is highest among American Indians/Alaska Natives (32%) followed by African Americans (23%), whites (22%), Hispanics (15%), and Asians (10%); it is highest among those with only a general education development (GED) diploma (46%) and among adults living below the poverty level (31%; CDC, 2007).

Among youth, smoking is highest among whites (23%), followed by Hispanics (17%). Factors associated with youth tobacco use include low socio-economic status, approval of tobacco use by peers or siblings, smoking by parents or guardians, accessibility and price of tobacco products, lack of parental support or involvement, and low levels of academic achievement. Studies also indicate that youth who smoke are more likely to perceive that tobacco use is the norm, lack skills to resist influences, have a lower self-image or self-esteem, and lack self-efficacy to refuse offers of tobacco. In addition, tobacco use in adolescence is associated with many other health risk behaviors, including higher-risk sexual behavior and use of alcohol and drugs (CDC, 2009).

Reducing Tobacco Use: Major Milestones and Strategies

In 1964, an Advisory Committee to the Surgeon General of the Public Health Service declared in a seminal report that "Cigarette smoking is a health hazard of sufficient importance in the United States to warrant appropriate remedial action" (IOM, 2007, p. ix). As described in *Ending the Tobacco Problem: A Blueprint for the Nation* (IOM, 2007), noteworthy milestones and strategies eventually contributing to this decline in the first decades following the 1964 Surgeon General's report include:

1964–1988: Initial milestones and strategies
- Initial public education publicizing frightening findings about tobacco's dangers.
- Advocacy by coalitions of voluntary health groups such as the American Cancer Society, American Lung Association, and American Heart Association.
- Pharmacological approaches to cessation.
- School-based prevention programs, sometimes as a part of alcohol or other substance abuse programs.
- American Medical Association testimonies before Congress regarding the dangers of tobacco use.
- Advertising policies including an early Federal Communications Commission (FCC) requirement that stations run one free counter-advertisement from health groups for every three cigarette commercials that they aired and a law in 1971 banning all cigarette advertising on television and radio.
- Warning labels progressing from "Warning: Cigarette Smoking May Be Hazardous To Your Health" to "SURGEON GENERAL'S WARNING: Smoking Causes Lung Cancer, Heart Disease, Emphysema, and May Complicate Pregnancy."

1988–2005: Progress once nicotine was declared an addictive agent
- A 1988 Surgeon General's report concluding that nicotine is an addictive agent, undermining the tobacco industry's position that smoking is a "free choice."
- Recognition that most smokers become addicted in their teens.
- U.S. Food and Drug Administration (FDA) control of cigarettes beginning in 1996, with new regulations limiting youth access and advertising targeting young people.
- States taking the lead in creating smoke-free spaces and new anti-tobacco coalitions in states beginning to affect important policy actions.
- The people of California passing Proposition 99, a referendum that increased the excise tax on tobacco from 10 to 35 cents per pack and earmarked 20 percent of the new revenues for a statewide anti-smoking campaign.
- State litigation, including the Master Settlement Agreement with the major tobacco companies that required companies to pay an estimated $206 billion to 46 states between 2000 and 2025 and to support a new charitable foundation—which became the American Legacy Foundation. (IOM, 2007, pp. 107–127)

Further Reductions in Tobacco Use: "A Blueprint for the Nation"

In 2007, the Committee on Reducing Tobacco Use presented 43 recommendations to achieve three distinct goals related to reducing tobacco use, published in *Ending the Tobacco Problem: A Blueprint for the Nation* (IOM, 2007, p. 3):

1. Reduce tobacco product use initiation.
2. Increase cessation.
3. Reduce exposure to environmental tobacco smoke.

This chapter focuses on two success stories—one related to the first goal of preventing initiation (the **truth® Campaign**) and the other to the second goal of increasing cessation (Washington State's **Quit Line**). More information on these 43 recommendations appears at the end of this chapter.

CASE STUDY 1
The truth® Campaign
Youth Tobacco Prevention: Empowering Teens With truth®

BACKGROUND, PURPOSE, AND FOCUS

truth®, launched in February 2000, is the largest national youth smoking prevention campaign in the United States and the only national prevention campaign not directed by the tobacco industry (see Figure 2-1).

The campaign was created by the American Legacy Foundation®, founded as a result of the 1998 Master Settlement Agreement between the tobacco industry and 46 states and 5 U.S. territories. The foundation's mission is to *build a world where young people reject tobacco and anyone can quit* (American Legacy Foundation, 2009). The

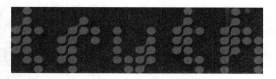

FIGURE 2-1 **truth**® Campaign Logo
Courtesy of the American Legacy Foundation

campaign exposes the tactics of the tobacco industry, the truth about addiction, and the health effects and social consequences of smoking. The focus is on inspiring teens to make informed choices about tobacco use by giving them the facts about the industry and its products and tools to enable them to "take control."

Source: Information and insights for this case were contributed by Patricia McLaughlin, the Legacy Foundation's Assistant Vice President of Communication.

TARGET MARKET PROFILE

The target market for the campaign is youth aged 12 to 17 years old who are defined as "sensation seekers" and thus most open to smoking. Nearly 80% of smokers begin using tobacco before the age of 18, so it is critical to reach this audience before they take up smoking and face a potential life of tobacco-related disease or even death (Mowery, Brick, & Farrelly, 2000). In 1999, a year prior to the campaign's launch, an estimated 35% of youth in 9th, 10th, 11th, and 12th grades used tobacco one or more times in the past 30 days. Rates increased by age from 28% of 9th-graders to 43% of 12th-graders (CDC, 2009).

MARKETING OBJECTIVES

Marketing strategies were developed with the following objectives in mind:

- *Behavior objectives:* Influence youth not to smoke and to express their concerns with the strategies, tactics, and lies of the tobacco industry.
- *Knowledge objectives:* For youth to know that the tobacco industry targeted them and to know the facts about the health effects, social cost, addictiveness, and ingredients/additives.
- *Belief objectives:* For youth to believe that not smoking is a way to express independence and that smoking is not the norm; they are in control and empowered to make the choice.

BARRIERS, BENEFITS, AND THE COMPETITION

Many youth find it hard not to at least try smoking, and several factors influence their desire to experiment, including peer pressure, older siblings and/or parents smoking around them, stress, and natural curiosity.

Benefits they imagine or they may assume include looking older, looking sexier, reducing stress, controlling weight, being independent, fitting in, being respected, expressing themselves, and being a rebel or a risk taker.

The competition, of course, is the tobacco industry, and the billions of dollars a year Big Tobacco spends to make its products accessible, visible, and seemingly cool—especially to youth. Other anti-smoking messages in the past came from the tobacco industry, and it was found that exposure was associated with more positive attitudes toward the industry and increased intentions toward future smoking.

POSITIONING

In the end, campaign planners want youth to see that the Big Tobacco companies are trying to manipulate them. As described on **truth®**'s Web site, "We're not anti-smoker, or anti-smoking. We're just anti-manipulations. With that in mind, we try to 'out' Big Tobacco's tactics so everyone knows what they're up to." The campaign's emphasis is on honest facts and information about tobacco products and the tobacco industry and gives teens tools that enable them to take control and make informed decisions about tobacco use. As also described on the foundation's Web site, "The power of our industry manipulation positioning is not only positioning **truth®** as a value-based brand, but in repositioning Big Tobacco. Our brand is the truth. Their brand lied."

STRATEGIES

The **truth®** Campaign uses evidence-based research, research with teen audiences, marketing and social science research, and lessons learned from the most successful anti-tobacco campaigns to inform its strategies. In the following presentation of strategies, a few that were *not* a direct strategy of the **truth®** Campaign are also mentioned. They are considered companion strategies, because they also target the youth market with similar objectives and positioning. Several of those that are included are ones highlighted and recommended by the Committee on Reducing Tobacco Use, helping to illustrate the use of the complete marketing mix in trying to achieve certain public health goals.

Product

- The *core product*, the benefit promised, is an opportunity for self-expression, healthy rebellion, and the health benefits of being a nonsmoker.
- The *actual product*, the desired behavior, is for youth to reject smoking.
- The *augmented product* includes a variety of opportunities for youth to express themselves, including sharing tobacco-related information with their friends through social networking sites and playing games that educate them about tobacco while entertaining and holding their interest.

Price

Although not a formal part of the **truth®** Campaign, the Committee on Reducing Tobacco Use says, "It is well established that an increase in price decreases cigarette use and that raising tobacco excise taxes is one of the most effective policies for reducing use, especially among adolescents" (IOM, 2007, p. 9). Although, of course, it is illegal in the United States for youth aged 12 to 17 to purchase cigarettes, increases in price have been a deterrent because such underage youth then have to pay others to purchase cigarettes for them.

Place

To illustrate the use of the "place" marketing tool, a recommendation from the Committee on Reducing Tobacco Use notes that a reasonably enforced youth-access restriction is an essential element of modern tobacco control. Age verification, as well as placing product displays behind the counter and banning self-service modes of access to tobacco work effectively to reduce youth access. The commission recommends, therefore, that (#11) all states should license retail sales outlets that sell tobacco products and (#12) all states should ban the sale of tobacco products directly to consumers through mail order, the Internet, or other electronic systems. Further, shipments of tobacco products should be permitted only to licensed wholesale or retail outlets (IOM, 2007, pp. 10–11).

Promotion

Messages

At the core of the **truth®** Campaign's promotional strategies are messages about the tobacco industry, as well as the health effects, social costs, addictiveness, and ingredients/additives of tobacco. The style and tone are "in-your-face" and hard-hitting, responding to teens' desire for powerful messages that display courage and honesty in a forceful way. To ensure that **truth**® is relevant to teens, teens are involved in testing advertising concepts and are encouraged to provide suggestions and feedback through the **truth**® Web site at http://www.thetruth.com/.

Messages supporting knowledge and belief objectives have included:

- Sodium hydroxide is a caustic compound found in hair removal products. It's also found in cigarettes.
- Tobacco companies' products kill 36,000 people every month. That's more lives thrown away than there are public garbage cans in New York City.
- Human sweat contains urea and ammonia. So do cigarettes.
- Benzene, arsenic, and cyanide are all poisons. They're all in cigarette smoke, too (NCI, 2001).
- There are more than 5 million deaths worldwide from smoking each year (WHO, 2005).

Messengers

Clearly, the key messengers for the **truth**® Campaign are youth, appearing in most ads, on Web sites, sharing information through social networking sites, and sharing information at grassroots events throughout the country. The campaign is designed to be peer-to-peer, so many of the campaign's elements can be passed on and shared with friends.

Media Channels

truth® advertising reaches a broad audience with multicultural messages. The **truth**® Campaign is everywhere in youth media—on television networks popular with teens like MTV, BET, G4, The N, Fuel, VH1, and fuse. **truth**® plays in cinemas, in advertising before movies. **truth**® also has a prominent presence on the Internet with its highly interactive and relevant-to-teens Web site, www.thetruth.com, that allows teens to engage with **truth**® on their own terms, as well as profiles on popular social networking sites like MySpace, Bebo, and Hi5. Box 2-1 provides a chronology of **truth**® Campaign themes.

BOX 2-1   A Chronology of truth® Campaigns, 2000–2008

- **truth®** (2000) launched at a youth summit attended by 1,000 teens from across the country.
- *Infect* **truth®** (2001, 2002) educated teens on the facts about cigarette design and engineering.
- The *Daily Dose* (2001) campaign laid the groundwork for all the **truth®** ads to come. Raw, no-frills ads featured real youth holding up long LED screens displaying **truth®**-related facts, providing information so that teens could begin to make their own educated choices about smoking.
- A look behind the *Orange Curtain* (2002, 2003) shed light on the tobacco industry's marketing tactics and included such topics as addiction and the health consequences of smoking.
- *Crazyworld* (2003) showed teens how tobacco companies play by a different set of rules than other companies. While many companies recall products at the first sign of danger to a consumer, the tobacco industry makes a product that kills 1,200 of its customers every day.
- *Connect* **truth®** (2004) used an orange dot icon to link together pieces of information to reveal the larger picture about the effects of smoking and the chain of events involving tobacco—from marketing to consumer illness and death.
- *Shards O'Glass* (2004) featured a fictitious company that manufactures freeze pops with glass shards in them, a dangerous product analogous to cigarettes. The ad is meant to raise consumer awareness about the harmful effects of smoking.
- *Seek* **truth®** (2004) used the Q&A (question-and-answer) format to encourage teens to ask questions and seek answers about the tobacco industry and its marketing and manufacturing practices.
- *Fair Enough* (2005) took a new approach to advertising with a sitcom-style television campaign that featured a cast and theme music. The commercials used tobacco industry documents to reveal marketing ideas.
- **truth®** *found* (2005–2006) pointed big orange arrows at some of the people and places targeted and affected by Big Tobacco.
- **truth®** *documentary* (2006) used a documentary filmmaking style to capture real people's reactions to the marketing tactics of the tobacco industry. The campaign, called **truth®** *documentary* for the style in which the ads were shot, featured one correspondent and a camera crew investigating the reasoning behind some ideas from Big Tobacco.

(continues)

BOX 2-1   **A Chronology of truth® Campaigns (continued)**

- *Infect* **truth®** (2006 update) called attention to the marketing tactics and health consequences of the tobacco industry in such a way as to "infect" people with that knowledge and encourage active peer-to-peer participation. *Infect* marked the debut of **truth®** on popular social networking sites like MySpace.
- **truth®** *documentary phase II* (2007) built on the approach of **truth®** *documentary* to continue to highlight the absurdity of statements found in tobacco industry documents.
- *The Sunny Side of* **truth®** (2008) is a tongue-in-cheek, darkly humorous song and dance that takes on tobacco industry words and actions. The campaign unleashes animation, music, dancing, and cartoons to reveal the "sunny side" of tobacco use and the tobacco industry.

Web and Interactive Elements

Social media and new technologies play an important role in how today's teens live, play, and work. The **truth®** Web site, www.thetruth.com, has distinct interactive elements designed to engage and amuse teens, while sharing important information about tobacco use.

Applications on the site allow teens to interact with each other and share information related to tobacco and **truth®**. Regular features of the site include games; interactive polls related to facts about tobacco; embedded videos of current **truth®** TV ads; and such downloadable items as posters, computer desktop kits, desktop wallpaper, and buddy icons. For example, an animated feature called "The Useful Cigarette" allowed visitors to point and click at an animated cigarette to learn how ingredients found in cigarettes and cigarette smoke can also be found in common household products such as pest repellant, floor wipes, and nail polish remover.

In addition to the main Web site, **truth®** homepages on popular social networking sites carry items such as e-mail cards, downloadable wallpapers, buddy icons, and screen savers. Having a presence on the social networking sites allows **truth®** to spread its messages quickly and economically throughout the teen community. The impact of the social networking sites on driving traffic back to the main Web site has been substantial, with thetruth.com experiencing its best sustained traffic.

Cinema

Going to the movies continues to be a popular form of entertainment for teenagers. Beginning in 2007, **truth®** advertising began playing in movie theaters as commercials before movies—another effective way in which to reach the teen audience. In 2008, The "Sunny Side of **truth®**" campaign was seen in more than 1,500 Screenvision theaters on nearly 10,000 screens in 48 states.

GRASSROOTS OUTREACH

Summer tours across the country allow teens to engage firsthand with the campaign. Signature orange **truth®** "trucks" rigged with DJ decks and video monitors allow teens to speak and interact firsthand with **truth®** "crew members" at popular events and music festivals where teens gather. At each tour stop, crew members hold fashion shows, dance contests, freestyle rap "battles," and DJ lessons. The fun and engaging atmosphere makes it easier for **truth®** crew members to discuss tobacco issues in a non-preachy manner. Teens also walk away from these interactions with **truth®** "gear" items like T-shirts, bags, hats, and wallets. The gear subtly reinforces facts about tobacco and incorporates cool graphics and designs, creating sought-after items that teens are proud to wear.

In addition, the tour is heavily featured on thetruth.com Web site throughout the summer, allowing teens to meet **truth®** crew members and read the crew members' blogs, view updates from tour stops, and get free tickets. The latest tour, in 2008, reached more than 500,000 teens in more than 30 cities across the country (see Figures 2-2 and 2-3).

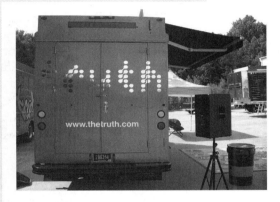

FIGURE 2-2   truth® Tour Truck
Courtesy of the American Legacy Foundation

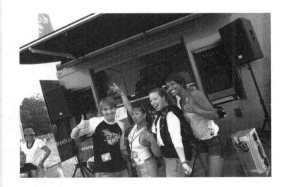

FIGURE 2-3   Summer Tours Engage Teens Firsthand with the Campaign
Courtesy of Joshua Cogan and the American Legacy Foundation

BUDGET

The American Legacy Foundation—and the **truth®** campaign—receive the majority of their funding as a result of the Master Settlement Agreement (MSA), which required the major tobacco companies to pay $206 billion over 25 years to compensate U.S. states for the cost of treating citizens with tobacco-related diseases. The American Legacy Foundation was created out of an MSA mandate that a national charitable foundation be created with the mission to help "prevent diseases associated with the use of tobacco products in the states."

A National Public Education Fund provided approximately 74% of the foundation's overall funding through 2005. This means that approximately $300 million in annual payments from the settling states to the American Legacy Foundation's National Public Education Fund have been suspended, thus producing a "funding cliff" that has dramatically affected the size and scope of the foundation's lifesaving programs.

Spending for the **truth®** Campaign reached a high in 2001, when the promotional budget was between $90 and $100 million. For 2008, the total promotional budget fell to between $35 and $40 million. Although that sounds like a lot of money, in comparison to what the tobacco industry spends it is actually very little. According to the Federal Trade Commission (FTC), the tobacco industry spent more than $13 billion in 2005 to market and promote its products in the United States alone—about $36 million per day—roughly equivalent to **truth®**'s budget for the year. **truth®** can never match that level of spending, so it strives to break through and be more cutting edge in order to effectively reach teens. With declining budgets, **truth®** is always looking for mutually beneficial partnerships that allow the campaign to further extend its lifesaving work and reach more teens.

The U.S. Centers for Disease Control and Prevention (CDC) is now (as of 2008) a key partner in further extending the reach of the **truth®** Campaign. Through a three-year, $3.6 million matching grant from the CDC awarded in 2006, the campaign increased its advertising in 18 states and 41 cities, reaching a broader range of youth, including young people in rural and surrounding smaller communities that typically have less exposure to the campaign because of low cable television penetration. The CDC renewed its grant with the foundation for a second phase of **truth®** advertising, allowing even more rural teens to be exposed to **truth®** advertising. A second component of the grant funds youth prevention-related grants at the community level.

OUTCOMES

A growing body of research has proven the efficacy of **truth®**. Research has found that the **truth®** Campaign accelerated the decline in youth smoking rates between 2000 and 2004. According to research published online in February 2009 by the *American Journal of Preventive Medicine* (AJPM), **truth®** was directly responsible for keeping 450,000 teens from starting to smoke during its first four years. A second study released through AJPM in February 2009 found that the campaign not only paid for itself in its first two years, but also saved between $1.9 and $5.4 billion in medical care costs to society.

In addition, research released in September 2007 found that the **truth®** Campaign may also be changing teens' perceptions about how common smoking is among their peers. A study conducted by RTI International and funded by the American Legacy Foundation indicated that teens exposed to the **truth®** Campaign have a more accurate view of the number of their peers who smoke. Teens with less exposure to the campaign believed smoking was more common among people their age. The study, "Association Between National Smoking Prevention Campaigns and Perceived Smoking Prevalence Among Youth in the United States," appeared in the *Journal of Adolescent Health*. The finding is good news for the **truth®** Campaign, because teens' perception of peer smoking has been shown to predict future smoking.

According to an article published on January 22, 2008, in *Health Education Research*, teens who were exposed to the American Legacy Foundation's national **truth®** youth smoking prevention campaign were more likely to harbor negative feelings toward the tobacco industry and more likely to intend not to smoke. The study expanded on previous research published in the *American Journal of Public Health* in 2002, *Getting to the Truth: Evaluation of National Tobacco Countermarketing Campaigns*, that looked at a 10-month period of the campaign. This 2008 study looks at an extended period of three years in which more than 35,000 young people aged 12 to 17 were polled on their attitudes toward **truth®**. The 2002 study showed that after only 10 months, exposure to the **truth®** Campaign increased young people's antitobacco attitudes and beliefs. This result was borne out again in the new study, which found that teens aware of the **truth®** Campaign were nearly twice as likely to say they did not intend to smoke in the future. The data showed that approximately 70% of teens were aware of the campaign over the three-year period. As in the prior study, the 2008 study examined nine tobacco-related beliefs and attitude items, including such points as "cigarette companies lie," "not smoking is a way to express independence," and "taking a stand against smoking is important to me." Exposure to the **truth®** Campaign was associated with steady, positive changes in attitudes, beliefs, and intentions to smoke.

In addition to proven research, the **truth®** Campaign has won more than 300 awards for advertising and public relations efficacy and has also been lauded by leading federal and state public health officials, the CDC, and the U.S. Department of Health and Human Services.

CASE STUDY 2
Washington State's Tobacco Quit Line

Like other states in the United States and consistent with the Centers for Disease Control and Prevention guidelines, Washington State is currently implementing a comprehensive tobacco control program with goals that include increasing cessation, preventing youth initiation, and reducing secondhand smoke exposure among the state's residents. A cornerstone of that program is the provision of a statewide toll-free telephone Quit Line, where any Washington resident may access trained counselors for tobacco cessation support. (See Figure 2-4.) National review panels have consistently recommended telephone counseling to help tobacco users to quit, and all states in the United States currently offer a tobacco quit line (Maher, Rohde, & Dent, 2007).

On November 14, 2007, the Washington Tobacco Quit Line, managed by the Washington State Department of Health, received its 100,000th call for help (Washington State Department of Health, 2008). This is the state's social marketing success story.

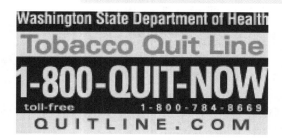

FIGURE 2-4   Quit Line Logo
Courtesy of Washington State Department of Health

BACKGROUND, PURPOSE, AND FOCUS

In 2000, there were an estimated 1 million adult tobacco users in Washington State. On November 15, 2000, the state launched a new service with a purpose to reduce this number and a focus on the estimated 70% (700,000) of smokers who had some desire to quit (Haase, 2002). As had been demonstrated by other states, a quit line approach is *effective* for a variety of reasons: it is more *cost-efficient*, with phone counseling as effective as face-to-face counseling yet less expensive to provide; it is *free* and *easily accessible* to residents throughout the state; it is more *convenient*, with no appointment necessary or need to travel; it is *confidential*; it offers *tailored protocols* for specific populations; and it has been shown to approximately double the typical (do-it-yourself) abstinence rates (Haase, 2002).

TARGET MARKET

The Quit Line's true target market—those most likely to call—were (and still are) tobacco users, aged 18 and over, who have decided they want to quit, those in the contemplation and preparation stages in the stages of change model (Prochaska, Norcross, & DiClemente, 1995). They have probably tried to quit in the past and may be feeling defeated. In terms of demographics, those who smoke are likely to be lower income, are less educated, live in rural areas, and may be less likely to have access to cessation support through traditional healthcare systems (BRFSS, 2006).

In terms of size of the target market, Washington's ongoing Behavioral Risk Factor Surveillance System (BRFSS) suggests the market is big, with two-thirds (68%) of smokers typically reporting that they want to quit, half (54%) seriously planning to quit within the next six months, and a third (33%) planning to quit within the next 30 days (BRFSS, 2006).

OBJECTIVES

The behavior objective for the campaign effort was (and still is) simple. The action program managers want from tobacco users who want to quit is to call the Quit Line.

BARRIERS, MOTIVATORS, AND COMPETITION

Formative research using focus groups prior to campaign development identified barriers to calling, those concerns that might keep someone from picking up the phone. Unanswered questions for this new service were the biggest barriers: How much does it cost? Will it be anonymous? Who will I talk to? What do they know about quitting? How many times can I talk with them? Can I get patches, pills, or other medications? Several fears were also expressed: *stigma* ("Others will think less of me"), *weakness* ("I should be able to do it myself"), *failure* ("If it works so great, I would have heard about it from other smokers"), and *judgment* ("If I called and didn't quit, I'd worry about what the person would think of me").

What might make smokers more likely to call? "Knowing what I am going to get when I call; knowing counselors are ex-smokers or have had experience with quitting; knowing the service would be free, friendly, and effective and tailored to me; and assurance that I can get ongoing support—not just a one-time call."

The greatest competition for this target market wanting to quit is trying to do it on their own. In addition, messages from others, often family members, who do not think they need to get help to quit smoking could keep them from picking up the phone.

POSITIONING

From these insights into barriers, motivators, and the competition, campaign planners crafted a positioning statement. "We want target audiences to believe that when they call the Quit Line, they will talk with counselors who will be empathetic and understanding of how difficult it is to quit. It has worked for others and is a better and easier option than trying to do it all by yourself." Importantly, planners did not (and still do not) want to make smokers feel bad, because they probably already have a heavy dose of guilt and feelings of helplessness.

Product

The Quit Line (1-800-QUIT-NOW, and in Spanish, 1-877-2NO-FUME) provides callers with a variety of services and information:

- One-on-one counseling and support from a trained specialist.
- A quit plan designed especially for each caller.
- Information about other resources, such as insurance benefits and additional programs available in local areas.
- Advice on designing a quit plan.
- Problem-solving ideas to help succeed.
- Skills to break old habits.
- Help deciding about products and medications that can help quitting be easier and more successful.
- Nicotine replacement therapy (patches, gum) for motivated quitters who are low-income or uninsured.
- Special services to help pregnant women quit smoking.

A free Quit Kit, which is mailed to those requesting one, is full of information on making a decision about quitting; getting ready to quit; knowing what to expect when quitting; coping with withdrawal symptoms and stress; and how to ask friends, family members, or co-workers for support.

Quit Line counselors have a bachelor's degree in health education, counseling, or a related field; are nonsmokers or ex-smokers with at least two years of abstinence; have previous experience with phone counseling, behavioral change programs, or addiction work; and participate in a rigorous initial orientation, as well as ongoing training.

Price

The Quit Line is a toll-free number, and there is no charge for the counselor. It is available for Washington residents, confirmed by the area code that shows up on the screen when the call is received, as well as the mailing address provided to the counselor for materials to be sent.

Place

Washington's Quit Line counselors are available for coaching seven days a week, from 5 a.m. to 9 p.m., with the exception of some major holidays when service begins at noon. A brief automated message thanks the caller for calling, mentions the call may be recorded for quality control purposes, and is then routed to a coach. After hours, callers can leave a message and a counselor will then return their call the next day. This accessibility is one of the most important advantages of a quit line, eliminating many of the barriers of traditional cessation classes such as having to wait for classes to form or needing to arrange for transportation. Quit lines are particularly helpful for people with limited mobility, as well as those who live in rural or remote areas. And due to their quasi-confidential nature, a phone service is more appealing to those reluctant to seek help in a face-to-face or group setting.

In addition, the Quit Line Web site, www.quitline.com, provides a downloadable worksheet for creating a quit plan, as well as a "Click to Call" button that prompts the user to enter his or her phone number and then receive a call back within five minutes. In addition, healthcare providers can refer a patient to the Quit Line by faxing them a form indicating the patient would like to be contacted by a Quit Line counselor, even what hours of the day would be most convenient.

Promotion

Messages were designed, messengers chosen, and media channels selected based on the target audience and the desired positioning, and are intended to highlight the product, price, and place.

Messages

Messages target those ready for action, apparent in this copy on the Quit Line Web site:

> Do you smoke cigarettes, cigars, or pipes? Chew tobacco? If you do and want to quit, or are thinking about it, the Quit Line is here to help. You may have tried quitting before. Maybe even more than once. Don't worry! That's why we developed the Washington State Quit Line. To help you successfully quit. The Web site provides tips to help you quit and all the information you need to know about calling the Quit Line. You can learn about Quit Line coaches who are ready to help you and hear a sample call. Check out the information below for phone numbers, hours and what to expect once you dial. After that, it's your call.

And brochure copy stresses the chances for success:

> Today more and more people are kicking the habit and quitting for good. You can be on your way to freedom by calling Washington's Tobacco Quit Line. New research shows that those who call the quit line double their chances of success.

Messengers

Key messengers include healthcare providers encouraging patients to call and Quit Line coaches assuring potential callers they understand and will help. Personal messages from counselors such as the following appear on the Web site as well:

> Tom: "I've been through the quit process and I can relate to it. It's rewarding to know I have an impact on people's lives. Callers say, 'Wow I didn't think of that. That really helps!' and it's nice to know I played a role in that. I just got off the phone with a guy who had been chewing and had successfully quit. He was so appreciative and just kept saying, 'I couldn't have done this without you!'"

> Merry: "I smoked for 25 years before I decided to quit. I understand how smokers feel and what it means to give up smoking, especially if you've been doing it for decades. That's why my most rewarding experiences have been helping long-time smokers. Some have smoked for more than 50 years! I draw on my experience and tell people that they have the ability to change, no matter how long they've been smoking."

Healthcare providers are important influencers as well, and those interested receive training and information about the Quit Line, as well as Quit Line wallet cards and brochures to give to patients.

Media Channels

A variety of media channels (including television, radio, print advertising, bar coasters, posters, postcards, transit ads, outdoor billboards, publicity, and the Web site) and grassroots targeting approaches (including flyers distributed at work sites, community colleges, and other community locations) are used to reach target audiences.

In June 2002, the Tobacco Program launched its first made-for-Washington advertising campaign promoting the Washington Tobacco Quit Line. A new television, radio, and print advertising campaign has promoted the Quit Line each year since this initial launch (see Figure 2-5).

In 2004, the campaign had the look and feel of an Alfred Hitchcock film. As reported in *The News Tribune* in Tacoma, Washington, "The anti-smoking spot starts with a woman who receives a telephone call at her office and encounters an eerie silence. Viewers see a cigarette on the other end of the telephone line. Next, while the woman drives in her car, she senses a presence. Viewers see a cigarette in the back seat, but the woman looks back and finds nothing. Finally, while the woman lies in bed, a cigarette appears frighteningly near her hand

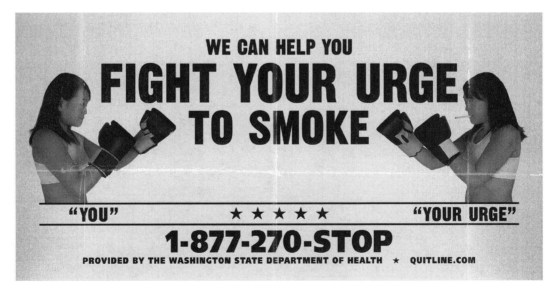

FIGURE 2-5 "Fight Your Urge to Smoke"
Courtesy of Washington State Department of Health

and she beats it to death with a shoe" (Voelpel, 2004). All to convince her, of course, that she can do it!

The latest campaign (2008) as this chapter was written, "Cold Turkey," emphasizes the importance of having a plan for organizing the quitting process. The star of the campaign is a real *cold turkey*, representing the difficulty of quitting "cold turkey" without a plan in place (see Figure 2-6).

In addition, the Tobacco Program hosts a Web site (Quitline.com) where visitors can listen to a sample call to the Quit Line, read stories from people who have quit tobacco, learn about the physical changes they can expect once they stop using tobacco, and meet some of the Washington Tobacco Quit Line specialists.

BUDGET

Funding for the Quit Line is from tobacco settlement dollars plus some enhanced funds from the Centers for Disease Control and Prevention (CDC) to run targeted promotions. The 2007–2008 budget for the service and promotion of the service was $2.8 million.

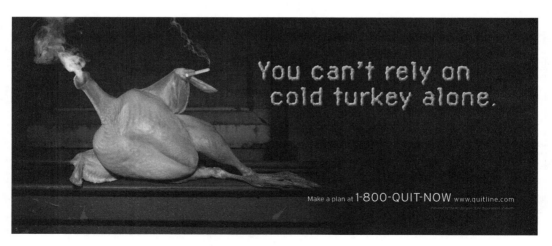

FIGURE 2-6   Graphic Image from 2008 Campaign Stressing the Need to Quit
Courtesy of David Emmite Photography

OUTCOMES

By 2006, the use of cigarettes in the state had decreased by approximately 24%, resulting in nearly 235,000 fewer smokers and moving the state to the fifth lowest prevalence of adult smoking in the nation—from 20th place in the year 2000. The Quit Line, launched in 2000, has certainly contributed to this outcome, receiving as mentioned earlier, its 100,000th call in November 2007 (Washington State Department of Health, 2007).

Profiles of Callers

An estimated 1% to 3% of Washington tobacco users have called the Quit Line, similar to overall national rates. Caller databases indicate that females are more likely to call than males (62% versus 38%), as well as those ages 41 to 50 (Haase, 2002; Quit Line, 2002). Telephone surveys conducted from October 2004 to October 2005 with Washington Quit Line callers shed light on additional demographics. Almost half of all callers (44%) were covered by private healthcare insurance or belonged to a health maintenance organization (HMO); a third (32%) received Medicaid; and a fourth (25%) were uninsured (Maher et al., 2007).

Quit Rates

Quit rate studies indicate that at six months, about 13% of callers have quit.

Hearing About the Quit Line

By 2006, nearly half of the smokers in the state had heard about the Quit Line (BRFSS, 2006), most commonly through television (37%), followed by a family member or friend (16%), healthcare provider (15%), or prior caller (12%), or through mention in the newspaper or magazine (6%; Quit Line, 2002).

Satisfaction With the Quit Line

A telephone survey with 356 callers, called back at two months after initial contact, indicated that the vast majority (86%) of callers were very or somewhat satisfied with the Quit Line; 87% were satisfied with their counselor; 89% with the materials they received; and 88% would recommend the Quit Line to a friend (Haase, 2002).

Cost-Effectiveness

Based on caller databases, telephone surveys, and budget records, the following costs were calculated; these can be used, in combination with expenditures, to determine a return on investment of resources:

- Estimated cost of the Quit Line service per Washington State smoker: $150.
- Estimated cost of the Quit Line per caller who made a serious attempt to quit: $140.
- Estimated cost of the Quit Line per caller who was tobacco free at six months: $830.

ADDITIONAL EVALUATION NOTES

Program managers for the Washington Quit Line offer a few additional insights for those considering adopting a similar service.

The Quit Line is most effective when used in combination with additional strategies, including tax increases, restrictions on smoking in public places such as restaurants and bars, and in combination with community-based activities such as recommendations from healthcare providers to call the Quit Line. They encourage others to advocate for cessation benefits to be included in health plans offered by employers to their employees, as well as by Medicaid and community health plans. Additionally, and though not formally tested, administrators have a "strong hunch" that offering a Quit Line and then having a highly visible campaign promoting it may help to "normalize" and increase quitting even among people who never call the line. After all, there are more than 25% fewer fellow smokers around in just seven years.

CONCLUDING NOTE: WE HAVE THE KNOW-HOW, BUT WILL WE DO IT?

Although much has been accomplished, the mission remains unfinished, with it unlikely that the United States will meet the Healthy People 2010 goal of 12% tobacco use for adults and 16% for high school youth (IOM, 2007, p. 124).

Concerns with waning momentum of tobacco control efforts and about declining attention to what remains the nation's largest public health problem, led the American Legacy Foundation (2004) to ask the Institute of Medicine (IOM) to conduct a major study of tobacco policy in the United States. The IOM then appointed a 14-member committee and charged it to assess past progress and future prospects in tobacco control and to develop a blueprint for reducing tobacco use in the United States. To carry out its charge, the committee conducted six meetings in 2004 and 2005, at which the members heard presentations from individuals representing academia, nonprofit organizations, and various state governments. The committee also reviewed an extensive literature from peer-reviewed journals, published reports, and news articles. The committee found it useful to set some boundaries on its work concerning the goal of "reducing tobacco use" and the time frame within which it should be achieved. To make its task manageable and well focused, the committee decided to focus its literature review and evidence gathering on reducing cigarette smoking (IOM, 2007, p. 31).

As referenced earlier in the chapter, this blueprint was published in 2007 in *Ending the Tobacco Problem: A Blueprint for the Nation*, which included 42 recommendations in these three categories (IOM, 2007, pp. 12–13):

- 22 measures to strengthen traditional tobacco control.
- 18 measures to change the regulatory landscape.
- 2 new frontiers in tobacco control:
  - Congress should direct the CDC to undertake a major program of tobacco control policy analysis and development and should provide sufficient funding to support the program.
  - The FDA should give priority to exploring the potential effectiveness of a long-term strategy for reducing the amount of nicotine in cigarettes and should commission the studies needed to assess the feasibility of implementing such an approach.

In the end, the committee projected that the following specific policies, if implemented effectively and collectively, were likely help the United States reach the original Healthy People 2010 smoking prevalence target of 12% by about 2020, with a 10% prevalence by 2025. Marketing mix tool labels have been added to reinforce the strategic blend this effort will require:

- *Product:* Full coverage of pharmacotherapy and behavioral therapy, training and coverage for tobacco brief interventions, multisession quit lines, Internet interventions, and free nicotine replacement therapy.
- *Product:* Universal implementation of school-based prevention sufficient to cut the rate of smoking initiation by 10%.
- *Price:* Tax increases of $1 or $2 per pack (depending on current state excise rates).

• *Place:* Heavy enforcement of youth-access laws, accompanied by publicity and high penalties.
• *Promotion:* Comprehensive media campaigns targeting youth and adults and funded at the levels recommended by the CDC (i.e., beyond the levels that have been used in the past) to prevent initiation and to increase quit attempts, heighten consumer demand for proven cessation programs, and increase smokers' health literacy about the value of using evidence-based treatments when trying to quit.

QUESTIONS FOR DISCUSSION

1. What component of the marketing process or element of the marketing mix do you think contributed most to the **truth®** Campaign's success?
2. What other factors and efforts do you think (or imagine) have also contributed to reduction in youth tobacco use in the United States?
3. For the Quit Line, several barriers were noted. What specific features of the product (Quit Line) addressed these barriers?
4. How would you go about calculating a rate of return on the Quit Line? What other data would you need?

REFERENCES

American Legacy Foundation. (2004). http://www.americanlegacy.org/

BBC News. (2008). Country profile: United States of America. Retrieved July 28, 2009, from http://newsvote.bbc.co.uk/mpapps/pagetools/print/news.bbc.co.uk/1/hi/world/americas/country_profiles/1217752.stm

Behavior Risk Factor Surveillance System (BRFSS). (2006). Behavior Risk Factor Surveillance System Adult Cigarette Use for Washington State. Atlanta, GA: Centers for Disease Control and Prevention (CDC).

Centers for Disease Control and Prevention (CDC). (2007). Fact sheet: Adult cigarette smoking in the United States: Current estimates. Retrieved July 28, 2009, from http://www.cdc.gov/mmwr/preview/mmwrhtml/mm5745a2.htm

Centers for Disease Control and Prevention (CDC). (2008). Morbidity and mortality weekly reports: Smoking & tobacco use. Retrieved March 19, 2009, from http://www.cdc.gov/mmwr/preview/mmwrhtml/mm5745a3.htm

Centers for Disease Control and Prevention (CDC). (2009). Fact sheet: Youth and tobacco use: Current estimates. Retrieved July 28, 2009, from http://www.cdc.gov/tobacco/data_statistics/fact_sheets/youth_data/tobacco_use/index.htm

Haase, T. T. (2002). *Effectiveness of the Washington Tobacco Quit Line.* Paper presented at the Joint Conference on Health, Wenatchee, WA. Retrieved July 28, 2009, from http://www.doh .wa.gov/tobacco/data_evaluation/Assessment/presentations/quit_line_final.pdf

Healthy People 2010. (2005). *Leading health indicators.* Retrieved July 28, 2009, from http:// www.healthypeople.gov/Document/HTML/uih/uih_4.htm

Institute of Medicine (IOM). (2007). *Ending the tobacco problem: A blueprint for the nation.* Washington, DC: National Academies Press.

Maher, J. E., Rohde, K., & Dent, C. W. (2007). *Is a statewide tobacco quit line an appropriate service for specific populations?* Retrieved July 28, 2009, from http://www.tobaccocontrol .bmj.com/cgi/content/abstract/16/Suppl_1/i65

Mowery, P. D., Brick, P. D., & Farrelly, M. C. (2000). Legacy first look report 3. *Pathways to established smoking: Results from the 1999 National Youth Tobacco Survey.* Washington, DC: American Legacy Foundation.

National Cancer Institute (NCI). (2001). Risks associated with smoking cigarettes with low machine-measured yields of tar and nicotine. *Smoking and Tobacco Control Monograph* 13, 1–236.

Prochaska, J. O., Norcross, J. C., & DiClemente, C. C. (1995). *Changing for good.* New York: Avon Books.

Quit Line. (2002). Adult tobacco telephone survey. Quit Line caller database, July 2001–June 2002.

Voelpel, D. (2004, December 5). Adman hopes to do for smoking what Hitchcock did for showering. *The News Tribune* (Tacoma, Washington), p. D1.

Washington State Department of Health. (2007). *Washington tobacco facts, January 2007.* Retrieved July 28, 2009, from http://www.doh.wa.gov/Tobacco/other/07tobfacts-public.pdf

Washington State Department of Health. (2008). *Washington Tobacco Quit Line receives 100,000th call for help.* Retrieved July 28, 2009, from http://www.prnewswire.com/ cgi-bin/stories.pl?ACCT=104&STORY=/www/story/11-14-2007/0004705649&EDATE =CBE/CSE Style:

World Health Organization (WHO). (2005). *Why is tobacco a public health priority?* Retrieved July 28, 2009, from http://www.who.int/tobacco/health_priority/en/index.html

CHAPTER 3

Saskatchewan in Motion

A Community-Based, Provincewide Social Marketing Initiative in Canada to Promote Physical Activity

François Lagarde, Cathie Kryzanowski, and James H. Mintz

CANADA: A COUNTRY OVERVIEW

Canada is the largest country in the Americas with 10 million square kilometers of land and a population of 33 million. About two-fifths of the country's population has origins other than British, French, or Aboriginal. It has a parliamentary democracy comprised of a federation of 10 provinces and three territories. English and French are the two official languages. Canada has an extensive social security network, including old-age pension, family allowance, employment insurance, and social assistance (Pan American Health Organization, 2008).

Healthcare System

Basic and publicly funded health care is provided to all Canadians through universal coverage of medically necessary healthcare services provided on the basis of need, rather than the ability to pay. These services are administered and delivered by the provincial and territorial governments and are provided free of charge with assistance from the federal government. The Canadian healthcare system has come under stress in recent years due to a number of factors, including changes in the way services are delivered, fiscal constraints, the aging of the baby-boom generation, and the high cost of new technology. Reforms are under way in most provinces and territories. Most reforms consider placing greater emphasis on promoting health, preventing illness and injury, and managing chronic diseases. The federal Public Health Agency of Canada acts as a focal point for disease prevention and control and for emergency response to infectious diseases; however, public health services are generally delivered at the provincial/territorial and local levels (Health Canada, 2005b).

Public Health Issues

Although Canadians are among the healthiest people in the world (Public Health Agency of Canada, 2007), they still face significant public health challenges:

- *Infectious disease factors:* In Canada, HIV rates have increased over the past five years, and sexually transmitted infections continue to spread. In addition, risks of a number of communicable diseases are increasing (e.g., West Nile virus), as well as possible emergencies and disasters associated with climate change and international terrorism.
- *Chronic disease burden:* More and more Canadians are directly associated with one or more risk factors, such as smoking, unhealthy eating, and physical inactivity, that often lead to the major chronic diseases, which account for two-thirds of all deaths in Canada: cardiovascular disease, cancer, diabetes, and respiratory disease. A number of initiatives have been implemented to address these issues. For example, the federal, provincial, and territorial health ministers have set a target to reduce obesity rates by 20% and an objective of increasing physical activity through public health policies and effective action. Recently, a Strategy for Cancer Control was developed and initiated.
- *Determinants of health and disparities:* Although Canadians are among the healthiest people in the world, some groups are not as healthy as others. Key health disparities in Canada are related to socioeconomic status, Aboriginal heritage, gender, and geographic location. Demonstrated changes to key indicators involve infant mortality, childhood obesity, poverty and child poverty, and road accidents, as well as the health and standard of living of Aboriginal people and visible minority immigrants. Recognizing that health is determined by complex interactions among social and economic factors, the physical environment, and individual behaviors, work to address health disparities and action on the determinants of health, in collaboration with

other sectors and partners, is considered central to public health. (Public Health Agency of Canada, 2007)

SOCIAL MARKETING AS A STRATEGY TO ADDRESS PUBLIC HEALTH ISSUES

As an early adopter of social marketing, Canada has integrated this unique form of marketing into many of its public health strategies for more than 30 years. Initially, social marketing was primarily used by national government departments, such as Health Canada (Mintz, 2004), and nongovernmental agencies like ParticipACTION, a national physical activity promotion agency (Edwards, 2004). Social marketing is now used in a more extensive and sustained way at all levels by an ever-growing constituency of trained professionals to address a broader range of public health issues.

Some Canadian public health issues and health determinants addressed through social marketing approaches in recent years include:

- Aboriginal diabetes (Health Canada, 2005a).
- Adult literacy (Turnley-Johnston, Lavack, & Clark, 2007).
- Air pollution (McDowell, 2008; McKenzie-Mohr, 2008).
- Alcohol abstinence among pregnant women (Deshpande et al., 2005).
- Drinking and driving (Mintz, 2004).
- Drug prevention (Mintz, 2004).
- Emergency preparedness (Mintz & Woolridge, 2008).
- Hand hygiene (Mah, Tam, & Deshpande, 2008).
- Healthy/environmentally friendly and affordable housing (Lagarde, 2007a, 2007b).
- Healthy living (Renaud, Caron-Bouchard, Beaulieu, & Martel, 2007).
- Injury prevention (Mintz, 2004).
- Nutrition (Duquette, 2008; Sali & Lavack, 2007).
- Occupational health and safety (Lavack et al., in press).
- Organ donation (Lagarde, 2005).
- Pesticides (Lévesque, 2008).
- Physical activity and healthy living (Edwards, 2004; Laberge, Bush, Chagnon, & Laforest, 2007).
- Smoking prevention and cessation (Lavack & Toth, 2004; Lagarde, Tremblay, & Des Marchais, 2007).
- Sudden infant death syndrome (Cotroneo, 2004).
- Youth development (Deshpande & Basil, 2006).

In an international survey on advanced-level social marketing training events (Deshpande & Lagarde, 2008), 174 of the 477 members of various social marketing and public-sector marketing listservs who responded to the survey were Canadians. While the findings from the survey cannot be generalized, because they are based on a small sample with a self-selection bias, the profile of Canadian respondents suggests that social marketing is being used extensively in public sector and nonprofit organizations at various levels of Canadian society:

- Most Canadians respondents worked for government (48%) or nongovernmental/nonprofit (29%) organizations.
- The job description of 30% of Canadian respondents specifically referred to social marketing.
- The field of practice most often mentioned was "protecting the environment" (35%) followed by "improved health" (22%).
- The geographical scope of Canadian respondents' work varied: 16% said citywide; 26% said county-/districtwide; 22% said provincewide; 22% said national; 10% said international; and 4% said nonapplicable.

The following Canadian Web sites are widely consulted by social marketing and health communications professionals in Canada and abroad:

- www.cbsm.com (Community-Based Social Marketing).
- www.hc-sc.gc.ca/ahc-asc/activit/marketsoc/index_e.html (Health Canada).
- www.thcu.ca (The Health Communication Unit, University of Toronto).
- www.toolsofchange.com (Tools of Change).

The case study in this chapter discusses the program launched in the province of Saskatchewan to encourage physical activity.

CASE STUDY
Saskatchewan in Motion

RATIONALE

Despite a large body of evidence stating that regular physical activity is critical to personal health and quality of life, the majority of Canadians remain inactive. According to the 2000 Physical Activity Monitor (Craig, Cameron,

Russel, & Beaulieu, 2001), a few years before *Saskatchewan in motion* was launched, 61% of Canadian adults were considered insufficiently active for optimal health benefits, and 43% of Canadian children and youth were insufficiently active for optimal growth and development.

Saskatchewan is a province with a population of 1 million, approximately 141,000 of whom are self-identified Aboriginals (Government of Saskatchewan, 2006). In studies such as the Canadian Fitness and Lifestyle Research Institute's Physical Activity Monitor and the Canadian Community Health Survey (CCHS), Saskatchewan consistently ranked among the most inactive provinces in Canada. In 2000, 69% of Saskatchewan adults were considered insufficiently active for optimal health benefits (Craig et al., 2001). Not surprisingly, the prevalence of diabetes in Saskatchewan increased by 41% from 1997 to 2001 (Canadian Diabetes Association, 2006). In addition, the incidence of obesity and overweight was above the national average (Tjepkema, 2004).

Saskatchewan in motion (SIM) was developed in 2002 by volunteer and public sector partners to increase physical activity by 10% by 2005 (see Figure 3-1). SIM is supported by the government of Saskatchewan to help achieve a similar target set by federal, provincial, and territorial ministers responsible for sport, recreation, and fitness to increase physical activity by 10% in every jurisdiction by 2010.

PURPOSE AND FOCUS

SIM is a provincewide movement aimed at increasing physical activity to generate health, social, environmental, and economic benefits. The intent is to ingrain understanding and behavior changes into the culture and fabric of Saskatchewan communities.

SIM adopted a social ecological model that suggests that successful movements require not only educational and promotional activities targeting the individual, but also efforts to reform organizations, develop policy, provide economic support, and inspire environmental changes—that is, a "people and

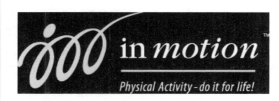

FIGURE 3-1   Saskatchewan in motion logo

Courtesy of Saskatchewan in motion

places" framework (Maibach, Abroms, & Marosits, 2007). SIM was designed as a comprehensive social marketing initiative that blends multimedia public awareness and education targeted at individuals with partnerships and community-based action (*Saskatchewan in motion*, 2008). The initiative focuses on creating conditions (physical and social environments) that support physical activity in a variety of settings. Communities are considered places as well as "interveners." "Communities need to be mobilized and take 'ownership' of a challenge for anything to take place" (Andreasen, 2006).

SITUATION ANALYSIS

Strengths

- Led by the Saskatoon Health Region in partnership with the University of Saskatchewan, the City of Saskatoon, and ParticipACTION, the community-level *in motion* concept was piloted in Saskatoon from 1998 to 2003. The pilot project was well researched and yielded very positive results. The project's success led provincial leaders to invest in a provincewide physical activity strategy.
- In Saskatchewan, the provincial lottery, managed by Sask Sport Inc., is the fundraiser for the volunteer sport, culture, and recreation system. This system is unique to Saskatchewan and has facilitated the development of a very strong, well-funded, vibrant sport, culture, and recreation delivery network throughout the province. The other important benefit of the lottery-funded network is the media-purchasing power it brings to the initiative. SIM partner Sask Sport Inc. purchases all lottery advertising and therefore carries significant weight when negotiating both airtime and public service contributions on behalf of SIM.

Weaknesses

- While the initial funding was generous, it was in the form of short-term grants. This created some challenges in establishing long-term partnerships and in developing plans, as well as recruiting and retaining qualified staff.

- While interest is high and passion is strong at the community level, the reality of day-to-day work continues to push the physical activity agenda to the corner of the desk or to fall on volunteer shoulders. Advocating for increased investment in human resources at the community level continues to be critical.

Opportunities and Challenges

- Prior to the SIM launch in 2003, there were no other physical activity strategies at the provincial level and very few community-based strategies. While initially identified as a weakness, it quickly became an opportunity as schools, communities, workplaces, neighborhoods, senior centers, and other settings all rallied behind the SIM brand and adopted it as their own.
- As mentioned earlier, Saskatchewan is a province of approximately 1 million people. The two largest cities each have a population of approximately 200,000, and the remaining 600,000 are spread among 800 communities ranging in size from 30,000 to 10. Many are isolated communities in the far north and other sparsely populated areas. Delivering a community-based strategy is more challenging when expertise and human capacity are limited outside of the two major centers. To address this issue, SIM placed significant emphasis on building community capacity and leadership training.
- At the time of the SIM launch, the province was leading up to its centennial in 2005, which provided many opportunities for new funding and programs. SIM was initially funded as part of the centennial celebrations to promote a sustainable future for the people of Saskatchewan.
- The people of Saskatchewan take great pride in being the lead province to establish the current national healthcare system. While highly valued, provincial healthcare spending continues to grow at a challenging rate. This situation lends a sense of urgency and commitment to explore new solutions with a wide range of partners.

Threats

The government of Saskatchewan provides short-term grant funding to SIM through a special fund from casino revenues. Although the investment has been significant, the short-term nature of the financial support poses a threat to the sustainability of the initiative:

- In the early years, some partners were slow to "join the movement." SIM was viewed as a short-term "flavor-of-the-month" initiative without sustained support for community action.
- It can be challenging to provide frequent reports and grant proposals showing significant short-term successes when addressing long-term societal change.

PAST AND SIMILAR EFFORTS

A wide range of excellent physical activity strategies began to emerge across Canada in communities and provinces in the late 1990s. SIM was unique in that it was the only strategy that embraced a comprehensive, multisetting social marketing approach. SIM looked to other successful health promotion strategies, such as tobacco reduction, seatbelt usage, and recycling, for guidance to build the strategy.

TARGET AUDIENCES

A wide range of public, stakeholder, and decision-maker audiences, summarized in Table 3-1, were considered in the SIM initiative.

The following demographic segments were identified as priorities:

- People aged 30 to 55 years (primarily because of their role as parents, as well as key influencers in communities, schools, workplaces, and families).
- Children.
- Youth.
- Aboriginal peoples.

TABLE 3-1 Saskatchewan in Motion Target Audiences by Category: Individuals, Stakeholders in Settings, Decision Makers

Individuals	Stakeholders in Settings	Decision Makers
• Adults aged 30–55	General	Provincial
• Children and youth	• Chronic disease organizations	• Elected officials
• Parents	Communities	• Deputy ministers
• Aboriginal people	• Recreation and sport professionals	Community
	• Community administrators	• Elected officials
	• Urban planners	• Senior administrators
	• Health promotion	• Key community leaders
	Schools	Education
	• Teachers	• Principals
	• Parent organizations	• School board officials
	Workplaces	Workplaces
	• Occupational health	• Chief executive officers
	• Human resources	• Managers

GOALS AND OBJECTIVES

SIM established a rallying and ambitious vision:

> The people of Saskatchewan will be among the healthiest, most physically active in Canada.

More specifically, SIM's goals are to:

- Be in the top three of Canada's most physically active provinces by 2012.
- Raise the "grade" for Saskatchewan children and youth as reported annually in Canada's Report Card on Physical Activity for Children and Youth.
- Celebrate the success of SIM based on measurements against clear outcomes.

Specific behavioral, knowledge, and belief objectives (where applicable) for the various audience categories are outlined in Tables 3-2, 3-3, and 3-4.

TABLE 3-2 Saskatchewan in Motion Behavioral Objectives

Audience Categories	Behavioral Objectives
Individuals	• More people in Saskatchewan will increase their level of physical activity to meet guidelines recommended by Canada's Guide to Healthy Active Living. Inactive individuals will increase activity to moderate levels, and moderately active individuals will reach the guidelines recommended by Canada's Guide to Healthy Active Living (i.e., adults—a minimum of 30 minutes a minimum of 5 days per week; children and youth—a minimum of 60 to 90 minutes every day of the week).
	• Individuals will speak out (advocate) about their physical activity needs and the needs of those they care about.
Stakeholders in settings	• Communities, schools, and workplaces will create the physical and social environments necessary to support individuals' desire to increase physical activity.
	• All Saskatchewan schools (elementary and secondary) will ensure that all students have access and opportunity for at least 30 minutes of physical activity every day.
	• Communities, schools, and workplaces throughout the province will consider and respond to the physical activity needs of Aboriginal people
	• First Nations communities will increase their capacity to engage citizens in physical activity opportunities.
	• Stakeholders will work together to create the conditions necessary for individuals to be more physically active.
	• Formal mechanisms will be in place to facilitate creative and cooperative partnerships at the community/delivery level.
	• Leaders will speak out (advocate) about their physical activity needs and the needs of those they care about.
	• Saskatchewan physical activity researchers will work together to establish a Center of Excellence for physical activity research. Researchers will gather, analyze, and report data that will tell a compelling story for SIM and guide the SIM strategic direction.
Decision makers	• The *in motion* movement will be supported with long-term, stable, and sustainable resources.
	• Decision makers at all levels will invest in physical activity.
	• School boards will implement a daily physical activity policy.
	• SIM leaders will be supported and recognized for their efforts to work together to develop, implement, and evaluate long-term, sustainable physical activity strategies.

TABLE 3-3   Saskatchewan in Motion Knowledge Objectives

Audience Categories	Knowledge Objectives
Individuals	• Saskatchewan adults will have increased awareness of how much physical activity is needed to achieve health benefits for themselves, children, and youth.
	• Saskatchewan adults will know where to go for credible information on physical activity for themselves and their families.
Stakeholders in settings	• Key stakeholders and delivery networks will have a clear understanding of their role in increasing physical activity.
	• Leaders in education (teachers, administrators, decision makers, and parent groups) will understand the physical inactivity issue and the role of schools in increasing physical activity for children, youth, and families.
Decision makers	• Decision makers in a variety of settings will understand their role in addressing physical inactivity.

TABLE 3-4   Saskatchewan in Motion Belief Objectives Among All Audiences

Belief Objectives
• Saskatchewan people will feel that they are part of a "movement" and that SIM is more than an organization or program (this feeling should translate to a strong and shared sense of belonging and accomplishment).
• SIM will be perceived as more than a short-term advertising campaign.
• An increased number of Saskatchewan people will recognize the SIM brand as a credible source for information about physical activity.
• A wide range of organizations will associate with and use the SIM brand and materials as their own.
• Physical activity will be considered the "norm" in Saskatchewan.

TARGET AUDIENCE BARRIERS, MOTIVATORS, AND COMPETITION

Barriers

Provincial research conducted by Fast Consulting (2003) and the University of Saskatchewan on behalf of SIM confirms national data (Craig & Cameron, 2004) that suggest the following barriers to individual participation in regular physical activity:

- Lack of time.
- Lack of interest or preference for more sedentary activities.
- Lack of access (to programs and/or facilities).

Other barriers identified included:

- Lack of skill.
- Concerns about personal safety.
- Winter climate.
- Lack of social support for participation.

Informal research and evaluation (past experience and interviews) suggest the following barriers to the development and delivery of community-based strategies:

- Lack of leadership capacity.
- Lack of financial resources.
- Lack of interest.
- Competing priorities.
- Lack of support from senior officials.
- Lack of a clear understanding of potential roles.

Motivators and Perceived Benefits

Literature review, focus group testing, and expert task force committees have guided the development of messages based on key motivators and perceived benefits (see Table 3-5).

Competition

The greatest competition for physical activity among adults, youth, and children is discretionary time over more desired, sedentary lifestyle choices (i.e., screen-time activities and increasing consumption of media; Maibach, 2007).

TABLE 3-5   Summary of Motivators and Perceived Benefits

Audiences	Motivators and Perceived Benefits
Individuals	• Although Saskatchewan adults understand the importance of physical activity for health benefits, health benefits alone were not enough to motivate action.
Adults	• Making physical activity fun, safe, easy, and convenient. • Spending time with friends and family. • Feeling good. • Maintaining a healthy body weight.
Children and youth	• Achieving fun/personal satisfaction. • Spending time with friends and family. • Pleasing others (teachers and parents).
Key stakeholders (all settings)	• Achieving professional goals. • Having an opportunity to influence the health of the people they care about.
Community setting	• Bringing partners together. • Adding new resources and expertise.
School setting	• Better managing classrooms and behavior. • Adding new resources and expertise. • Increasing readiness to learn among students.
Workplace setting	• Increasing employee morale. • Adding convenience.
Decision makers (all settings)	• Achieving professional goals. • Having an opportunity to influence the health of the people they care about. • Reducing (healthcare) costs. • Establishing a healthy and vibrant society.
Community setting	• Achieving environmental targets. • Attracting new families/workplaces. • Obtaining economic benefits.
School setting	• Providing support for teachers. • Sharing responsibility (with community and family). • Assisting with academic achievement.
Workplace setting	• Increasing productivity. • Reducing absenteeism. • Bettering employee recruitment and retention.

Saskatchewan is a motor vehicle–based society. The small population (1 million) is spread out over a large land mass (651,900 km²), even in large communities. Community growth trends have also moved shopping, services, and major recreation facilities to the edges of communities, forcing people to almost exclusively choose motor vehicles over more active modes of transportation.

For many stakeholders, physical activity strategies are add-on activities. Alongside healthy eating, substance abuse, and crisis management in hospitals, physical activity is just another issue competing for investment by decision makers.

POSITIONING STATEMENTS

SIM wants people in Saskatchewan to see physical activity as:

- Fun, easy, and safe—providing energy and a sense of well-being, feeling and looking good, as well as a sense of pride by being a good role model for children.
- Providing a break in our busy lives.
- Being adopted by a growing number of people in Saskatchewan (being part of a movement).

Calls to action to stakeholders and decision makers should be perceived as realistic. As an initiative, SIM was designed as a provincewide (nongovernmental) "movement" to promote physical activity (not owned by one organization) supported by thousands of community leaders (including Aboriginal leaders), schools, workplaces, and health professionals to create conditions that are conducive to physical activity where people live, learn, work, and play. In short, SIM wants the people of Saskatchewan to increase physical activity for themselves and those they care about.

STRATEGIES

Mobilizing Settings Around the 4Ps

The "settings" approach of SIM is specifically aimed at addressing various product, price, place, and promotion considerations related to physical activity. In keeping with the roles recommended by Maibach (2003) for state-level organizations, SIM systematically approaches settings through a number of mobilization and advocacy interventions:

- Communities are approached using many of the recommended steps in the Active Living by Design program (Active Living by Design, 2008). Communities are initially invited to submit a proposal to host a one-day "Moving Together" symposium. They receive a CAN$5,000 grant for facilities, meals, and other expenses. SIM provides expert speakers and a facilitator. To be eligible, communities must ensure that the mayor (and at least one other councilor), senior community officials, senior health officials, and influential community members are in the room for at least one hour first thing in the morning. SIM works with the organizers to prepare an agenda. At the symposium, a motivational speaker talks about the issue and the need to make changes to the community environment. A representative from Active Living by Design from Minnesota then talks about how it works in his or her community, which is followed by a community discussion about the next steps. Although decision makers are only expected to listen to the speakers, at least 50% of them will typically stay for the day once they hear the speaker in the morning.
- Community school councils are charged with an accountability framework for schools. SIM is offering to work with them to determine what schools should be accountable for over the coming years and ensure physical activity is not omitted (i.e., committing to the goal of a minimum of 30 minutes of physical activity every day per student). This goal is accomplished through a combination of physical education, physical activity breaks/programs, intramural activities, sports programs, and special events.

The following are sample calls to action aimed at various stakeholders and decision makers in order to address product, price, place, and promotion issues regarding physical activity (for more, see www.saskatchewaninmotion.ca). These calls to action are based on varying degrees of evidence (see Brownson, Haire-Joshu, & Luke, 2006; Gordon, McDermott, Stead, & Angus, 2006; Lagarde & LeBlanc, 2008):

- *Community setting:*
  - Product:
    - Start a running/walking, biking, in-line skating, or dance club.
    - Search for unused space and turn it into a group activity area.
    - Offer secure bicycle racks so people can bike around the community.
    - Coordinate physical activity challenges to coincide with local and major sporting events.
  - Price:
    - Offer incentives for distance parking.
    - Offer activities and programs based on people's skills.

- Place:
  - Develop indoor and outdoor walking paths.
  - Convert local halls into walking areas.
  - Groom a cross-country skiing trail near your community.
  - Ensure environments and facilities are available and accessible to people with disabilities.
  - Develop and encourage active and safe routes to school.
  - Offer safe, attractive, and accessible trails for bicycling, walking, and wheelchair activity.
- Promotion:
  - Promote active transportation. Make people aware of the various opportunities to run, walk, bike, or in-line skate to commute within your community or for short trips.
  - Place a physical activity board in high pedestrian traffic or business areas.
  - Hold recognition activities for people making efforts to adopt healthier lifestyles.
- *School setting:*
  - Product:
    - Add a "Move" memory game—Play a memory game in which students memorize movements instead of words.
    - Fitness breaks—Take two-minute breaks between lessons. Ask students to lead or just play music and let them dance!
    - Add "verb fun"—Students act out verbs such as skip, hop, and jump. Have students modify actions by adding adverbs, such as rapidly, powerfully, and enthusiastically.
  - Price:
    - Request used sports equipment donations to make activity buckets for use at recess and other breaks.
  - Place:
    - Adjust school schedule to optimize gym use during recess.
  - Promotion:
    - Create an active environment by posting a bulletin board full of photos of teachers, students, and administrators being active.
- *Workplace setting:*
  - Product:
    - Start a walking club.
    - Start an active commuter program with your colleagues to get to and from work.
    - Participate in or start a recreation league at your company.

- Allow flextime for people to participate in physical activities.
- Try a group stretch routine instead of sitting down for a coffee break.
- Integrate a physical activity program into your human resources strategy.
- Host recreational events, such as golf tournaments, horseshoe-pitching, dances, and sports days.
- Price:
  - Share the costs of employee memberships in physical activity programs or clubs.
- Place:
  - Ensure that employees have access to bike racks, showers, changing rooms, and so on.
  - Stay at hotels with fitness areas while on trips.
- Promotion:
  - Use bulletin boards to provide general and local physical activity information for employees and their families.
  - Send e-briefs and newsletters with physical activity tips and prompts.

To address the unique needs of northern and Aboriginal peoples, additional school policy resources were developed, jointly with the Northern Healthy Communities Partnership. It contains numerous product-, price-, and place-related strategies.

Mass Media and Advocacy Campaigns

Although each setting strategy includes promotional elements, two additional streams of communication activities were designed: (1) a mass-media campaign to reach individuals and, more specifically, the main segment of the target population (people aged 30 to 55) and (2) an advocacy campaign to reach key stakeholders and decision makers. These streams were consciously designed to take into account the various complementary models of behavior change implicit in public health communications campaigns: the individual effects model (focusing on individual knowledge, attitudes, and behaviors), the social diffusion model (focusing on social norms), and the institutional diffusion model (focusing on policy changes; Hornik, 2002).

The mass media campaign and messages were designed in a number of phases as follows:

- *Phase 1—captivate and motivate:*
  - Introducing the brand and tagline ("Join the Movement").
  - Let people know getting active is fun, easier than they think, and they'll feel good!

- Show a variety of people being active in a wide range of ways.
- Encourage people to call a toll-free number or visit a Web site for 100 easy ways to be active and other information (see Figure 3-2).
- *Phase 2—demonstrate and motivate:*
  - Show people examples of specific ways to get active and what "counts" toward being physically active at least "30 minutes a day, five days a week" for health benefits.
  - Show that physical activity is catching on and becoming the norm.
  - Talk about the benefits and rewards of physical activity, particularly those that appeal to human aspirations, such as wanting to feel great.
  - Continue to drive people to the Web site for more information.
  - Start incorporating success stories/testimonials/comments on the Web site so people can see what others are doing and be encouraged to follow suit.
  - Encourage people to ask others to "Join the Movement."
- *Phase 3—celebrate and motivate:*
  - Keep using a highly recognizable look, feel, and music, but introduce real-life success stories as proof that Saskatchewan *really is in motion*.
  - Continue to encourage those who have not joined the movement to do so by asking, "Have you joined the movement?"
  - Link to Saskatchewan's centennial as a time for celebration.
- *Phase 4—reach out to others:*
  - Provide messages focused on being active with your family and those you care about.

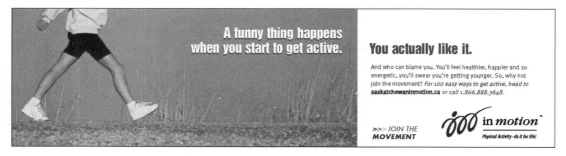

FIGURE 3-2　"You actually like it" ad
Courtesy of Saskatchewan in motion

- Address the disconnection between perceived physical activity levels and real physical activity levels.
- Encourage parents to pay attention to how much activity their kids are really getting.

The communication channels used include mass media (television, radio, newspapers, outdoor, movie theaters, and posters), schools, workplaces, public events, prompts in public settings, and the Internet. Messengers are peers (testimonials), actors to whom individuals can relate, and ambassadors (influential individuals from a variety of settings).

Key messages for the advocacy campaign are essentially the following (see Figure 3-3):

- We are facing a physical inactivity epidemic with consequences relevant to your work/school/community (depending on interest or focus).
- It will require long-term sustainable investment in efforts that are upstream, cooperative, innovative, and community/setting-based.
- You have a role to play to address this crisis.
- It is a shared role; others will join your efforts.
- *In motion* can help with tools, resources, human resource capacity, and training.
- Join the movement.
- Be a leader.

The communication channels used as part of the advocacy components include meetings, sector-specific delivery networks, conferences, trade shows, presentations, articles, direct mail, tools and resources, and the SIM Web site. Messengers are sector leaders, ambassadors, and peers.

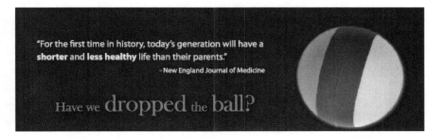

FIGURE 3-3 Advocacy banner
Courtesy of Saskatchewan in motion

BUDGET AND TIME FRAME

The budget for the first three years (April 2003–March 2006) was CAN$2 million per year:

- Advertising and promotion: CAN$800,000.
- Community grants: CAN$700,000.
- Resource development and training: CAN$300,000.
- Targeted strategies: CAN$100,000.
- Research: CAN$100,000.

The budget for the next two years (April 2006–March 2008) was CAN$1.6 million per year:

- Mobilizing communities (training, resources, grants): CAN$700,000.
- Raising awareness (advertising and communications): CAN$600,000.
- Building partnerships: CAN$125,000.
- Research: CAN$175,000.

In addition to the preceding resources, the following investments were made:

- The University of Saskatchewan, a SIM research partner, has invested several million dollars in research projects funded both internally and by national research partners.
- Saskatchewan media have invested, on average, CAN$6 for every dollar spent on advertising. From April 2003 to March 2008, approximately CAN$2.3 million was spent, with media values estimated to be more than CAN$13.8 million.
- SIM strategic partners have invested close to CAN$300,000 per year in in-kind contributions.
- Efforts are in place to measure the significant investments made at the community level and in various settings.

EVALUATION

The process evaluation for SIM was conducted at the conclusion of the initial three-year phase (March 2006) by an independent firm (Meyers Norris Penny, 2005). Consultations during the process evaluation led to the following conclusions and lessons learned:

- The *in motion* brand was appropriate to use and should continue to be the brand for Saskatchewan's physical activity strategy.
- Community ownership was critical to community uptake, and communities with an identifiable leader were the most successful. Three recurring factors (strong leadership, committed volunteers, and broad-based community involvement) were key to success.
- *In motion* received significant media attention focused on obesity and inactivity. Communities had a heightened degree of interest, but readiness in terms of necessary skills and competencies was lacking. The degree of training, mentorship, consultative support and resource development required was vastly underestimated.
- Interviewees identified a need for professional staff at the regional level.
- Program resources were deemed sufficient for the project. The short-term funding was, however, insufficient to develop, launch, and implement a project aimed at achieving a 10% behavior change within three years.
- The initiative was deemed a success based on the skills sets and experience of those involved, as well as the involvement of national experts to help develop strategies.
- The mass media campaign benefited greatly from existing relationships between partner organizations and media agencies.
- Interviewees generally agreed that a mass media campaign combined with a community mobilization strategy is a necessary and effective way to inspire change.
- The timely distribution of communication materials and resources was a challenge throughout the project.

In terms of outputs as of 2008, SIM has grown in five years to a movement made up of thousands of individuals, 158 community action teams, 400 schools (approximately half), 473 workplaces, and more than 800 champions and leaders in 252 communities (accounting for approximately 80% of the population).

Research projects to monitor changes related to the product, price, and place components of the social marketing mix in the various settings are under way, and findings are not yet fully available. One such research project conducted by the University of Saskatchewan is measuring the impact of SIM on community capacity building before and after launching the SIM initiative. Measures include a range of factors, such as improved organizational structure, leadership, program management and assessment, resource mobilization, participation, and adoption of desired actions (see the behavioral objectives for stakeholders in settings in Table 3-2). Initial results show positive overall results.

As a proximal measure of its mass media campaign, SIM's campaign/brand awareness was monitored by an independent firm (Checkmate Strategic Planning, 2005). One year after its launch, SIM achieved 49% prompted brand awareness among the main audience of the mass media campaign (adults aged 30 to 55). Brand awareness increased to 58% in 2005 and to 69% in 2007. Such outcome compares with the median (70%) observed in an international review of physical activity campaigns (Cavill & Bauman, 2004).

A baseline survey was conducted prior to the launch of the SIM initiative to determine physical activity levels and attitudes toward physical activity among Saskatchewanians. The survey was conducted by a research company (Fast Consulting, 2003) in partnership with the University of Saskatchewan. It was designed to be compatible with the Canadian Fitness and Lifestyle Research Institute Physical Activity Monitor to enable national comparisons. In a follow-up survey conducted in 2005 (Fast Consulting, 2005), data showed an increase in self-reported physical activity among adults (from 48% to 56%). However, no significant changes were noted among children, youth, and Aboriginal peoples. Based on these outcomes, SIM is redirecting some of its efforts toward children and youth as well as considering alternative evaluation methods to parent reporting on children's levels of activity. There is also an appreciation that noticeable change will require sustained efforts for many years ahead.

CONCLUSION

As an illustration of how social marketing practices have evolved in Canada, *Saskatchewan in motion* has adopted a multifaceted approach to behavioral change and has formalized a systematic process to promote and advocate for community-based action. In addition to a mass media campaign, a central component of SIM is the commitment of community partners (municipalities, schools, and workplaces) to create and adopt the necessary programs and physical and social environments, as well as policies to make physical activity more attractive, barrier-free, and sustainable. The ultimate impact of SIM on physical activity levels will likely be observed only over a longer period because experience has shown that social and behavioral change is gradual and the result of long-term and sustained efforts (Hastings, 2007; Siegel & Doner Lotenberg, 2007). However, the involvement of a growing number of stakeholders and initial results are encouraging. They form the basis for a dynamic societal movement in support of physical activity in Saskatchewan.

QUESTIONS FOR DISCUSSION

1. How is SIM's approach consistent with a comprehensive social marketing framework?
2. Can you give some examples of calls to action aimed at various stakeholders and decision makers to address product, price, place, and promotion issues related to physical activity?
3. How was the SIM message strategy used to highlight that physical activity is becoming the norm?

REFERENCES

Active Living by Design. (2008). Retrieved July 28, 2009, from http://www.activelivingby design.org

Andreasen, A. (2006). *Social marketing in the 21st century*. Thousand Oaks, CA: Sage Publications.

Brownson, R. C., Haire-Joshu, D., & Luke, D. A. (2006). Shaping the context of health: A review of environmental and policy approaches in the prevention of chronic diseases. *Annual Review of Public Health* 27, 341–370.

Canadian Diabetes Association. (2006). *Regional advocacy workshops—Saskatchewan back-grounder*. Retrieved July 28, 2009, from http://www.diabetes.ca/Files/2006-sask-backgrounder.doc

Cavill, N., & Bauman, A. (2004). Changing the way people think about health-enhancing physical activity: Do mass media campaigns have a role? *Journal of Sports Sciences* 22(8), 771–790.

Checkmate Strategic Planning. (2005). *In motion—Public awareness survey 2005* (unpublished).

Cotroneo, S. (2004). *Back to sleep—Health Canada SIDS social marketing campaign.* Retrieved July 28, 2009, from http://www.toolsofchange.com/English/CaseStudies/default.asp?ID=161

Craig, C. L., & Cameron, C. (2004). *Increasing physical activity: Assessing trends from 1998–2003*. Ottawa, Ontario, Canada: Canadian Fitness & Lifestyle Research Institute.

Craig, C. L., Cameron, C., Russel, S. J., & Beaulieu, A. (2001). *Increasing physical activity: Supporting children's participation*. Ottawa, Ontario, Canada: Canadian Fitness & Lifestyle Research Institute.

Deshpande, S., & Basil, M. (2006). Lessons from research on social marketing for mobilizing adults for positive youth development. In E. G. Clary & J. E. Rhodes (Eds.), *Mobilizing adults for positive youth development: Lessons from the behavioral sciences on promoting socially valued activities* (pp. 211–231). New York: Kluwer/Plenum.

Deshpande, S., Basil, M., Basford, L., Thorpe, K., Piquette-Tomei, N., Droessler, J., et al. (2005). Promoting alcohol abstinence among pregnant women: Potential social change strategies. *Health Marketing Quarterly* 23(2), 45–67.

Deshpande, S., & Lagarde, F. (2008). International survey on advanced-level social marketing training events. *Social Marketing Quarterly* 14(2), 50–66.

Duquette, M. P. (2008). *Montreal dietary dispensary.* Retrieved July 28, 2009, from http://www.toolsofchange.com/English/CaseStudies/default.asp?ID=37

Edwards, P. (2004). No country mouse: Thirty years of effective marketing and health communications. *Canadian Journal of Public Health* 95 (Suppl. 2), S6–S13.

Fast Consulting. (2003). *In motion* physical activity baseline survey for the provincial *in motion* strategy. Unpublished report presented to *Saskatchewan in motion*.

Fast Consulting. (2005). *In motion* physical activity survey for the provincial *in motion* strategy. Unpublished report presented to *Saskatchewan in motion*.

Gordon, R., McDermott, L., Stead, M., & Angus, K. (2006). The effectiveness of social marketing interventions for health improvement: What's the evidence? *Public Health* 120, 1133–1139.

Government of Saskatchewan. (2006). *Saskatchewan Aboriginal peoples*. Retrieved July 29, 2008, from http://www.stats.gov.sk.ca/pop/2006%20Census%20Aboriginal%20Peoples.pdf

Hastings, G. (2007). *Social marketing: Why should the devil have all the best tunes?* Oxford, UK: Butterworth Heinemann.

Health Canada. (2005a). *Aboriginal Diabetes Initiative (ADI)—Eat right. Be active. Have fun. You can prevent diabetes campaign*. Retrieved July 28, 2009, from http://www.hc-sc.gc.ca/ahc-asc/activit/marketsoc/camp/adi-ida_e.html

Health Canada. (2005b). *Canada's health care system*. Ottawa, Ontario: Government of Canada. Retrieved July 28, 2009, from http://www.hc-sc.gc.ca/hcssss/alt_formats/hpbdgps/pdf/pubs/2005-hcs-sss/2005-hcs-sss_e.pdf

Hornik, R. C. (2002). Public health communication: Making sense of contradictory evidence. In R. C. Hornik (Ed.), *Public health communication: Evidence for behaviour change* (pp. 1–19). Mahwah, NJ: Lawrence Erlbaum Associates.

Laberge, S., Bush, P., Chagnon, M., & Laforest, S. (2007). *Promotion de l'activité physique et impact de l'activité physique sur certains facteurs favorisant l'apprentissage*. Montréal, Quebec, Canada: Comité de gestion de la taxe scolaire de l'île de Montréal.

Lagarde, F. (2005). *Guide for planning public awareness and education initiatives to promote organ and tissue donation*. Canadian Council for Donation and Transplantation. Retrieved July 28, 2009, from http://www.ccdt.ca/english/publications/final-pdfs/Guide-Public-Awareness.pdf

Lagarde, F. (2007a). *Equilibrium 2007 & 2008 integrated strategic orientation*. Ottawa, Ontario: Canada Mortgage and Housing Corporation.

Lagarde, F. (2007b). *The social marketing of affordable housing solutions*. Ottawa, Ontario: Canada Mortgage and Housing Corporation.

Lagarde, F., & Leblanc, C. M. A. (2008). *Physical activity in schools*. Background paper for the June 2007 Satellite Expert Roundtable on the WHO Global Strategy on Diet, Physical Activity and Health: A School Policy Framework.

Lagarde, F., Tremblay, M., & Des Marchais, V. (2007). Physicians taking action against smoking. In G. Hastings, *Social marketing: Why should the devil have all the best tunes?* (pp. 292–296). Oxford, UK: Butterworth Heinemann.

Lavack, A., & Toth, G. (2004). *Reducing the social acceptability of smoking: A role for government?* Case Study 4.05, Case Studies in Public Administration Program, Institute of Public Administration of Canada.

Lavack, A. M., Magnuson, S., Deshpande, S., Basil, D., Basil, M., & Mintz, J. H. (in press). Enhancing occupational health and safety in young workers: The role of social marketing. *International Journal of Nonprofit and Voluntary Sector Marketing*.

Lévesque, M. (2008). *Reducing pesticide use in Hudson, St. Lazare, and Notre Dame de L'Ile Perrot*. Retrieved July 28, 2009, from http://www.toolsofchange.com/English/CaseStudies/default.asp?ID=172

Mah, M., Tam, Y. C., & Deshpande, S. (2008). A social marketing analysis of 20 years of hand hygiene promotion. *Infection Control and Hospital Epidemiology* 29(3), 262–270.

Maibach, E. W. (2003). Recreating communities to support active living: A new role for social marketing. *American Journal of Health Promotion* 18(1), 114–119.

Maibach, E. W. (2007). The influence of the media environment on physical activity: Looking for the big picture. *American Journal of Health Promotion* 21(4), 353–362.

Maibach, E. W., Abroms, L. C., & Marosits, M. (2007). Communication and marketing as tools to cultivate the public's health: A proposed "people and places" framework. *BMC Public Health* 7, 88. [Electronic version]

McDowell, J. (2008). *20/20—The way to clean air*. Retrieved July 28, 2009, from http://www.toolsofchange.com/English/CaseStudies/default.asp?ID=188

McKenzie-Mohr, D. (2008). Turn it off: An anti-idling campaign (2007). In P. Kotler & N. R. Lee (Eds.), *Social marketing: Influencing behaviors for good* (3rd ed., pp. 360–362). Thousand Oaks, CA: Sage Publications.

Meyers Norris, Penny. (2005). *Saskatchewan in motion* process evaluation. Submitted to *Saskatchewan in motion*.

Mintz, J. H. (2004). *Social marketing in health promotion . . . The Canadian experience*. Retrieved July 28, 2009, from http://www.hc-sc.gc.ca/ahc-asc/alt_formats/cmcd-dcmc/pdf/marketsoc/experience_e.pdf

Mintz, J. H., & Woolridge, T. (2008). Is your family prepared? (Public Safety Canada 2006–2007). In P. Kotler & N. R. Lee (Eds.), *Social marketing: Influencing behaviors for good* (3rd ed., pp. 156–160). Thousand Oaks, CA: Sage Publications.

Pan American Health Organization. (2008). *Canada: Health situation analysis and trends summary*. Retrieved July 28, 2009, from http://www.paho.org/English/DD/AIS/cp_124.htm#problemas

Public Health Agency of Canada. (2007). *Public Health Agency of Canada 2007–2008 report on plans and priorities*. Retrieved July 28, 2009, from http://www.tbs-sct.gc.ca/rpp/0708/phac-aspc/phac-aspc_e.pdf

Renaud, L., Caron-Bouchard, M., Beaulieu, S., & Martel, G. (2007). Étude de l'impact de la campagne de sensibilisation aux bienfaits de la saine alimentation et de l'activité physique: le Défi Santé 5/30. In L. Renaud (Ed.), *Les médias et le façonnement des normes en matière de santé* (pp. 195–204). Québec: Presses de l'Université du Québec.

Sali, N., & Lavack, A. M. (2007). 5-to-10-a-day program. In H. MacKenzie (Ed.), *Contemporary Canadian marketing cases* (3rd ed., pp. 296–303). Toronto, Ontario, Canada: Pearson Prentice Hall.

Saskatchewan in motion. (2008). Retrieved July 28, 2009, from http://www.saskatchewaninmotion.ca/

Siegel, M., & Doner Lotenberg, L. (2007). *Marketing public health: Strategies to promote social change* (2nd ed.). Sudbury, MA: Jones and Bartlett Publishers.

Tjepkema, M. (2004). *Measured obesity—Adult obesity in Canada: Measured height and weight (Nutrition: Findings from the Canadian Community Health Survey—Issue no. 1)*. Ottawa, Ontario: Statistics Canada (Catalogue no. 82-620-MWE2005001).

Turnley-Johnston, N., Lavack, A. M., & Clark, G. (2007). Literacy partners of Manitoba. In H. MacKenzie (Ed.), *Contemporary Canadian marketing cases* (3rd ed., pp. 277–293). Toronto, Ontario, Canada: Pearson Prentice Hall.

CHAPTER 4

Love, Sex, and HIV/AIDS

Using Social Marketing to Redefine Gender Norms Among Mexican Youth

Ruth Massingill

La mentira dura hasta que la verdad llega. [*A lie prevails until the truth arrives.*]

—Ballesteros, 1979

"If you *really* loved me, you would . . ."

Between raging hormones and peer pressure—an intoxicating combination—teens often become sexually active before they are emotionally mature. To add to the equation, in many cultures a "boys-will-be-boys" attitude gives tacit permission for young males to act irresponsibly, especially in sexual matters. This has always created social and health problems, but with the onslaught of HIV/AIDS, such cultural norms have helped fuel the global spread of the disease.

Since first diagnosed in the early 1980s, HIV/AIDS has become one of the most deadly health issues worldwide. More than 33 million people—2.5 million of them children younger than 15—now live with the disease (UNAIDS, 2007). About half of the infected are women, contrary to popular perception, and heterosexual transmission is the most common means of infection worldwide (UNAIDS, 2007). Often called an "underground epidemic," the associated stigma and discrimination associated with HIV/AIDS discourage people from getting tested or accessing care (HIV infection and AIDS in the Americas, 2003).

Mexico's leaders are using social marketing initiatives to change ingrained cultural behaviors among adolescents and young adults and thereby reverse the trend of increasing HIV/AIDS inflections.

MEXICO: A COUNTRY OVERVIEW

The United Mexican States is a land of contrasts where affluence and poverty live cheek by jowl and a wealth of natural splendors coexist with urban blight. Likewise, the climate varies from tropical to desert; the terrain ranges from beachfronts to deserts to mountain peaks.

With about 110 million inhabitants, Mexico is the most populous Spanish-speaking country in the world. Although its territory is almost triple the size of Texas, its northern neighbor, and spans three time zones, Mexico is primarily an urban culture. Three-quarters of the population lives in cities, with 20 million crowded into the capital (U.S. Department of State, 2008), where the contrast between riches and rags is painfully evident. Mexico City, in the heart of the country, is a modern international business and arts center surrounded by sprawling shantytowns and plagued by political turmoil and environmental concerns.

During its turbulent human history, the country has seen the rise and fall of many regimes. Mexico had long been the site of advanced Amerindian civilizations when it came under Spanish rule in the early 1500s. Hard-won independence did not come until the early 19th century. From the 1930s until 2000, the nationalist Institutional Revolutionary Party, or PRI, dominated Mexico's politics. The election (in 2000) of Vicente Fox of the opposition party, center-right Partido Acción Nacional (PAN), set a new political course that continued when PAN's Felipe Calderón took office six years later (Mexico factsheet, 2008).

With the country's political situation in transition, a multitude of social and economic problems have surfaced. Perhaps foremost is the contrast between the haves and the have-nots. Mexico is one of the world's most open economies, but it is heavily dependent on trade, especially with the United States, which purchased more than 80% of its exports in 2007 (U.S. Department of State, 2008). Although Mexico is a major oil producer and exporter—petroleum accounts for nearly one-third of government revenue—prosperity is only a dream for most Mexicans; poverty and disease are the realities. Unemployment is less than 4%, but one-fourth of the population is underemployed (Country profile: Mexico, 2008).

A popular response is to search for work in the United States. More than a million poor Mexicans are arrested each year trying to cross the U.S. border illegally, and hundreds die in the attempt (Country profile: Mexico, 2008). They leave behind towns and villages virtually empty of able-bodied men to be husbands and fathers. Even within the country, migration is an established pattern; many women also leave rural homes to take jobs in inner-city factories, only to fall victim to violent crime, exploitation, or illness.

HIV/AIDS ENTERS THE PICTURE

With the majority of the populace crowded into industrialized urban areas in less than ideal circumstances, it is not surprising that air and water pollution are major concerns, leading to a variety of health problems such as hepatitis A, typhoid fever, and bacterial diarrhea. Many of the affected are children; almost 30% of Mexico's population is under 15, with about 700,000 more males than females. Overall, however, life expectancies remain relatively high: 73 years for men and almost 79 years for women (U.S. Department of State, 2008).

Average life spans could drop, Mexican health officials fear, as the newest offspring of poverty and ignorance—the AIDS epidemic—affects more and more vulnerable populations. In many Latin American countries, the HIV epidemic is the main threat to social sustainability, with recent reports showing the disease is increasingly affecting the youngest and most productive populations as well as poor and marginalized groups. Sadly, the 2007 national census revealed that half of new HIV/AIDS cases in Mexico are occurring among those between 10 and 24 years old (Tizcareño, 2008). Unless it is curbed, this trend bodes ill for the future and predicts additional diversion of resources from other health, welfare, and education priorities. Mexico ranks 13th globally and 3rd in the Americas in the total number of HIV cases reported, but the increase has been continuous since 1981. With an estimated average of 4,000 new cases annually, AIDS has become the fourth leading cause of death for Mexican men aged 25 to 44 (WHO, PAHO, & UNAIDS, 2006, pp. 2–7).

AIDS has been reported in all 31 states of the Mexican Republic, with more than half of the infected living in the Federal District. Although the epidemic is largely concentrated among men who have sex with men, higher rates of HIV infection are also being documented among injecting drug users and women. Of the estimated 180,000 people living with HIV/AIDS in Mexico, almost one-fourth are women (International HIV/AIDS Alliance, 2008). Unfortunately, as male partners infect more women, heterosexual transmission is on the rise and, in some parts of the country, is now the predominant mode of transmission. Official estimates of the adult prevalence rate are still relatively low, ranging from 0.3% to 0.4%, but the disease is responsible for about 6,200 deaths a year (International HIV/AIDS Alliance, 2008). Persuading the infected to seek testing and treatment is expensive and difficult, so prevention is viewed as the superior social and financial choice.

Although Mexico has had HIV/AIDS programs since the early 1980s, only recently has there been a more unified national response in recognition that the disease has become a complex healthcare challenge, with psychological, social, ethical, economic, and political dimensions. Policy makers have realized it is critical to coordinate interdisciplinary responses from diverse organizations (Stewart et al. 2001, p. 5), which is a cornerstone of social marketing, a key tactic in combating HIV/AIDS in developing and industrialized countries for the past 20 years.

MAKING A CASE FOR SOCIAL MARKETING

As the link between public health and commerce, social marketing is the primary method international organizations such as UNAIDS use to combat global health issues (Hastings & Saren, 2003). When social marketing can build partnerships that include governments, nongovernmental organizations (NGOs), international agencies, and private businesses—so-called upstream audiences—working in conjunction with downstream targets, then the entire social fabric of a community can be permanently altered (Andreasen, 2006).

National and local organizations often adopt the techniques being used by global groups, and that is the case in Mexico where HIV is a growing concern. Because the AIDS epidemic in Mexico is still concentrated in vulnerable populations, political and healthcare leaders are faced with both the challenge and the opportunity to step up prevention measures before the disease spreads to the general population as it has in many parts of the world. There are, however, cultural obstacles to be overcome, in addition to political and economic hurdles.

According to Mexico's National Center for Prevention and Control of HIV/AIDS (Censida), changing how Mexicans view gender roles and erasing widespread prejudice against gays will be necessary to combat the disease effectively. Censida's director, Jorge Saavedra, has said repeatedly that machismo and homophobia are fueling the country's HIV/AIDS epidemic. Saavedra emphasized that machismo undermines prevention messages and "puts women, as well as men, at risk" (Machismo, 2006).

In addition to Mexico's new political regime, an army of international groups and national activist organizations are publicly committed to making treatment available to the infected and to changing cultural norms that contribute to the spread of the disease. Dozens of social marketing campaigns directed to specific target groups are under way across the country.

Mexico's commitment to this problem is a matter of public record. Regional heads of state endorsed the Neuvo Leon Declaration in 2004, a pledge to focus on HIV/AIDS treatment and prevention (USAID, 2005). The 2008 Secretary of Health, Jose Angel Cordova Villalobos, has said the decline in new HIV cases will be achieved mainly through education and awareness. To that end, Villalobos is collaborating with international global leaders to focus on "feminization of the epidemic"—strategies with a gender perspective (Sanchez, 2008).

Two successful examples of initiatives with gender perspectives are the focus of this chapter. Programas Hombres and Mujeres are companion campaigns designed to change how young men and women view gender roles and to urge them to consider the costs of stereotypical definitions of masculinity and femininity as well as the benefits of changing health-threatening behaviors.

CASE STUDY
Gender Norms Redefined in an Anti-HIV/AIDS Campaign

BACKGROUND

Addressing gender norms—societal messages that dictate what is appropriate or expected behavior for males and females—is increasingly recognized as a key strategy to prevent the spread of HIV infection, particularly among young people. Those links between gender attitudes and the spread of AIDS prompted a partnership of Latin American NGOs (see Figure 4-1) to develop Program H ("H" for *homens*, or men, in Portuguese, and *hombres* in Spanish). This social marketing initiative, first tested in Brazil and Mexico in 1999, has since been successfully used in more than 15 countries on three continents to persuade young men to question traditional norms related to manhood (Barker, 2007).

Building on their success in educating young men about the social and health costs of machismo culture, in 2005 the Program H partners and World Education launched Program M ("M" for *mulheres*, women in Portuguese, and *mujeres* in Spanish) to empower young women to take control of their sexual and reproductive health. It includes educational and

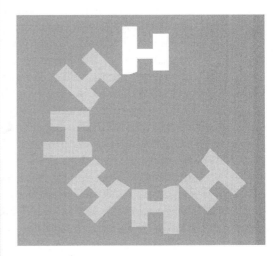

FIGURE 4-1   The H Alliance is an international consortium of NGOs, U.N. agencies, and the private sector working to promote gender equity among youth.

Photo courtesy of Instituto Promundo

campaign strategies that engage young women in critical reflections about life choices, health, and sexuality. Skills training, role models, and support from peers are important components of both initiatives.

Both programs are strongly research based. Program H's conceptual framework began with a "mapping" of masculinity to understand how men and women view what it means to be male. Men who were inclined to be more gender-equitable in their attitudes provided insights into the best ways to change the prevailing views about manhood. Likewise, Program M was built on research that explored women's concepts of empowerment and the key factors that contribute to their feelings of autonomy and self-worth.

Instituto Promundo, a Brazilian NGO that includes among its partners Salud y Género, a Mexico-based NGO, designed the programs. Promundo's mission is to "contribute to social equity through the testing and implementation of social technologies that promote the holistic development of children and youth . . . utilizing their participation throughout the process" (Instituto Promundo, 2008a). Salud y Género, with a respected track record of gender equity research and initiatives, has been the driving force behind Programas Hombres and Mujeres in Mexico (Salud y Género, 2008; Esplen, 2006, pp. 47–48).

Their efforts are reinforced by international initiatives that aim to erase behavior change barriers and thereby reduce HIV/AIDS infections. For example, USAID, the largest bilateral HIV/AIDS donor to Mexico, integrates gender issues into HIV prevention programs by recommending policy changes and training women in advocacy and leadership roles. USAID also focuses on upstream audiences to reduce HIV/AIDS stigma and discrimination among healthcare providers and decision makers in the legal environment and the mass media (USAID, 2005).

Likewise, Population Services International, the first international organization to use social marketing to combat AIDS, uses targeted behavior change communications (BCC) in Mexico to focus on gender equity and prevention messages. An innovative example of PSI's initiatives is a campaign called *Menos Etiquetas*, which relies heavily on "peer educators" but reinforces that strategy with BTL (below-the-line) techniques such as blogs, an array of promotional materials in places frequented by youths, and creative Bluetooth viral marketing (O. Le Touze, PSI Mexico, personal communication, April 7, 2008).

Programs H and M helped lay the groundwork for this mosaic of social change initiatives. In less than a decade, initiatives targeting Mexican youth have documented successes in motivating lifestyle changes that promise more gender-equitable behaviors and a reduced prevalence of HIV/AIDS.

TARGET AUDIENCE

Programs Hombres and Mujeres target young men and women aged 15 to 24, mostly from low-income populations. Many of these Mexican teens are already sexually experienced according to a 2001 report on reducing HIV infection among youth. This study of 2,064 Mexican students found that 24% of the males and 7% of the females were sexually active, with more than 90% of those teens reporting sexual debut before age 15 (Stewart et al. 2001, p. 12).

Both campaigns were informed by substantial target market research. To establish a baseline for future evaluation of Program H, researchers first analyzed behavioral data from a representative sample of young men to determine the extent to which respondents were at risk of HIV. They found young men typically engaged in a number of risky sexual behaviors, with an average age of 13 for sexual initiation. Almost one-third of sexually experienced youth had had more than one sexual partner in the previous month. Although condoms were used almost two-thirds of the time, 25% of respondents reported at least one sexually transmitted disease or infection (STI) symptom during the three months prior to the survey. Fewer than 10% had ever taken an HIV test (Hutchinson, Weiss, Barker, Segundo, & Pulerwitz, 2004, pp. 4–5).

Program M was based on research that began with a review of Latin American literature to define the concept of female empowerment. Focus group discussions with groups of young women aged 14 to 24 who lived in marginalized communities outside Queretaro, Mexico, and interviews with empowered young women defined the cultural expectations that were common in the target audience (Levack, 2003). One focus group participant is representative of a common conflict among the young women: "When I was younger, I thought about getting married and having children. Today, I think more about myself and chasing after my goals" (Instituto Promundo, 2008b).

CAMPAIGN OBJECTIVES

Although social marketing is not a theory, it informs and structures its framework using psychology, sociology, anthropology, and communications (Kotler & Zaltman, 1971, p. 3). The transtheoretical (stages of change) behavioral change model is one of the persuasive approaches that underlies Programs H and M because much of the target audience must be moved through early stages of indecision. The programs begin with knowledge objectives, eventually resulting in a shift of basic beliefs about gender equity, and thereby leading to behavior changes.

Knowledge Objectives

The initiatives were designed to first provide opportunity and information that would spark a thoughtful assessment of life choices. For the hombres, that involved encouraging them to (1) question traditional social norms related to manhood, (2) reflect on the advantages of more gender-equitable behaviors, and (3) rethink what it means to be a man. Mujeres, on the other hand, were encouraged to (1) reflect on gender norms and rights and (2) consider their self-efficacy and empowerment.

Belief Objectives

Because research indicated that young men generally decide and control how and when young women have sex, promoting gender equity, with a strong focus on sexual health, was crucial.

Program H was designed to change traditional beliefs that

- Men should initiate sexual activity early in life.
- Men should have multiple sexual partners.
- Men should maintain control over their female partners.
- Unsafe sex is more enjoyable than safer sex.

Program M was designed to change prevailing beliefs that

- Women should not know much about sexuality, including how to protect themselves from HIV and other STIs.
- Women should not negotiate protective behaviors with their male partners, such as condom use or monogamy. (Instituto Promundo, 2008b)

Behavior Objectives

Translating these cultural shifts into new behaviors was the key to both short- and long-term successes for the programs. Specifically, both initiatives sought to reduce the number of sexual partners and increase the use of condoms when both partners agreed to have sex. In the long term, however, Programs H and M aim to create a culture where both sexes (1) adopt more gender-equitable lifestyles, (2) make healthy life choices, and (3) build respectful relationships.

Clearly, the overreaching goal of this initiative is much broader than changing the lives of the individual young men and women who participate in Programas Hombres or Mujeres. It is an assault on gender expectations that extends across generations.

BARRIERS, OPPORTUNITIES (BENEFITS), AND COMPETITION

Making such revolutionary and deep-seated societal changes is an ambitious project with a host of obstacles, ranging from political to religious to economic. With Mexico's political climate in transition, both barriers and opportunities for change exist. The business-friendly PAN has responded to pressure from diverse interests to tackle discrimination that contributes to the spread of HIV/AIDS. Then-president Vicente Fox signed a constitutional amendment in 2001 that outlawed discrimination, including bias based on sexuality. Since 2003, federal agencies in Mexico have been required to fund tolerance campaigns (Campbell, 2005).

But early socialization that establishes inequitable gender roles as the norm may encourage risky behaviors among both young men and women. Instituto Promundo's research indicates gender inequity in relationships—when men have greater power than women—can also lead to sexual coercion and physical violence, circumstances in which HIV-protective behaviors are impossible to initiate and maintain (Pulerwitz, Barker, Segundo, & Nascimento, 2006, p. 4).

For both audiences, the tenets of machismo—if practiced by young men and accepted by young women—dictate lifelong patterns that distort personal relationships and endanger the health of future generations. (See Figure 4-2.)

The benefits of reversing these traditional beliefs are self-evident, but timing is critical because attitudes formed in adolescence often crystallize into lifelong behavior patterns. Marcos Nascimento, now Promundo co-director, noted that international research with teens indicates "viewing women as sexual objects, using coercion to obtain sex, and viewing sex from a performance-oriented perspective" may become established behavior unless the pattern is

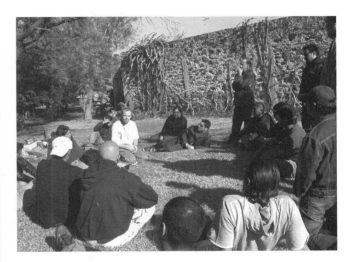

FIGURE 4-2   Peer educators facilitate conversations about traditional male attitudes as part of Programa Hombres in Mexico. For many young men, these workshops are the first time they have discussed the costs of machismo.

Photo courtesy of Salud y Género

broken before adulthood (Nascimento, 2005). (See examples in Box 4-1.) Without intervention, young women, too, can become trapped in situations where their life choices are curtailed.

Some might argue that the strongest competition to the messages promulgated by Programs H and M is a mix of emotional blackmail ("If you really loved me . . .") and peer pressure, the lure of immediate sexual gratification, and entertainment media's reinforcement of machismo's many manifestations.

POSITIONING

For the young men targeted by Program H, the challenge is to redefine "what it means to be a man." Programa Hombres repositions manliness to include responsible monogamous relationships, safe and loving sex, and respect for women.

Likewise, Program M seeks to reposition young women's perception of their role in relationships from subservient to equal and to expand their sense of self-efficacy.

BOX 4-1 **Machismo Defined**

Traditional attitudes about masculinity—sometimes called *machismo*—include beliefs that

- Men have more sexual urges than women.
- Men have the right to decide when and where to have sex.
- Sexual and reproductive health issues are women's concerns.
- Men have the right to outside partners or relationships while women do not.
- Child care or parenting is primarily a woman's issue.

These traditional beliefs sustain and support the behaviors of men who have internalized such norms, and in turn, act on them, by

- Not using condoms.
- Not seeking health services.
- Relegating reproductive health issues to women.
- Not taking an active role in caring for children they father.

Source: Nascimento, 2005.

CAMPAIGN STRATEGIES, IMPLEMENTATION, AND EVALUATION

Successful campaigns speak to the target in culturally sensitive ways. In this situation, the challenge was to present the messages in words and images that honor the culture while working to change the very pillars of centuries-old societal norms.

Although federally funded tolerance campaigns with slogans such as "Homosexuality is not a disease; homophobia is," primarily target homophobia, their controversial nature also sparks a public dialogue about the stigma of HIV/AIDS (Cevallos, 2009). This kind of conversation is critical to the success of Programs H and M, which rely on open discussions about having sex, using condoms, and the risk of AIDS. In a country where 90% of the population is Roman Catholic (U.S. Department of State, 2008), the church's positions on diversity, gender norms, sex outside of marriage, and birth control are strong influences that must be addressed.

Involving Program H and M's target audiences at every stage was a key strategy on the path to accomplish this tricky cultural balancing act. As previously explained, young men and women were central to the research that informed the campaigns. In addition, youths from two low-income communities of Rio de Janeiro developed the campaign materials, which have been adapted for use in other Latin American countries as well as in India and Tanzania and, more recently, the Balkan region in Europe.

From radio spots to postcards and from YouTube videos to special events, campaign materials promote a new male identity that is "cool," responsible, open to conversation, and respectful toward his partner. The companion Mujeres program employs a similar range of collateral materials to help women visualize having more autonomy and negotiation power. Members of the target audience who already questioned rigid models of masculinity or femininity became "peer promoters" in the interventions, spearheading implementation and attracting other youths to the programs. A diverse network of allied groups extended the campaigns' reach and a representative sample of youths provided feedback for evaluation.

Intervention activities for each campaign consisted of two main components: (1) a field-tested curriculum with a manual and an educational video for promoting attitude and behavior change and (2) a lifestyle social marketing campaign for promoting changes in community or social norms (Nascimento, 2005).

A Curriculum Product to Promote Change

The educational techniques, manuals, and accompanying videos that make up the curricula for Programs H and M are termed "social technologies," a concept developed by Instituto Promundo and defined as "all educational material, methodological procedures or tested techniques, validated and with a proven social impact created with the aim of solving a social problem" (Instituto Promundo, 2008c).

The Program H curriculum was developed in 1999 by four Latin American NGOs and coordinated by Instituto Promundo, including Salud y Género (Queretaro and Xalapa, Mexico), Ecos (São Paulo, Brazil), and Instituto PAPAI (Recife, Brazil). The curriculum provides a framework to examine gender issues, a 20-minute cartoon video, and 70 activities organized under five themes (see Box 4-2). Activities include role-plays, brainstorming exercises, discussion sessions, and individual reflections for small groups. The intervention is designed to be used over a six-month period for a total of 120 hours. To serve as gender-equitable role models for the young men, adult men facilitated the exercises (Pulerwitz et al., 2006, pp. 12–13).

Using the same approach, Program M's educational materials include a cartoon (see Box 4-3), which tells the story of "Maria," a girl who begins to question the "do's and don'ts of the world around her and how they influence the way she thinks and acts" (Once upon a girl, 2006). A discussion guide for use with small groups poses candid questions about socialization, sexuality, drugs, and

---

BOX 4-2 **Intervention Activity–Curriculum**

(Designed to promote attitude/behavior change)

Program H manuals
Each manual in the five-volume set contains a theoretical introduction, group activities (such as brainstorming, dramatizations, discussions, and individual reflection), and references for further research, including local organizations, videos, and Web sites. The themes of the manuals are:

1. Sexuality and reproductive health.
2. Fatherhood and caregiving.
3. From violence to peaceful coexistence.
4. Reasons and emotions (including communication skills, substance abuse, and mental health).
5. Preventing and living with HIV/AIDS.

Source: Instituto Promundo, 2008d.

BOX 4-3   **Cartoon Videos**

Boys play football. Girls play with dolls. Boys should be tough. Girls should be sweet and always look nice.

Debunking such stereotypes is the mission of two 20-minute videos for Program H (Once Upon a Boy; see Figure 4-3) and Program M (Once Upon a Girl; see Figure 4-4). Designed for universal understanding by using only visuals with no words, the films generate discussion among facilitated groups of young men or women and seek to deconstruct gender

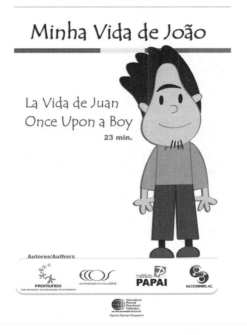

FIGURE 4-3   Once Upon a Boy: Created to provide an overview of the key questions around male development, the film features a boy named Juan and the challenges he faces as he becomes a man: domestic violence, his first sexual experience, his girlfriend's pregnancy, and his first job.

Photo courtesy of Instituto Promundo

BOX 4-3 **Cartoon Videos (Continued)**

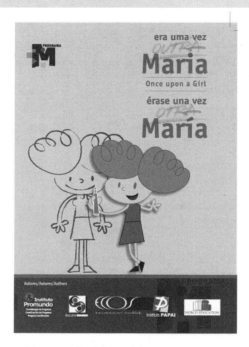

FIGURE 4-4 Once Upon a Girl: Touching on topics as varied as household roles and intimate relationships, this video features Maria's road to womanhood and the challenges young women face growing up.
Photo courtesy of Instituto Promundo

stereotypes. They are also tools for health or education professionals to hone their skills in working with youths on gender and health issues.

A university teacher who works with youth said:

> I presented the cartoon "Once Upon a Girl" to a group of adolescents and got them to discuss some of the points raised. It's incredible to see how the girls themselves have a very rigid view of how a woman should behave. Many still believe women should be passive, subservient. The video helped me deal with these issues. (Instituto Promundo, 2005, p. 27)

pregnancy. A participant who now works as a social promoter to disseminate program methodologies described her experience:

> Program M activities are very involving; everyone participates. I learned how to use contraceptive methods, had access to information on sexual and reproductive health, and on preventing STDs. Some young women in the community were shy; many didn't even talk to one another. They are more at ease now; they talk about their lives and have become friends. (Instituto Promundo, 2005, p. 13)

A manual similar to the one for Program H is in production for Program M. Both initiatives are designed to create safe spaces in which young men and women can question traditional views. (See Figure 4-5.) Questioning is always presented in a positive manner, never as an imposition.

Pricing Strategies

Making the program materials as widely available as possible, especially to high-risk groups of hombres and mujeres, is the overriding consideration in setting prices. The five-volume manual, available in English, Spanish, and Portuguese, can be downloaded at no charge from Instituto Promundo's Web site, or it can be ordered in a bound volume for US$50. The 20-minute cartoons for both programs, with their accompanying discussion guides, are offered on VHS for US$15 or on DVD for US$20.

Hora H condoms, which are used in the social marketing lifestyle campaigns (see "Promotion Strategies"), are distributed at cost under an arrangement with the manufacturer.

Place Strategies

With more than 77% of Mexico's population living in cities, most national HIV prevention programs focus on urban populations (USAID, 2005). Young men are less likely

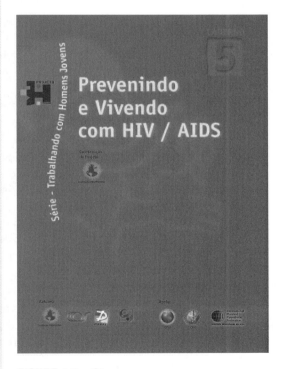

FIGURE 4-5 Since young men on average have more sexual partners than young women, ensuring that new generations develop more gender-equitable and safer sex is critical to reduce HIV transmission.

Photo courtesy of Instituto Promundo

than young women to seek health services, making it difficult to reach them with information and other services, so Program H takes information to them in the communities where they live. Entertainment venues such as bars, community dances, and parties proved to be effective ways to reach the target audience. In addition, the Mexican Ministry of Health adopted Program H, and 10,000 copies were printed with the government's seal, lending official credibility to the initiative.

According to Gerardo Ayala, of Salud y Género, healthcare providers have used Program H's methodology to reach more than 10,000 young people in six states—Chiapas, Baja California Sur, Sonora, Distrito Federal, Veracruz, and Querétaro. "The way in which we spread and implemented Program H in Mexico is very diverse and tends to be massive," Ayala elaborated (quoted in de Botton, 2007).

Promotion Strategies

Unlike many developing countries, where social marketing is used to combat HIV/AIDS, Mexico has a high average literacy rate: almost 93% for men and 90% for women (U.S. Department of State, 2008).

As might be expected, young people are more likely to use the Internet, although of Mexico's 110 million people, only about 20% have access to the Web (Internet World Stats, 2007). The Latin culture is family/relationship oriented, so personal communication is often more effective—and more credible—than mediated communication channels. Nevertheless, social marketers are increasingly incorporating new media tools to stretch their budgets while expanding their reach to young computer-savvy audiences. As part of that outreach, comprehensive information about Programs H and M is available online and the cartoon videos can be viewed on YouTube.

In addition to the curriculum, Alliance H—Promundo and its partner organizations—developed a "lifestyle social marketing" process to promote gender-equitable lifestyles among young men and women. (See Figure 4-6.) For Program H, young men in the target audience identified their preferred sources of information and cultural outlets in the community. Messages that it is "cool and hip" to be a more "gender-equitable" man were presented via radio spots, billboards, posters, postcards, and dances.

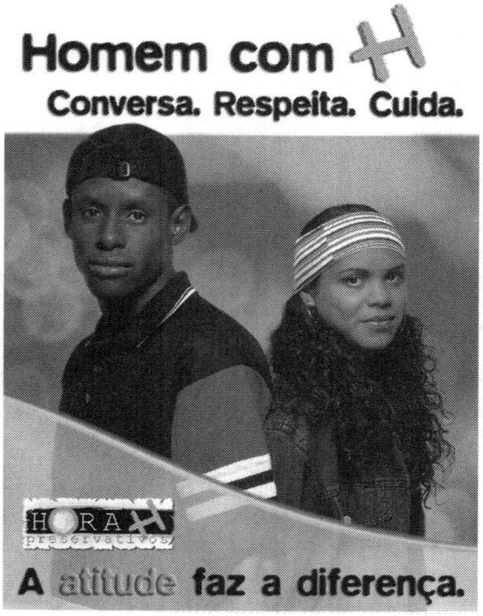

Homem com H
Conversa. Respeita. Cuida.

A atitude faz a diferença.

FIGURE 4-6   Poster used in lifestyle social marketing campaign: "Talk. Respect. Care. Attitude makes a difference."

Photo courtesy of Instituto Promundo

Promundo also partnered with SSL International, makers of Durex condoms, who provided a branded condom, Hora H, at production cost. Hora H condoms were distributed in nontraditional venues and shops such as funk balls and cafés as a central part of the campaign. Promoting the use of condoms is such an integral part of HIV/AIDS social marketing that the practice has its own acronym— condom social marketing (CSM)—and manufacturers' agreements such as the one with SSL International are common. Population Services International, however, has discontinued CSM in Mexico due to administrative and political hurdles and because Mexico, unlike poorer countries, has many condom brands vying for market share (O. Le Touze, PSI Mexico, personal communication, 2008).

The Program H campaign was called "In the Heat of the Moment," a theme chosen because young men said they frequently heard their peers say, "Everybody knows you should use a condom, but in the heat of the moment . . ." (Pulerwitz et al., 2006, p. 14). The campaign's theme and media mix, combined with easy access to condoms, present a persuasive message encouraging young men to respect their partners, to avoid using violence against women, and to practice safer sex.

Because changing young men's attitudes and their consequent actions is the first priority in this staged behavior change communication effort, Program M's media strategy has not yet been launched. In the meantime, however, other campaigns, such as PSI Mexico's "Menos Etiquetas" gender-equity initiative, are incorporating the research and successful techniques of Programas H and M to reach young people at risk. Like Program H, Menos uses peer educators to initially broach themes that include gender norms, HIV/AIDS, and stigma. A traditional media mix including posters, postcards, stickers, and flyers (see Figures 4-7 and 4-8) is teamed with social media such as blogs and Bluetooth viral marketing (PSI Mexico, 2008).

Other Strategies

An intriguing political response to the problem of attracting substantial support is the "positioning" of women as the primary victims—"the innocents"—in the battle against AIDS. This widespread rhetoric is designed to gain broad political support from faith-based organizations as well as from political leaders looking for the most acceptable route to public approval. Because women comprise about half of those infected worldwide, this marketing approach lends itself to a wide range of emotional/rational appeals.

In a 2007 EU summit, Bill Gates, a major contributor of funds to fight AIDS, appealed to the G-8 countries to pledge new resources to "beat AIDS" and urged:

> A top priority must be to address the prevention needs of women and girls . . . biologically, women are twice as likely as men to contract HIV. And many

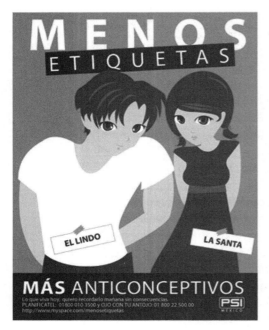

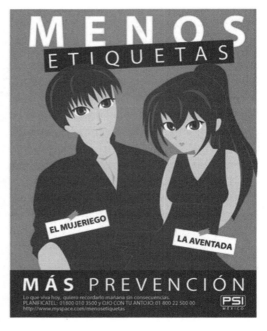

FIGURE 4-7   Population Services International's Menos Etiquetas campaign promoting gender equity launched with this eye-catching poster, *Más Anticonceptivos* ("More Contreceptives").

Photo courtesy of PSI Mexico

FIGURE 4-8   The Menos Etiquetas Campaign merged traditional techniques such as this poster advocating *Más Prevención* ("More Prevention") with new media.

Photo courtesy of PSI Mexico

women—including those who are married—have little power to ensure their partners are faithful or use condoms. (Gates, 2007)

Mexican activists recognize the power of public sympathy for women and are pushing for funding to protect women's health.

FINDING FUNDING

Quoting precise budgets for Programs H and M is virtually impossible due to the many organizations—international, national, and local—and the hundreds of volunteers who are working individually with young men and women. Funding for the members of Alliance H comes variously from international foundations, multilateral organizations, government agencies, private companies, and individual donors.

NGO Salud y Género estimates that it alone has spent about 150,000 pesos (about US$14,555) a year on Program H curriculum interventions in Mexico, but explains that due to the uncertain nature of funds and resources, it is not possible to establish precise budgets for the workshops. As the need is manifested, the organizations search for ways to meet that need (G. Ayala, Salud y Género, personal communication, May 27, 2008).

The success of Programs H and M rely mightily on the diversity of their partners and their combined strengths. The positive outcomes of Program H encouraged the Alliance partners to invest in Program M and even attracted additional partners, including the MacArthur Foundation, World Education (in the United States), and the Special Secretariat of Women's Policies (in Brazil). In these projects—as in most social marketing initiatives—partnerships are the key to success because social marketers, although employing the 4Ps of marketing, usually lack the infrastructure and the marketplace environment commercial marketers take for granted.

EVALUATION

In the case of Programs H and M, evaluation methodologies were put into place even before the campaigns were field-tested. (See Box 4-4.)

These workshops were the first time many participants had discussed the societal ramifications of being a man. Márcio Segundo of Instituto Promundo was the study's research coordinator. He said Program H's creative participatory activities sparked critical thinking about "issues that affect their lives, such as sex, HIV, relationships, violence, drugs, and fatherhood" (Hutchinson et al., 2004, p. 5). In one of the communities evaluated, the use of condoms increased from 58% to 87% after participating in Program H. That survey also revealed that the percentage of men who agreed with the statement, "the most important role of a woman is to take care of the house and cook" shrank from 40% to 29% (de Botton, 2007).

Altered attitudes translated into new behaviors. One young man said, "Before [the workshops] I had sex with a girl, I had an orgasm, and then left her. If she got pregnant, I had nothing to do with it. But now, I think before I act" (Pulerwitz, et al., 2006, p. 20).

Overall, Program H evaluations show group discussions that prompt critical reflection about the costs of traditional manhood, and a media campaign that demonstrates gender-equitable behaviors encourage young men to make changes that protect themselves and their partners from HIV infection. Findings also indicate improvements in both condom use and a reduction in reported STI symptoms with groups that participated in Program H training.

BOX 4-4 Evaluating Program H

To assess Program H's impact in Mexico, researchers adapted Promundo's Gender Equity in Men (GEM) Scale to fit the cultural context of young men in Mexico. The adapted scale measured traditional attitudes about gender roles related to HIV/AIDS and pregnancy prevention, violence, sexual relationships, domestic chores and caregiving, and homosexuality. Informants also provided information on HIV-related risk, such as STI symptoms, condom use, and number of sexual partners. A total of 270 young men aged 14 to 24 participated in a Program H workshop, and another 270 young men selected as a control arm received a four-hour orientation on safer sex and awareness of gender-based violence. Both groups completed a survey before the intervention, immediately afterward, and three months later (Levack, 2003).

Respondents were asked whether they agreed, partially agreed, or disagreed with each statement.

Sample Items From the GEM Scale
- Men are always ready to have sex.
- Women who carry condoms with them are "easy."
- I would never have a gay friend.
- Changing diapers, giving the kids a bath, and feeding the kids are the mother's responsibility.
- I would be outraged if my wife asked me to use a condom.
- A woman should tolerate violence in order to keep her family together.
- There are times when a woman deserves to be beaten. (Pulerwitz et al., 2006, pp. 15–16)

"The scale quantitatively measures changes in support for prevailing gender norms," explained Dr. Julie Pulerwitz of Horizons/PATH, one of the study's principal investigators. When combined with qualitative information, this data help researchers identify shifts in gender roles within a community (Hutchinson et al., 2004, p. 4).

Assessment for Program M is not complete, but anecdotal evidence indicates the curriculum interventions are having positive results. The outcomes are so positive, in fact, that the program has been adapted for use with young women in India, where similar cultural norms exist.

SUMMARY

What is the measure of success for a social marketing initiative? If demonstrated behavioral change by the downstream audiences and policy changes and approbation by upstream decision makers are valid indicators, Programs H and M are extremely successful.

For the young men and women targeted by the interventions, the conclusion is that addressing unequal gender norms, especially machismo attitudes, is a vital part of HIV-prevention strategies. These changes can conceivably extend into future generations, leading to a culture with stronger, healthier personal relationships.

"Young men don't learn behaviors in isolation," said Dr. Gary Barker, former executive director of Promundo and one of Program H's creators. The kind of individual reflection Program H and M generates is a first step in changing what is expected behavior for men and women (Hutchinson et al., 2004, p.7).

Program H's results are receiving international notice. In their 2006 annual reports, the UN Children's Fund (UNICEF) and the World Bank lauded Program H as a promising intervention leading to gender equity. More recently, the International Center for Research on Women presented its 2008 Innovation Award to Salud y Género for its "cutting edge work with men and boys to challenge assumptions about proper masculine roles, reduce violence against women and improve men's support of women's reproductive health (ICRW awards, 2008). (See Figure 4-9.)

If imitation is the greatest flattery of all, Program H adaptations in 15 countries so far surely denotes global success. "Program H was conceived since the beginning with the idea that its methodology could be fit to scale and reproduced in any place, any group or number of people, and in different languages," explained Gary Barker (quoted in de Botton, 2007).

Inspired by Programs H and M's materials and experiences, Instituto Promundo launched a multimedia campaign known as JPEG (the acronym in Portuguese for Youth for Gender Equity). According to Christine Ricardo, co-director of Promundo, JPEG's centerpiece is a radio-based soap opera, "Between Us," about a young couple. JPEG also uses the peer-educator format that proved so successful in Programs H and M. The next step, Ricardo said, is a large, sustained collaboration to "scale up the use of

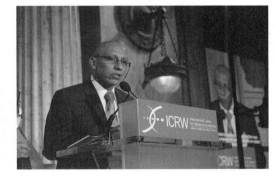

FIGURE 4-9 Gerardo Ayala of Salud y Género accepts the 2008 Innovation Award in Washington, D.C., on the eve of International Women's Day.

Courtesy of ICRW/photo by K. Sardari

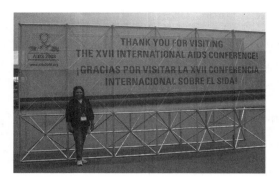

FIGURE 4-10   Mexico City welcomed more than 20,000 delegates to the global dialogue about curbing HIV/AIDS.

Photo courtesy of Ruta Reproductions

the JPEG campaign and Programs H and M in the public education sector in Brazil and India" (Christine Ricardo, Instituto Promundo, personal communication, August 20, 2008).

Although the alliance members are pleased that results of gender-equality programs indicate that cultural change and subsequent HIV prevention are possible, they agree there is much to be done to continue the momentum of this global movement.

In Mexico, the country's leaders put that nation in the forefront of the global HIV/AIDS dialogue by hosting the biannual XVII International AIDS Conference that attracted more than 20,000 to Mexico City in August 2008. (See Figure 4-10.) This was both a political and an economic commitment for Mexico, which was only the third developing country to host the conference. The Mexican government contributed $4 million of the $25 million cost of the conference, almost twice as much as the Canadian government donated for the 2006 conference in Toronto (Sanchez, 2008).

In a country like Mexico, where pesos are precious, this budget is a significant admission that HIV/AIDS is a critical issue that must be publicly addressed before the "underground epidemic" claims more victims. Investing in social marketing initiatives has yielded promising results, but there is still much more to do to ensure that love plus sex does not equal AIDS for Mexico's youth.

QUESTIONS FOR DISCUSSION

1. How are machismo and homophobia fueling Mexico's HIV/AIDS epidemic? Is this true in other countries as well?
2. What are below-the-line communication techniques? Try to think of some specific ways BTL might be effective in social marketing campaigns aimed at Mexican youth.
3. Which components of Programs H and M make the campaigns adaptable for use in other countries and cultures?
4. How many of the cultural norms discussed in this chapter are traditions in your own family or social circle? How have these beliefs affected the life choices of people you know?

REFERENCES

Andreasen, A. R. (2006). *Social marketing in the 21st century*. Thousand Oaks, CA: Sage Publications.

Ballesteros, O. A. (1979). *Mexican proverbs: The philosophy, wisdom and humor of a people*. Austin, TX: Eakin Press.

Barker, G. (2007, January 8). *The Instituto Promundo story*. Policy Innovations. Retrieved July 28, 2009, from http://www.policyinnovations.org/ideas/innovations/data/InstitutoPromundo Story

Campbell, M. (2005, June 9). Mexico tackles discrimination to fight AIDS. *The Christian Science Monitor*. Retrieved July 28, 2009, from http://www.csmonitor.com/2005/0609/p06s01-woam.htm

Cevallos, D. (2009, May 17). Latin America: For a day against homophobia. *Inter Press Service News Agency*. Retrieved July 28, 2009, from http://ipsnews.net/news.asp?idnews=37776

Country profile: Mexico. (2008). *BBC News*. Retrieved July 28, 2009, from http://news.bbc.co.uk/2/hi/americas/country_profiles/1205074.stm

de Botton, S. (2007, October 8). Not all men are the same. *Comunidad segura*. Retrieved July 28, 2009, from http://www.comunidadesegura.org/?q=en/node/35603

Esplen, E. (2006, October). *Engaging men in gender equality: Positive strategies and approaches*. Institute of Development Studies, University of Sussex. Retrieved July 28, 2009, from http://www.bridge.ids.ac.uk/reports/BB15Masculinities.pdf

Gates, B. (2007, June 6). How to beat AIDS. *Guardian Unlimited*. Retrieved July 28, 2009, from http://commentisfree.guardian.co.uk/bill_gates/

Hastings, G., & Saren, M. (2003). The critical contribution of social marketing. *Marketing Theory* 3(3), 305–322.

HIV Infection and AIDS in the Americas: Lessons and challenges for the future. (2003, April). Provisional report. Epidemiology Network for Latin America and the Caribbean. Retrieved February 13, 2009, from http://www.mapnetwork.org/MAPLACDraftAprill9,2003%20to%20print.doc

Hutchinson, S., Weiss, E., Barker, G., Segundo, M., & Pulerwitz, J. (2004, December). Involving young men in HIV prevention programs. *Horizons Report*. Retrieved July 28, 2009, from http://www.populationcouncil.org/horizons/newsletter/horizons(9)_1.html

Instituto Promundo. (2005). *Annual Report*. Retrieved July 28, 2009, from http://www.promundo.org.br/Relatorios/RA_promundo_INGLES.pdf

Instituto Promundo Web site. (2008a). *FAQs*. Retrieved July 28, 2009, from http://www.promundo.org

Instituto Promundo Web site. (2008b). *Activities*. Retrieved July 28, 2009, from http://www.promundo.org

Instituto Promundo Web site. (2008c). *Social Technologies*. Retrieved July 28, 2009, from http://www.promundo.org

Instituto Promundo Web site. (2008d). *Publications*. Retrieved July 28, 2009, from http://www.promundo.org

International Center for Research on Women (ICRW). (2008, March 5). *ICRW awards gala honors global leaders for advancing the well-being and economic progress of women and girls*.

Press release. Retrieved July 28, 2009, from http://www.icrw.org/html/news/pressreleases/2008/GalaPressRelease030508.pdf

International HIV/AIDS Alliance. (2008). *Mexico: Alliance linking organization: Colectivo Sol.* Retrieved July 28, 2009, from http://www.aidsalliance.org/sw7241.asp

Internet world stats. (2007, June 30). *Mexico and Central America.* Retrieved July 28, 2009, from http://www.internetworldstats.com/central.htm

Kotler, P., & Zaltman, G. (1971). Social marketing: An approach to planned social change. *Journal of Marketing* 35(3), 3–12.

Levack, A. (2003). *Improving the quality of sexual heath and gender-based violence prevention programs in Mexico: Development of plans for formative research and program evaluation.* Report for Department of Health Services, University of Washington.

Machismo, homophobia undermine HIV-prevention efforts in Mexico, advocates say. (2006, February 13). *The Body.* Retrieved July 28, 2009, from http://www.thebody.com/content/art7762.html

Mexico factsheet. (2008, April 9). Economist.com. Retrieved July 28, 2009, from http://www.economist.com/countries/Mexico/profile.cfm?folder=Profile-FactSheet

Nascimento, M. (2005). Working with young men to promote gender equality: An experience in Brazil and Latin America. *Eldis Document Store.* Retrieved July 28, 2009, from http://www.eldis.org/fulltext/working-with-young-men-Jan2006.pdf

Once upon a girl: Discussion guide. (2006). Instituto Promundo. Retrieved July 28, 2009, from http://www.promundo.org.br/materiais%20de%20apoio/publicacoes/MANUAL%20M.pdf

Population Services International (PSI) Mexico. (2008, March). *Progress report: ASRH campaign in Chetumal.* The Summit Foundation.

Pulerwitz, J., Barker, G., Segundo, M., & Nascimento, M. (2006). *Promoting more gender-equitable norms and behaviors among young men as an HIV/AIDS prevention strategy.* Horizons Program and Instituto Promundo. Retrieved July 28, 2009, from http://www.popcouncil.org/pdfs/horizons/brgendernorms.pdf

Salud y Género. (2008). Retrieved July 28, 2009, from http://www.saludygenero.org.mx/

Sanchez, R. (2008, May 14). Inauguration government office to support AIDS 2008. *NotieSe.* Retrieved July 28, 2009, from http://www.notiese.org/

Stewart, H., McCauley, A., Baker, S., Givaudan, M., James, S., Leenen, I., et al. (2001). Reducing HIV infection among youth: What can schools do? Key baseline findings from Mexico, South Africa, and Thailand. *Horizons Report.* Retrieved July 28, 2009, from http://pdf.usaid.gov/pdf_docs/Pnacq831.pdf

Tizcareño, C. E. (2008, May). Half of new HIV/AIDS cases are between 10 and 24 years old. *NotieSe.* Retrieved July 28, 2009, from http://www.notiese.org

UNAIDS. (2007, December). *AIDS epidemic update.* Retrieved July 28, 2009, from http://data.unaids.org/pub/EPISlides/2007/2007_epiupdate_en.pdf

USAID. (2005). *Health Profile: Mexico.* Retrieved July 28, 2009, from http://www.usaid.gov/our_work/global_health/aids/Countries/lac/mexico_05.pdf

U.S. Department of State. (2008). *Profile: United Mexican States.* Retrieved July 28, 2009, from http://www.state.gov/r/pa/ei/bgn/35749.htm

World Health Organization, Pan American Health Organization, and UNAIDS. (2006, December). *Epidemiological fact sheets on HIV/AIDS and sexually transmitted infections.* Retrieved July 28, 2009, from http://www.who.int/GlobalAtlas/predefinedReports/EFS2006/EFS_PDFs/EFS2006_MX.pdf

CHAPTER 5

Tuberculosis
Keys to Success in Peru

Nancy R. Lee

Just recently, a TB patient from a village called Morne Michel hadn't shown up for his monthly doctor's appointment. So—this was one of the rules— someone had to go and find him. The annals of international health contain many stories of adequately financed projects that failed because "noncompliant" patients didn't take all their medicines. (Paul) Farmer said, "The only non-compliant people are physicians. If the patient doesn't get better, it's your own fault. Fix it."

—Kidder, 2004, p. 36

Paul Farmer is a physician, a director at Johns Hopkins, a professor at the Harvard School of Medicine, an anthropologist, and, according to at least one of his former patients in Haiti, "he's a god" (National Public Radio, 2003). Farmer specializes in infectious disease and has made it his mission to transform health care on a global scale, focusing on the world's poorest and sickest communities. (Perhaps that explains the passion and sense of urgency in this chapter's opening quote.) In 1987, he founded a nonprofit organization called Partners in Health, which now treats about 1,000 patients daily for free in the Haitian countryside. They also work to cure tuberculosis in Peru, the public health issue and country of focus for this chapter.

The tuberculosis challenge is a natural for social marketing. There are specific behaviors to be influenced for audiences downstream as well as upstream. There are SMART goals (specific, measurable, achievable, relevant, and time-bound) that have been set for countries by organizations such as the United Nations that established targets for tuberculosis control included in one of the Millennium Development Goals.

There are opportunities for application of all 4Ps in the marketing mix, ones actually needed to reach these ambitious goals. And there are mechanisms in place to monitor and evaluate progress. This chapter begins with a brief description of the world's tuberculosis problem, provides a country overview, and then presents key elements of a successful marketing effort to reduce the incidence and prevalence of tuberculosis in Peru.

THE WORLD'S TUBERCULOSIS PROBLEM

Tuberculosis (TB) is a contagious disease. Like the common cold, it spreads through the air. Only people who are sick with TB in their lungs are infectious, but when these people cough, sneeze, talk, or spit, they propel TB germs, known as *bacilli*, into the air. Unfortunately, a person needs only to inhale a small number of these to then be infected. Left untreated, each person with active TB disease will infect on average between 10 and 15 people every year. But people infected with TB bacilli will not necessarily become sick with the disease because the immune system "walls off" the TB bacilli which, protected by a thick waxy coat, can lie dormant for years. When someone's immune system is weakened, the chances of becoming sick are greater (WHO, 2007). Nearly 2 billion people around the world are infected with the rod-shaped bacterium that causes tuberculosis (WHO, 2007). This is almost one out of three human beings. If TB disease is detected early and fully treated, people with the disease quickly become noninfectious and are eventually cured (WHO, 2008a). Twenty-two countries account for 80% of the TB cases in the world, with the largest incidence and prevalence of cases in Southeast Asia and Africa (2005 data; Stop TB Partnership, 2008; WHO, 2007).

In 2006, there were an estimated 9.2 million new cases of TB, including 700,000 cases among people living with HIV, and 500,000 cases of multi-drug-resistant TB (MDR-TB). An estimated 1.5 million people died from TB in 2006. In addition, another 200,000 people with HIV died from HIV-associated TB (WHO, 2008a).

On March 17, 2008, the World Health Organization (WHO) reported that worldwide efforts to confront tuberculosis are making progress, but too slowly. Their Global Tuberculosis Control report (WHO, 2008a) finds that the pace of the progress to control the tuberculosis epidemic slowed slightly in 2006 (the most recent year for which data were available). The new information documents a slowdown in progress on diagnosing people with TB, a key strategy to preventing its spread and increasing treatment. Between 2001 and 2005, the average rate that new TB cases were detected was increasing by 6% per year. Between 2005 and 2006, however, that rate of increase was cut in half, to 3%. Moreover, in most African countries there has been no increase in the detection of TB cases through national programs. The reason for this slowing of progress in rates of detection is that some national programs that were making rapid strides during the last five years have been unable to continue at the same pace in 2006 (WHO, 2008a).

The Global Tuberculosis Control report highlights two aspects of the epidemic that could further slow progress on TB. The first is the increase in multi-drug-resistant tuberculosis (MDR-TB), reported by WHO in March 2008 to have reached the highest levels ever recorded. To date, however, the response to this epidemic has been inadequate. Given limited laboratory and treatment capacity, countries were projecting they will provide treatment only to an estimated 10% of people with MDR-TB worldwide in 2008 (WHO, 2008b). The second threat is the lethal combination of TB and HIV, with slow progress toward testing TB patients for HIV. In 2006, although 700,000 were tested, the target goal was 1.6 million (WHO, 2008a).

The main constraints to achieving the global targets appear to be lack of political commitment, poor health systems, an irregular supply of anti-TB drugs, and weak communication components in TB control programs (Llanos-Zavalaga, Poppe, Tawfik, & Church-Balin, 2004). The WHO report also documents a shortage in funding. Despite an increase in resources, especially from The Global Fund and some middle-income countries, TB budgets are projected to remain flat in 2008 in almost all of the countries most heavily burdened by the disease. Ninety countries in which 91% of the world's TB cases occur provided complete financial data for the report. To meet the 2008 targets of the Global Plan to Stop TB, the funding shortfall for these 90 countries is about US$1 billion.

Peru is internationally recognized for its success in reducing the incidence of tuberculosis by an estimated 7% per year between 1990 and 2000, from about 190 per 100,000 to 140 per 100,000 (The Global Fund, 2003). Its story, which follows, illustrates the role social marketing efforts played in this success and should inspire those working to achieve the 2015 Millennium Development Goal #6 to reduce TB prevalence and death rates by 50% relative to 1990 (WHO, 2007).

A vast majority of the information for this highlighted case was provided by Fernandez Llanos-Zavalaga, Patricia Poppe, Youssef Tawfik, and Cathleen Church-Balin in a report they wrote in September 2004 for *Communications Insights*: "The Role of Communication in Peru's Fight Against Tuberculosis." *Communication Insights* is published by the Health Communication Partnership based at Johns Hopkins Bloomberg School of Public Health/Center for Communications Programs.

PERU: A COUNTRY OVERVIEW

With a population of 27.9 million, Peru is the 41st most populated country in the world (Census, 2007) and 4th most populated in South America. Almost the size of

Alaska (five-sixths), Peru is divided by the Andes Mountains into three sharply differentiated zones: western coastlines, central mountains, and eastern forested slopes. Extending 1,500 miles along the Pacific, Peru is an important link between Asia and Brazil, and its rich and varied heritage includes the ancient Incan capital of Cuzco and the lost city of Machu Picchu. Main exports are fish and fish products, copper, zinc, gold, crude petroleum, lead, coffee, sugar, and cotton (*BBC News*, 2008). The 1993 constitution established a presidential democracy with a powerful executive, elected for five years. A 120-member legislature, elected at the same time as the president, also sits for five years. The major religion is Christianity, with more than 80% of citizens Roman Catholic. Although the official languages are Spanish and Quechua, Aymara is also spoken (CIA, 2009).

In the early 1990s, internal terrorism in the country was creating political, economic, and social destabilization. By 2000, Peru's economy suffered substantial losses, and many families became even more impoverished. By 2002, more than half (54%) lived below the poverty line, with 15% living in extreme poverty (Llanos-Zavalaga et al., 2004). Today, the country is seeing growth, but the lot of the rural poor is little improved.

Literacy rates are high, with 88% of adults able to read and write (Infoplease.com, 2008), and according to the World Bank, 99.9% of children complete primary education and 92.4% complete secondary education (The World Bank, 2008).

Life expectancy for men is 71 years, and for women, 76 years (UN, 2009). The infant mortality rate is 33 deaths for every 1,000 live births (Llanos-Zavalaga et al., 2004), and the mortality rate for children under five is 25.2 per 1,000 live births. Health concerns in Peru are compounded by a lack of basic health education among the majority of the rural population, as well as physical and financial access to medical care. Nutrition and sanitation tend to be the main causes of chronic health issues (Foundation for Sustainable Development, 2008).

CASE STUDY
Tuberculosis Prevention and Treatment in Peru

PLAN BACKGROUND, PURPOSE, AND FOCUS

In 1991, when Peru accounted for about 15% of TB cases in the Americas even though it had only 3% of the population, there were approximately 190 cases per 100,000 adults of TB in the country. The abandonment rate of drug therapy was at 12.1% (Llanos-Zavalaga et al., 2004). Only 50% of people diagnosed with TB were able to get treatment and, of those, only half were cured (WHO, 2008c). Drugs were in short supply, record systems nonexistent, and health workers overworked. Public outcry, including spontaneous street demonstrations by TB patients calling for access to effective drugs, led to high-level commitment and action. The country's incoming government declared TB a significant and widespread public health problem and allocated additional resources to their National Tuberculosis Control Program (NTCP), increasing the annual budget from US$600,000 to US$5 million (Llanos-Zavalaga et al., 2004; WHO, 2008c). The country clearly not only recognized the impact the disease was having on its citizens, but also on the country's economy. With TB affecting primarily the most economically productive age group, and a 1999 study showing the economic cost of TB between US$67 and US$108 million, most considered this significant increase a "good investment"(Llanos-Zavalaga et al., 2004).

The *purpose* of this bolstered effort of course was to decrease the incidence of TB, with two areas of *focus*. One was on Directly Observed Treatment—Short Course (DOTS), an internationally recommended approach for TB control programs where a trained healthcare worker monitors the patient taking each dose of anti-tuberculosis medication. The treatment comprises initial daily doses, followed by twice-weekly doses, directly observed to ensure compliance. Without this focus and service, many patients were not completing their regime or taking medications in a timely manner, leading to prolonged illnesses and increased infections in communities. (Although DOTS is the focus of global tuberculosis control, this short course therapy does not cure MDR-TB. In settings of high transmission of multi-drug-resistant tuberculosis, "DOTS-plus," a complementary DOTS-based strategy with provisions for treating multi-drug-resistant tuberculosis, is recommended.) The second important area of focus was on the identification of patients currently infected so that treatment could begin.

TARGET MARKET PROFILE

Getting more people identified who are currently infected and then getting those diagnosed to accept and complete recommended drug therapies required a plan working with key markets downstream, midstream, and upstream. The strategies used are discussed later, but here, first, are the target markets for the plan.

Downstream efforts for diagnosis were to focus on reaching high-risk groups, especially the urban poor in crowded, urban areas known as "TB pockets" or "hot spots." The capital city of Lima was one such target, with 60% of all cases in the country, but only 29% of the population (Llanos-Zavalaga et al., 2004). As noted earlier, TB mainly affects the most economically productive age group, those between 15 and 54 years of age (Llanos-Zavalaga et al., 2004). "Closed populations," because of their high TB prevalence, were also a priority for outreach and included prisoners, patients in mental institutions, retirement home dwellers, and homeless people sleeping in shelters. As patients were identified, they then became the target for drug therapy, as well as those currently taking the medications, to ensure a complete and timely completion.

Midstream efforts, reaching out to those with the ability to influence others in the target markets' community, recognized the need for community involvement in detecting new cases, including family members, neighbors, co-workers, and friends of those at risk. As will be shared in the strategy section, community-based surveillance groups were established on a more formal basis to organize activities to identify and support patients and their families. Working with healthcare providers and their staffs was essential as well, with efforts focused on strategies that would increase the identification of those infected, as well as getting those identified into programs that would help treat and cure the disease.

Upstream efforts recognized the importance of policy makers, communities, the media, and the commercial sector. Policy makers at the national as well as local levels were critical in order to secure funding to ensure the availability of drugs, laboratory supplies, and communication outreach programs. The media would be instrumental in creating high visibility for major events and to stimulate public and political will. Pharmaceutical drug representatives were also considered a target, recognized as a potential distribution channel for communications, as well as a partner for potential price reductions or free drugs.

MARKETING GOALS AND OBJECTIVES

Marketing goals and objectives for the effort were clear and bold. In 1991, when the NTCP adopted the WHO Global Targets, the road ahead looked long and steep, and Peru was one of a handful of high-burden TB countries to take it on. Peru committed to diagnose 70% of pulmonary TB cases and, once diagnosed, accepted the challenge to cure at least 85% of cases; at the time, they were curing only 50%, representing a 70% increase. Peru also wanted to decrease the treatment abandonment; at the time, 12.1% of those being treated were abandoning their treatment (Llanos-Zavalaga et al., 2004).

BEHAVIOR OBJECTIVES

Downstream there were four clear behavior strategies to accomplish with target markets:

- Influence those with symptoms to get diagnosed.
- Influence those who have been diagnosed to accept treatment.

- Influence those receiving treatment to complete the regime.
- Influence those successfully treated to become advocates.

Midstream efforts that focused on families, co-workers, neighbors, friends, and healthcare workers were also specific in desired behavior outcomes:

- Encourage friends and family members with symptoms to get diagnosed and accept treatment, and support them in completing treatment.
- Participate, when needed, in the DOTS program by observing the patient take the medication.
- Additionally, for healthcare workers:
  - Integrate TB services into the primary healthcare system.
  - Upgrade provincial hospitals, district-level hospitals, and primary healthcare clinics.
  - Provide more effective diagnostic services, counseling, and treatment.
  - Strengthen human resource capacity by training staff at all levels in clinical, laboratory, and counseling skills, helping to overcome biases.
  - Conduct DOTS.

Upstream efforts were intended to persuade:

- Policy makers to:
  - Provide support for expanded and improved clinical services.
  - Help ensure availability of drugs and laboratory supplies.
  - Work to develop partnerships and contributions from international and local authorities, community-based organizations, and the private sector.
  - Media to attend and cover special events, as well as report on key TB-related facts and program activities.

Knowledge objectives were educational in nature, recognizing that behavior change would depend on target audiences knowing what symptoms to watch for, how the disease is spread (and not), the effectiveness of treatment, that treatment is free, and that fully completing treatment was necessary in order to be cured. *Belief objectives* took on reducing stigma and correcting misconceptions among all target audiences, as well as the general public.

BARRIERS

Formative research was conducted by the NTCP to assess the public's, as well as healthcare workers' current knowledge and attitudes regarding TB. Findings confirmed suspicions of widespread stigma, misconceptions, and lack of the facts about the disease. It also highlighted concerns with access to diagnosis, drugs, and coordinated care.

Downstream, many of those infected were unaware that their persistent cough was a signal they should get tested. Others, who suspected they were infected and knew they should be tested, did not know where they should go or imagined they would not be able to afford it. Those being treated were not always convinced they needed to be taking their drugs as prescribed, believing that since they felt better they were cured, or seeing the burden of traveling on foot to a clinic several times a week as too exhausting. These barriers of stigma and access were magnified several-fold for those who were homeless, in prison, or in mental institutions. In addition, those with MDR-TB were having difficulty accessing or paying for the type of drugs needed.

Midstream barriers were the greatest for healthcare workers, where stigmas as well as misconceptions were even more pronounced. Some believed, for example, that they could get TB by shaking hands with an infected patient, even by sitting on a chair that an infected person sat on. As a result, healthcare workers would take protective measures such as setting up two desks between themselves and the TB patient or by asking the patient not to face them while they talked. Some even expressed that they perceived an assignment to work on TB at a clinic as a punishment. The healthcare system's capacity for diagnosis, clinical services, and lack of coordination threatened success if patients downstream responded in large numbers.

Upstream policy makers were distracted, especially in 1990, by changes in leadership and other national priorities including crime, illegal drugs, internal terrorism, and poverty. A priority to revamp the healthcare systems and increased funding for TB would be challenging, with the national TB program functioning at the time only on the periphery of the primary healthcare system.

POSITIONING

Given these barriers to getting tested, completing regimens, "being around" patients, and competing country priorities, planners wanted "everyone" to have a sense of urgency about the impact tuberculosis was having on citizens, as well as their country. At the same time, they wanted "everyone" to be hopeful: for patients to know that there are cures and that free help is available; for family members, friends, and healthcare workers to realize that their help is needed; for the media to see TB as a major issue of public interest and concern; and for policy makers to see their efforts as a good investment.

MARKETING MIX STRATEGY

In Peru, all 4Ps in the marketing mix were needed to "get the job done."

Product: DOTS, Adequate Drug Supplies, Clinical Services, Training, and Information Systems

Downstream product strategies focused on DOTS. Mentioned earlier, this service usually involves a healthcare worker who directly administers, observes, and then documents the patient's ingestion or injection of the tuberculosis medication (see Box 5-1 for Paul Farmer's DOTS story). Product quality efforts were to ensure that when citizens arrived for testing, and when patients arrived for drugs, there would be ample supplies and assistance. It was fully recognized that clinical services would need to be in place in order to serve the demand communications were anticipated to create: if patients or potential patients were unable to receive high-quality services and drugs, as promised, they might not return or complete treatment. Collaboration with international and national pharmaceutical companies, along with technical assistance from international agencies, helped ensure a sufficient drug supply, and a centralized procurement system increased efficiencies and cost-effectiveness of their distribution. Funding from the government and international donors increased the number of microscopes and other supplies for laboratories. Serving these populations well would also require the integration of TB services into the primary healthcare system, as well as upgrading hospitals and clinics to provide more effective diagnostic services, counseling, and treatment.

Midstream efforts were intended to strengthen interpersonal skills and expand service capacity, with staff at all levels receiving training in clinical, laboratory, and counseling skills. Training curricula were developed with technical assistance from WHO and the Pan American Health Organization, focused on healthcare workers' first contact with patients, and included components to counter healthcare providers' perceptions about TB (as well as about TB patients). Workers were taught how to avoid TB while still being inviting and welcoming. Computers were provided and used to upgrade health management information systems, and staff were trained to record and analyze data using software specifically designed for the TB program. And for the political leaders and media *upstream*, informational seminars were provided with presentations by international experts.

Price: Free Services and Monetary and Nonmonetary Incentives

Downstream, not only did patients receive free testing, treatment, and counseling, they were also offered incentives. To encourage completing treatment,

BOX 5-1 **DOTS Therapy**

(This brief story expands on the opening chapter quote from Paul Farmer and highlights a journey he took to visit the patient in Morne Michel.)
The one-way trip to Morne Michel usually took him two hours (on foot). About three hours after we'd set out, we arrived at the hut of the non-compliant patient, another shack made of rough-sawn palm wood with a roof of banana fronds and a cooking fire of the kind Haitians call "three rocks."

Farmer asked the patient, a young man, if he disliked his TB medicines.

"Are you kidding?" he replied. "I wouldn't be here without them."

It turned out that he'd been given confusing instructions the last time he was in Cange, and he hadn't received the standard cash stipend. He hadn't missed any doses of his TB drugs, however. Good news for Farmer. Mission accomplished. He'd made sure that the patient's cure wasn't being interrupted. . . .

"Some people would argue this wasn't worth a five-hour walk," he said over his shoulder. "But you can never invest too much in making sure this stuff works. . . . The objective is to inculcate in the doctors and nurses the spirit to dedicate themselves to the patients, and especially to having an outcome-oriented view on TB." . . .

We started on again, Farmer saying over his shoulder, "And if it takes five-hour treks or giving patients milk or nail clippers or raisins, radios, watches, then do it. We can spend sixty-eight thousand dollars per TB patient in New York City, but if you start giving watches or radios to patients here, suddenly the international health community jumps on you for creating *nonsustainable projects.* If a patient says, I really need a Bible or nail clippers, well, for God's sake!"

Source: Kidder, 2004, pp. 41–42.

low-income patients received food packages as an incentive, and some received reimbursement for transportation costs to the health clinic and free lodging for those in need. In addition, the NTCP started a micro-credit loan program to help patients start a small business and leave disease and poverty behind. For example, Socios En Salud (SES), a sister organization of Partners in Health and one of the largest nongovernmental organization (NGO) healthcare organizations in Peru, helped women in the community earn an income by providing membership in a cooperative workshop that participates in crafts fairs in Peru and has sold handicrafts as far away as the United States, Japan, and Switzerland (Partners in Health, 2006). (See Figure 5-1.)

Midstream, not only did the NTCP recognize health directors at public gatherings when they reached program targets, they actually published the outcomes of all clinics in an annual report, further rewarding those who had made their targets and intending to motivate those who had not to "work even harder." And healthcare workers were also provided incentives, with contests for posters and awards given for the best poster design. And for country leaders *upstream*, the World

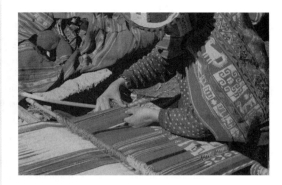

FIGURE 5-1　A craft business benefiting from a microloan.

Health Organization showcased Peru's commitment and progress toward reducing the country's incidence of TB as an international success story.

Place: Making Access to Services More Convenient

Access to diagnosis and treatment was significantly enhanced, including extending hours into the evenings, home visits, and expansion of DOTS to all areas of the country, providing the infrastructure necessary to ensure services to all citizens. This improved access was made possible by the Ministry of Health's integration of TB services into the primary healthcare system and the upgrade of provincial hospitals, district-level hospitals, and primary healthcare clinics.

Promotion: Persuasive Communications

Persuasive communications were developed and disseminated to the public, community, and political leaders through a variety of media channels, both wide and narrow, providing information about the causes of TB, sources of infection, how it is transmitted, symptoms, treatment, and prevention.

Messages

Key messages were clear, simple, consistent, and included three major slogans:

- "Treatment for one is prevention for all" was the slogan for the campaign, intended to motivate the community to become involved in the program.
- "If you cough for more than 15 days, you should go to the health center" was developed to encourage patients as well as the general

public to help family members, neighbors, and other community members seek care.

- "All TB services are for free" was designed to appeal to low-income groups and motivate them to seek care.

Additional messages focused on correcting misconceptions about the disease and the importance of timely and complete treatment. The NTCP logo appeared at all TB service sites and was widely disseminated on mass media, as well print materials, posters, and billboards.

Messengers

Healthcare workers were key to establishing the credibility of messages, and family members and community organization volunteers were key to overcoming barriers through personal persuasiveness.

Media Channels

To ensure effectiveness, consistent messages were conveyed through a mix of mass media, printed materials, popular media, social networks, advocacy, and special promotions.

Mass Media

NTCP aired several television and radio spots to raise community awareness, correct misconceptions, motivate patients to seek care, and encourage the public to advocate for resources. NTCP also worked with local authorities to air messages in theaters, on local radio stations, and on select billboards. With Peru's high literacy rate, print media especially became an important tool for improving knowledge about tuberculosis—what symptoms to watch for, how it is spread, and how important completing treatment is to achieve a total cure.

Print Materials

In addition to mass media, local authorities designed print materials, including letters, question-and-answer cards, fact sheets, leaflets, newsletters, posters in the local Quechua and Aymara languages, and a manual for street theater productions with strong messages about dealing with tuberculosis.

Special Events

One major event, World TB Day, was an opportune time to organize high-visibility events and included parades and other public gatherings to advocate for continued support for the TB control programs. A week-long campaign used the campaign's slogan as a theme, "Treatment for one is prevention for all," and included more articles in the newspapers and on the Internet, and radio programs aired regular slots on TB. A short documentary about the achievements in the fight against TB in Peru was shown on TV; seminars for health workers and medical staff addressed planning and mobilization strategies; and awareness-raising events took place in the main squares of the major cities with activities including theatre, street drama, and placing stickers on cars. Street theaters, card games with question and answers, and focused group discussions using flipcharts were also used frequently through-out the years to bring messages directly to hard-to-reach audiences such as those in shanty towns and other hotspots.

Videos

The program replaced the traditional flipchart presentations with video spots that were developed for healthcare providers to show in healthcare facility wait-ing areas.

One-on-One Communications

Health workers were considered the linchpin of the TB strategy. They were trained to provide an informative and welcoming first contact for those seeking diagnosis and were encouraged to reach out to other visitors in the health facil-ity as well, helping to spread communications regarding tuberculosis symptoms and treatment available. In addition, private practitioners were instructed that when they found a patient with TB, they should send him or her to the TB clinic with a written note so that the patient would be treated.

Community Mobilization

In 1995, NTCP established community organizations called "Community Surveillance Units" to help detect TB and follow up on treatment, playing an important role in linking the health team to the community. Other important community groups included mothers' groups, churches, patient and family sup-port groups, and Family Parents Associations.

Advocacy

The program used advocacy to secure political commitment and involvement at all levels and to keep the TB issue in the national spotlight. Local groups were formed to mobilize patients and their families, provide peer education, learn pa-tient rights and responsibilities, defend them with political leaders, and then gain coverage for them in media. Political leaders and the media were invited to attend seminars and presentations organized with international experts.

Table 5-1 summarizes marketing mix strategies for downstream target markets.

TABLE 5-1   Summary of Marketing Mix Strategies for Target Markets Downstream

The 4Ps	Strategies Targeting TB Patients
Product	
Core:	*Core:*
Benefits for the behavior	From testing: peace of mind
	From taking drugs: getting well
Actual:	*Actual:*
Behaviors and features of behavior	Get tested and take all drugs
Augmented:	*Augmented:*
Tangible objects and services	DOTS therapy
	Adequate supplies of drugs
	Counseling
	Patient and family support groups
Price	
Monetary and nonmonetary incentives	Free testing
	Free drugs for those who need them
	Microcredit loans
	Reimbursement for travel
	Free lodging
	Food packages for low-income families
Place	
Access to tangible objects and services	Extended clinic hours
	Home visits for DOTS
	Transportation for those in need
Promotion	
Key messages	*Key messages*
	"All TB services are free."
	"If you cough for more than 15 days you should go to the health center."
	"Treatment for one is prevention for all."

TABLE 5-1 (Continued)

The 4Ps	Strategies Targeting TB Patients
Key messengers	*Key messengers*
	Healthcare workers
	Family members
	Community organization volunteers
Key media channels	*Key media channels*
	Mass media: television, radio, billboards, print media
	Print materials: posters, letters, fact sheets
	Special events: World TB Day, street theaters
	Videos: healthcare facility waiting areas
	Personal communications: health workers
	Community mobilization: surveillance groups
	Advocacy: local groups targeting families and political leaders

PARTNERSHIPS

Partnerships were created at all levels of the program, from the top levels of government to the community levels, with both international as well as national organizations, and with public, private, and NGO sectors.

Important international partners included the Pan American Health Organization (providing technical support and training for capacity building), the Japan International Cooperation Agency (expansion of laboratory services), the Peru-Canada Agreement (information system support), USAID (supporting the communication strategy development), the international NGO Socios en Salud (improving the diagnosis and treatment of patients with MDR-TB), and the BASIC Health and Nutrition Project (assistance in implementing educational and counseling activities; Llanos-Zavalaga et al., 2004). In addition, collaboration with international pharmaceutical companies helped ensure a sufficient drug supply (Llanos-Zavalaga et al., 2004).

National partners collaborated with NTCP to secure endorsement from Peru's medical leaders, facilitate participation of medical leaders in seminars, and include up-to-date information in TB medical curricula. The

Association of Tuberculosis Patients was an important partner in advocacy, and national pharmaceutical industry and private medical practitioners facilitated pooled purchasing of TB drugs at the national level (Llanos-Zavalaga et al., 2004).

Nongovernmental organizations also played an active role, with local churches and community-based organizations providing outreach to the community and a link to health clinics. As mentioned earlier, in 1995 NTCP established community organizations called Community Surveillance Units (CSUs) to help detect TB and follow up on treatment. The CSUs played an important role in linking the health team to the community. By 2000, 22,672 CSUs with 48,420 volunteers were serving 751,771 families. Other important community groups included mother groups, patient and family support groups, and Family Parents Associations. These groups allowed the community to feel ownerships of the program and played an important role in case detection and ensuring treatment compliance (Llanos-Zavalaga et al., 2004).

OUTCOMES

In 2000, WHO reported promising results in Peru, touting its TB program as "one of the world's most successful DOTS programs in the world . . . one of only a handful of high-burden countries to have met the WHO targets for TB control of 70% case detection rates and 85% cure rates." By 1998, in fact, an estimated 94% of TB cases were being detected and 90% of patients were being cured, preventing close to 70,000 cases and deaths.

The number of health centers participating in the program soared from 1,000 in 1991 to more than 6,000 by 1999. And as efforts to detect new cases intensified, the number of laboratories capable of carrying out smear tests rose from 300 in 1989 to more than 1,000 by 1999 (WHO, 2008c).

POSTNOTE

While Peru succeeded in the late 1990s in meeting the targets set by WHO, the country now faces new challenges: MDR-TB and co-infection with HIV/AIDS. Many believe that new commitments have been made to address this, and efforts have been redoubled. For example, a grant from The Global Fund will help finance the treatment of MDR-TB for 2,000 patients and their families. The grant will also aid Peru in its goal to increase its tuberculosis detection rate to 100%. The program will focus on the high-risk populations, including prisoners and residents of the urban areas of Lima and Callao. This financing will enable the Ministry of Health to develop more community-based surveillance programs, to initiate compulsory testing for tuberculosis for all prisoners, and to then administer first- and second-line treatment to those diagnosed with the disease. Through the collaborative work of WHO, Harvard Medical School, and others, successful negotiations with pharmaceutical companies are giving countries like Peru an opportunity to purchase second-line drugs for tuberculosis at deeply discounted prices, once the countries demonstrate that they have the infrastructures for distribution. This is lowering the price of the course of drugs from more than US$10,000 per patient to US$3,000 per patient (The Global Fund, 2003).

SUMMARY AND IMPLICATIONS

Authors of the "The Role of Communication in Peru's Fight Against Tuberculosis" mentioned at the beginning of the chapter, shared 10 lessons they believe are valuable to other countries developing TB communication strategies:

1. Political commitment is essential, especially when combined with increased resources.
2. Communication activities should be strategically timed to correspond with improvements in clinical services.
3. Integrate communication activities into all program activities at all levels.
4. Formative research can unlock key communication challenges.
5. Communication programs are more effective when consistent messages are conveyed through a mix of mass media and interpersonal communication.
6. Involve the community and local healthcare providers, including private practitioners, in the TB control program.
7. Create partnerships at all levels.
8. Put some effort into reaching the hard-to-reach, especially if they have high prevalence rates.
9. Create a positive and encouraging culture.
10. Simple and consistent messages can help the public recognize TB cases. (Llanos-Zavalaga et al., 2004)

From a social marketing perspective, several strengths of this effort are noteworthy, contributing to its success:

- Program planners recognized there were multiple and unique target markets to influence: patients, their families and friends, healthcare workers, media, pharmaceutical companies, and political leaders.

- Formative research provided important insights regarding audience barriers to adopting desired behaviors, ones beyond those that could be addressed by communications alone.
- Existing data made it possible to establish SMART goals, allocate necessary resources to monitor progress, and make adjustments as needed.
- An agreement on an overarching positioning for the campaign guided communication planning and led to an integrated approach.
- The need for all 4Ps in the marketing mix were recognized and supported. Product strategies recognized the need for adequate drug supplies, counseling services, and direct observation of drug compliance. Price strategies recognized that costs were a key hurdle for many and that incentives, even small ones like food baskets, could be powerful motivators. Place strategies recognized that convenient access in terms of hours and locations would affect testing as well as compliance. And promotional strategies recognized the need for an integrated approach of key messages in a variety of media channels, especially the critical role of personal, one-on-one communications to persuade audiences downstream and advocacy to persuade those upstream.

QUESTIONS FOR DISCUSSION

1. The author believes that the other 3Ps (product, price, and place) were important elements of success in this case. Do you agree? Why?
2. What elements of this model do you think are most important for other countries to adopt?
3. What other marketing strategies could Peru have used to accomplish even greater outcomes?

REFERENCES

BBC News. (2008). Country profile: Peru. Retrieved July 28, 2009 from http://newsvote.bbc.co .uk/mpapps/pagetools/print/news.bbc.co.uk/1/hi/world/americas/country_profiles/ 1224656.stm

CIA. (2009). *The CIA world factbook: Peru.* Retrieved July 28, 2009, from https://www.cia.gov/ library/publications/the-world-factbook/geos/pe.html

Census. (2007). *Countries and areas ranked by population.* Retrieved July 28, 2009, from http://census.gov/cgi-bin/ipc/idbrank.pl

Foundation for Sustainable Development. (2008). *Health issues in Peru.* Retrieved July 28, 2009, from http://www.fsdinternational.org/?q=ntlopps/country/peru/healthissues

The Global Fund. (2003). *Stopping tuberculosis in Peru.* Retrieved July 28, 2009, from http://www.theglobalfund.org/en/in_action/peru/tb1/

Infoplease.com. (2008). *Peru.* Retrieved July 28, 2009, from http://www.infoplease.com/ipa/A0107883.html

Kidder, T. (2004). *Mountains beyond mountains: The quest of Dr. Paul Farmer, a man who would cure the world.* New York: Random House.

Llanos-Zavalaga, F., Poppe, P., Tawfik, Y., & Church-Balin, C. (2004). *The role of communication in Peru's fight against tuberculosis.* Baltimore: Johns Hopkins Bloomberg School of Public Health, Center for Communication Programs.

National Public Radio. (2003, September 25). *The quest of Dr. Paul Farmer.* Retrieved July 28, 2009, from http://www.npr.org/templates/story/story.php?storyId=1472188

Partners in Health. (2006). *Peru/socios en salud.* Retrieved July 28, 2009, from http://www.pih.org/where/Peru/Peru.html

Stop TB Partnership. (2008). *Tuberculosis in countries.* Retrieved July 28, 2009, from http://www.stoptb.org/countries/

The United Nations (UN). (2009). *Indicators on health.* Retrieved July 28, 2009, from http://unstats.un.org/unsd/Demographic/products/socind/health.htm

The World Bank. (2008). *Peru data profile.* Retrieved July 28, 2009, from http://devdata.worldbank.org/external/CPProfile.asp?PTYPE=CP&CCODE=PER

World Health Organization (WHO). (2007). *Tuberculosis fact sheet.* Retrieved July 28, 2009, from http://www.who.int/mediacentre/factsheets/fs104/en/print.html

World Health Organization (WHO). (2008a). *Worldwide efforts to confront tuberculosis are making progress but too slowly.* Retrieved July 28, 2009, from http://www.who.int/tb/features_archive/global_tb_control_report08/en/index.html

World Health Organization (WHO). (2008b). *A world free of TB.* Retrieved July 28, 2009, from http://www.who.int/tb/en/

World Health Organization (WHO). (2008c). *Health a key to prosperity: Success stories in developing countries. Peru set to halve new TB cases every 10 years.* Retrieved July 28, 2009, from http://wholint/inf-new/tuber1.htm

CHAPTER 6

Increasing School Meal Uptake in a Deprived Region in England
Overcoming the Barriers

Rowena Merritt, Aiden Truss, Lucy Reynolds, and Emma Heesom

School meals in primary schools make a vital contribution to the dietary intake of schoolchildren in England (Nelson et al., 2005). However, the number of school meals purchased has fallen in 75% of schools (Ofsted[1], 2007). The substantial decline began after changes were rapidly made to school meals, in a bid to make them more nutritionally balanced. While the reasons for the decline are complex, the lack of consultation with pupils and parents and the poor promotion of new menus were all singled out as contributing factors to the fall. This chapter discusses a social marketing intervention developed to arrest and

[1]Ofsted—the Office for Standards in Education, Children's Services and Skills—is the official body for inspecting schools in England.

then reverse this decline and to maintain and increase the uptake of healthy school meals by children in a deprived part of England. This project was initiated by the North East Centre of Excellence (NECE), as part of a program of activity that aims to improve the efficiency and sustainability of public sector food procurement.

UNITED KINGDOM: A COUNTRY OVERVIEW

The United Kingdom (UK) is situated in western Europe and is comprised of four countries: England, Scotland, Wales, and Northern Ireland. While England is not a large country (130,395 square kilometers), it has a relatively large, and growing, population. In mid-2006 the resident population of the UK was 60,587,000, of which 50,763,000 lived in England. Life expectancy for both men and women has continued to rise. In 2002, life expectancy at birth for females born in the UK was 81 years, compared with 76 years for males (Office for National Statistics, 2008a).

In the 2001 census, 92.1% of the population classified themselves as White. Christianity is the main religion in Great Britain. There were 41 million Christians in 2001, making up almost three-quarters (72%) of the population. People with no religion form the second largest group, comprising 15% of the population (Office for National Statistics, 2001).

In the UK, there are three distinct branches of government: the executive, the legislature, and the judiciary. The executive in the UK comprises the Prime Minister and his ministers. The legislature in the UK consists of the two Houses of Parliament. The executive (government) presents to the legislature bills that it wants to pass into law, and then it is up to Parliament to debate these bills, amending them if it thinks fit, and finally deciding whether to pass the bill and make it an Act of Parliament or not. The role of the judiciary is to interpret the laws passed by Parliament. Because the UK does not have a written constitution, the judiciary cannot hold that a particular Act of Parliament or any action of the executive is contrary to the constitution and accordingly unlawful. The UK has had a political system in which two parties have dominated for at least three centuries. The parties presently dominating the political scene are the Labour Party and the Conservative (Tory) Party.

In England, healthcare services have been the responsibility of central government for more than 50 years. The Department of Health has made many changes throughout its history to support the public to lead healthy lives. The department's overall purpose is to ensure better health and well-being, better care, and better value for all. It is responsible for standards of health care in the country, including the National Health Service (NHS), setting the strategic framework for adult social care and influencing local authority spending on social care. It also sets the direction on promoting and protecting the public's health, taking the lead on issues like environmental hazards to health, infectious diseases, health promotion and education, the safety of medicines, and ethical issues.

Throughout its history, the department has evolved to make it better equipped to lead the health and social care system. The most recent changes to its structure took place in 2003, leading to a smaller department with six ministers, 2,245 staff, and three executive agencies (Department of Health, 2009).

As a consequence of this restructuring, the Department of Health in England devolved its spending decisions to the regional areas. The types of subject areas given priority by the Department of Health include smoking cessation, teenage pregnancy, child and adolescent mental health, substance misuse, sexual health, falls prevention, physical activity, and obesity control (Department of Health, 2009).

SOCIAL MARKETING IN ENGLAND

In 2006, an independent national review of health-related campaigns, commissioned by the Department of Health in England, highlighted the use of social marketing to improve the impact and effectiveness of health promotion in England at national, regional, and local levels.

To help develop skills and capacity in this area, the National Social Marketing Centre (NSM Centre) was established in a strategic partnership between the Department of Health in England and the National Consumer Council (re-launched as *Consumer Focus* in October 2008). Part of this partnership saw the establishment of 10 learning demonstration projects. The learning demonstration sites are positioned across England and address a range of health behavior issues, from breastfeeding and healthy eating to smoking cessation and anti-social drinking. The following case study is taken from one of the sites, one addressing school meals in a deprived region in the country.

School Meals in England

SETTING THE SCENE

As a result of rapidly increasing rates of childhood obesity and other weight-related diseases, there is increasing concern about the quality of children's diets and a growing demand for a change to the school meal offer and uptake, supported through government policy.

As noted in "School Meals in Primary Schools" (Nelson et al., 2005), "school meals make a vital contribution to the dietary intake of school children in England" (p. 16). Every day, more than 3 million school meals are served. There are 7.6 million English primary and secondary school pupils, and 43% of them take a school meal. However, despite the volume of school meals currently being served, there are patterns of poor health and eating behavior among children that are cause for concern and a sense that children are increasingly powerful consumers—able to choose what they do or do not eat to a growing degree.

Whether a child does or does not eat a healthy meal at school is now recognized as being fundamental to that child's behavioral, educational, and social development. As a result of this recognition, coupled with rapidly increasing rates of childhood obesity and other diet-related diseases, the UK government has committed to increasing the number of children eating school dinners and to improving the school meal offer in terms of health and nutritional value (School Meals Review Panel, 2005).

As the School Meals Review Panel (2005) observed in "Turning the Tables," a report on transforming school food:

> The health advantages of well-cooked, well-presented meals, made from good-quality ingredients to accepted nutritional standards, by school caterers who are confident in their skills and valued by the school community, are inestimable. The benefits of good school meals go beyond high-quality catering. They also produce social, educational, and economic advantages. (p. 5)

SCHOOL MEALS ON THE POLITICAL AGENDA

England's Department of Health and Department for Education and Skills (DfES) are working closely to implement change and have introduced a range of interventions to boost school meal uptake and improve nutritional health. In

2004, the Department of Health issued a milestone white paper, "Choosing Health," in which it committed to "improve nutrition in school meals" by revising school meal standards to reduce salt and fat consumption and enhance fruit and vegetable intake, to be enforced through Ofsted inspections; applying new healthy eating standards to cover food across the whole school day; and supporting schools to provide the best meal service possible (Department of Health, 2004).

In an attempt to improve the standard of school meals, the Department for Education and Skills set up the School Food Trust, a nondepartmental public body, in 2005. Its mission is to transform school food and food skills and promote the education and health of children and young people by improving the quality of food supplied and consumed in schools. Following the report published by the School Meals Review Panel in October 2005, the trust was tasked with taking forward the panel's recommendations to transform school food and food skills to improve health and education for school-age children and young people. Whilst the School Food Trust works closely with DfES, it is an independent organization providing information, advice, and guidance to anyone involved in school food. In terms of interventions, it covers three main areas: (1) information and support, (2) training and conferences, and (3) funding.

DEPRIVATION IN NORTHEAST ENGLAND

This case study was piloted in Northeast England, which has large areas of deprivation. The statistics given here highlight the extent of the deprivation:

- The unemployment rate in the region was 6.5% in 2006, the second highest in the UK (Office for National Statistics, 2008b).
- The average price for dwellings in the Northeast was £132,000 in 2005, which remains the lowest in England and Wales. This is £60,000 below the national average (Office for National Statistics, 2008b).
- Of the 215,430 pupils on roll in the Northeast in 2006, 37,930 (17.6%) were taking free school meals. This is substantially higher than the UK average of 13.3% (School Meal Arrangements, 2006).

Health inequalities are a major concern for the Department of Health in England. A recent report found the gap in life expectancy between the bottom fifth and the population as a whole had widened by 2% for males and 5% for females between 1997–1999 and 2001–2003 (BBC, 2005). In England, health inequalities are measured by life expectancy and infant mortality. Northeast England is one of the priority regions with a disproportionate share of health inequalities. The health inequalities gap in Northeast England is attributed mainly to a historic legacy of industrial and mining industries.

THE SOCIAL MARKETING PROCESS

Conducting the Scoping Work

During the scoping phase, the following work was done:

- A steering group to manage the project was set up.
- A stakeholder strategy was developed, and key stakeholders were identified and engaged.
- Due to the limited budget for this project, an audit of other resources, which could be tapped into, was done.
- A review of the secondary literature was conducted by a researcher. This review looked at key policy drivers and examined other interventions that had been developed to tackle this problem internationally, nationally, and locally.
- After the review of the secondary data, knowledge gaps still remained, so primary research was conducted with head teachers, parents, and children.
- The qualitative research highlighted distinct differences among the head teachers. Based on these insights, head teachers, who were the primary target audience, were segmented further.
- Behavioral goals were set.
- The marketing mix was developed and pretested with the primary target audience.

Establishment of the Steering Group

The steering group was made up of people who were passionate about the issue being addressed and who also had time to dedicate to the project. Other people who were interested in the project but did not have any time available to carry out work for the project were involved through the stakeholder strategy.

Specifically, external partners with a vested interest in addressing the issue and the authority to represent their respective organizations were invited to a prospective steering group *briefing*, where the issue being addressed was presented and the social marketing process explained. In addition, expectations for the steering group and commitment needed from it were made clear. From this initial meeting, a steering group of six people was established, which included three local catering managers, one representative from the School Food Trust, and one project manager from the NSM Centre. The group chair, who managed the project's budget, worked for the NECE, the organization that instigated the project.

SWOT Analysis

Once the steering group was established, it conducted a SWOT analysis. By identifying both the internal (strengths and weaknesses) and external (opportunities and threats) factors to the project (see Table 6-1), this analysis helped the steering group develop a clear plan of action. Due to school meals being high on the political agenda, the SWOT analysis was updated every three months to ensure that the project stayed abreast of the changing political environment.

Based on the SWOT analysis, various actions were put in place to try to minimize the threats and utilize the strengths. For example, to ensure join-up with national work, an employee of the School Food Trust was asked to be a member of the steering committee, and training on social marketing was given to the steering group and their colleagues.

Stakeholder Engagement

In an early meeting, the steering group created a list of key stakeholders. Many of the stakeholders identified worked closely with the catering staff in schools and therefore knew the problems firsthand. Other stakeholders were identified due to their influence in this area, and the resources they had could be tapped into for this project. Once the list of key stakeholders was drawn up, they were plotted by the group onto a power and interest matrix. This helped the group identify those stakeholders who were most important to engage and those who required a less proactive approach.

Once the stakeholders were plotted on the matrix (see Figure 6-1), a strategy for handling each of the matrix quads was developed. For example, representatives from the different groups in the "key players" and "keep satisfied" areas were invited to attend the Solution Group, which developed the interventions.

Reviewing the Secondary Evidence

Secondary evidence looking at past and current interventions that have addressed the issue and their target audience was collated and reviewed by a researcher. Local, national, and international interventions were considered. The interventions were found through a desk search.

Various interventions were reviewed, which have had, or are intended to have, an impact on school meal uptake and the promotion of healthy eating among children. These include both local and national initiatives to improve the school meal offer and increase uptake, and they represent a mixture of top-down and bottom-up interventions. This information was used to help the steering group brainstorm and plan their next steps.

TABLE 6-1 SWOT Analysis for the Project

Factors/Variables	Internal	External
Positive	*Strengths* • Every school has a school meals service, the majority of which operate on site. • The steering group feels passionately about this topic and has extensive experience of working with head teachers and cooks in the local area.	*Opportunities* • The government has made a commitment to increase the number of children eating school meals. • School meals have become more nutritious, and a lot is being done in the region to improve the dining room experience, such as new chairs and tables and a salad bar where the children can help themselves.
Negative	*Weaknesses* • There is a lot of pressure on the time of those on the steering group. • Catering managers are under great pressure; if they cannot increase the school meal uptake, more job losses for their staff are inevitable. • There is sometimes a great disconnect between national and regional work, which leads to discontentment and local areas inadvertently competing with national projects. • Caterers, for the most part, have no control over the dining space or facilities. • Financial constraints from local authorities exist due to the economic downturn.	*Threats* • Home-packed lunch food can be purchased very cheaply, and parents feel it caters better for fussy eaters. • Distrust of government and the School Food Trust is due to the speed of changes and a perceived lack of empathy. • Media backlash of the "Jamie Oliver effect" fuels parents feeling that they know best (Jamie's School Dinners, 2005). • The increase in food prices, labor costs, and fuel prices leads to a fear of price increases and lower numbers.

It became evident from the review that a host of interventions were being implemented to boost school meal uptake and encourage sustainable healthy eating habits among schoolchildren. At a national level, there were funding pools, healthy schools initiatives, food nutrient standards, FSA (Food Standards Agency) targets, national conferences, partnerships, training opportunities, and information forums—all of which combined together either to enforce or to encourage change. These strategic interventions were then translated into ground-level initiatives, which ranged from choice control within schools to parental involvement schemes, dining room improvements, head teacher communication initiatives, parental education incentives, menu improvements, curriculum initiatives, cookery lessons, packed lunch regulation, and so on. Furthermore, the evidence base suggested that a whole school approach—which offers a combined package of enforcement, support, and education (including management change, curriculum planning, teaching and learning, school environment, and provision of pupil support services)—would be the most successful means of achieving behavior change (see

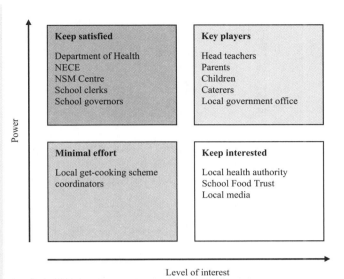

FIGURE 6-1   Power and interest matrix for the Northeast project.

http://www.healthyschools.gov.uk/About-Whole-School-Approach.aspx).

What also emerged from this overview, however, was a profusion of information initiatives, support services, regulations, guidelines, Web sites, marketing campaigns, case studies, debates, conferences, awards, and incentive schemes. Although all the information, legislation, and advice was aimed at promoting school meal uptake, it could overwhelm the target audience.

In other words, while this wealth of interventions reflected the weight being given to the school meals debate and marked a positive climate for change, there was a potential for confusion, overabundance, and fragmentation within the sector and a need to be alert to proliferation and duplication as a potential barrier to clear communication of messages, behavior goals, and targets.

IDENTIFYING THE TARGET AUDIENCE(S)

Primary research and interviews with key stakeholders identified that the two most important influencers of school meal uptake are head teachers and parents. Primary research with local head teachers was completed, and individual interviews and focus groups with parents and children were also conducted. These interviews were used to identify the barriers, guide the design of interventions, and prioritize target audiences.

Primary Audience: Head Teachers

Head teachers are the essential cog in a school and, as such, are the people who need to be engaged in order to unlock the other stakeholders. By encouraging a whole school approach on school food—packed-lunch policies; direct involvement in the dining hall ambience, layout, and structure; and better communication with caterers and parents—school meal uptake will increase.

Secondary Audience: Parents

Parents are also a vital customer. In key stage 2 they still control the choice, in the vast majority of cases, and their misconceptions over choice, value, and environment of school meals and the dining hall has direct bearing on uptake.

Secondary Audience: Children

Children at key stage 2 increasingly influence their parents and can impart misinformation from the type of food offered to their desires to eat what they choose, which means that they can "bribe" or influence parents.

Due to financial limitations, the marketing strategy was broken down into two phases. During phase 1, the target audience was head teachers because they were identified as the key influencer by all stakeholders and in all of the research. Phase 2 will focus on children and parents (due to start in 2010, subject to financial support). Further segmentation work was done with teachers, based on the findings from the qualitative research. Four main customer groups were identified for head teachers. These were:

- Too busy.
- Disengaged and confused.
- Trying within their field.
- Engaged and passionate.

A typical *too busy* head teacher will not engage with the school meals agenda, the caterer will find it difficult to secure a face-to-face meeting, and he or she will be unlikely to respond to e-mail or written communication. This head teacher will see little benefit in being hands-on in the school meals agenda; will have other, "more urgent" priorities to attend to; and commonly finds the "Jamie Oliver effect"[2] an annoyance as things were much simpler before.

> "I think the school meals service should be taking the initiative with this, rather than ourselves."
>
> "Really, I feel that if I make a stand, here, I've got absolutely no backing from the government or from the governors."

A typical *disengaged and confused* head teacher will not understand his or her role in the school meals provision and may often pass on inaccurate information to parents. This teacher will not be aware of all the national standards and may be confused as to who is responsible for the management of school meals and kitchen staff in the school. This head teacher will feel that school meals have changed for the better but feel unsupported against tricky parents and will not always immediately see the benefits of school meals. The communication with the catering provider may only occur when there is an issue or problem to resolve. However, this teacher will be open to communication if it is clear, concise, and easily available.

> "Limit packed-lunch places? I think I'd have parents with placards at the school gates if I did that."

A head teacher who is *trying within their field* believes that the changes in school meals were needed and feels school meals offer a good service to their school. He or she will have sporadic communication with the catering provider, but this communication will generally be positive. This teacher knows his or her mission and promotes school meals to parents as far as practicable. He or she is keen to learn from other head teachers and to share examples of what has worked. There will be further opportunity to engage this head teacher in deeper and more connected communications; he or she would be open to new ideas and would probably welcome more formal engagement, through a school food group, for example, with the school cook and caterer.

> "I just need to work a little bit more with a couple of members of the kitchen staff."

The *engaged and passionate* head teacher is at the forefront of the school meals debate in the region and will probably have prioritized school meals

---

[2]Jamie Oliver is a celebrity chef. He produced a documentary-style TV program looking at school meals in the UK. The program highlighted how nutritionally poor they were. The program caused a lot of tabloid press activity, and in rapid response the government changed school meals dramatically, making them more balanced nutritionally, but taking away many of the foods which the children ate.

before the "Jamie Oliver campaign." Commonly, there will be packed-lunch policies and school gardens in this head teacher's school, and there is an open door for the caterer. This head teacher is commonly asked to pilot new ideas or marketing promotions. This head teacher will have an effective "Golden Table," and the cook and dinner nannies (the colloquial name for school dining hall supervisors) will sometimes take part in other activities in the school.

> "25's the maximum [number of packed-lunch places allowed]—I've set a number . . . it's understood now, we've had 8 or 9 years of that."
> "I do dinner duty *every* day. If I don't my deputy does."

The steering group agreed to concentrate on only two segments initially: *disengaged and confused* and *trying within their field*.

AIMS AND OBJECTIVES

The overall aim of this project was to arrest and then reverse the decline in pupils' uptake of healthy school meals, and to maintain and increase their uptake at key stage 2 (aged 7 to 11). The SMART objectives set for the project were:

1. Increase by 3% in a two-month period the number children in key stage 2 eating school meals one to three days a week.
2. Increase the number of head teachers who receive and read the newsletter by 15% by July 2009.
3. Increase the number of head teachers who attend a meeting with their local catering manager by 10% by September 2009.
4. By the end of summer term 2009, most head teachers who received the intervention will have a better understanding of their role in school meals, to be measured by qualitative research.
5. By the end of summer term 2009, most head teachers who received the intervention will have better knowledge of the nutrition standards and know which myths are false, to be measured by qualitative research.
6. By the end of winter term 2009, the dinner nannies who have attended the training will have the following proficiencies:
   - Customer service skills.
   - Positive behavioral management/motivation techniques.
   - Basic first aid.
   - Food and nutrition knowledge.
7. By the end of summer term 2009, the amount of food and packaging waste will have decreased by at least 5%.

TARGET AUDIENCE BARRIERS, MOTIVATORS (BENEFITS), AND COMPETITION

Barriers to Performing the Behavior

Head Teachers

A purposive sample of head teachers from the region was identified and selected to participate in the study with the help of three members of the project's steering group. The head teachers all managed primary schools. Sampling was based on area, size of school, and current uptake of school meals (classified as high, medium, or low by members of the steering group). The main barriers identified by the head teachers were:

- Communication clutter—due to school meals being a government priority, head teachers have been bombarded with information, legislation, and advice. Confusion exists, however, as to who manages the catering services within a school (the heads themselves or the local education authority?) and what exactly can and cannot be included in school meals (e.g., can an individual school deviate from the government menus if it still meets nutritional guidelines?).
- Quality of the food (poor cooking skills of the cooks) and a lack of availability of popular items for the children served last.
- Concerns over the composition of the food the children eat for lunch (e.g., children were often reported to choose only carbohydrates).
- Lack of dining hall management, understanding of nutritional standards, and customer service skills of the dinner nannies.
- Children's lack of cooking skills and knowledge of the different food products (e.g., many head teachers commented on how their children did not know what certain vegetables and fruits were, such as kiwi fruits and parsnips).

Research conducted with parents and children also identified a range of barriers.

Parents

Barriers identified by the parents included:

- Loss of ability to give their children something they know they will eat.
- Worries over lack of availability of popular items for the children served last.

- Concerns over the composition of the food their children are allowed with school meals, for example, gravy on their salad, pasta with potatoes (too many carbohydrates).
- Cost of school meals in families with more than one child (especially in the light of future price rises caused by increasing food costs).
- Desire for an easy life means that parents give in to what their children want and they cannot face the daily battle over food with their children.

Children

Research with children identified the following barriers:

- Because the menu changes were enforced, many of the most popular options (e.g., chicken nuggets and chips) are no longer served. Children are confronted with food that is often unfamiliar, unpopular, and unlike what they are given at home.
- School meals take longer than packed lunches to serve and eat. Children have to queue up and then sit down for two courses. This cuts into their playtime.
- Due to lax or nonexistent regulation of packed-lunch content, children bring confectionary and convenience products into the dining hall. These appealing items can seem a much more attractive offer than the new nutritionally balanced school meals.
- If the food does not look appealing, children will not want it. Similarly, if it is served on a tray in compartments that run over into one another, it will not be appealing. Quite often, the way food is served and looks is a major barrier to uptake.

Competition

The qualitative research conducted with head teachers, parents, and children identified pack lunches as being the primary competition for the following reasons:

- *Choice.* Pack lunches can cater to "fussy eaters," allowing children to pick and choose their own, often unhealthy, options.
- *Price.* Especially for families with more than one child who are managing a tight budget, pack lunches offer a cheaper option and one they know their children will eat (value for money).
- *Fullness.* Parents would much rather their children are full, even if what they have eaten is not strictly healthy, than sign them up for school meals, which they often claim not to have eaten.

- *Peer popularity.* Pack lunches are still seen as "cool," especially when they contain popular recognized brands, which can be swapped and traded among friends.
- *Freedom.* Pack lunches can be eaten outside in the summer. They can also be scarfed down quickly so that children can get out to play sooner.

MARKETING STRATEGY–PHASE 1

As mentioned previously, due to the economic slowdown and pressures on local government funding, it was only possible to continue, in the short term, with interventions aimed predominantly at head teachers. Therefore, the main barriers addressed by this marketing strategy are those presented mainly by the head teachers. However, some of the interventions also addressed some of the barriers identified by parents and children.

After the scoping work was completed, a solution group was set up to help the steering group decide upon and develop the interventions. This group was made up of catering managers, school cooks and dinner nannies, head teachers, and health promotion specialists from the local health authority. The findings from both secondary and primary research were presented to the solution group. The group then helped develop the multipronged intervention marketing strategy described later.

Product

- The *core product*, the benefit promised, is one nutritionally balanced meal and the long-term health benefits attached to eating at least one nutritious meal a day. However, because in phase 1 we were focusing on head teachers, due to their strong influence on parents and children, the core product is also:
  - Improved behavior and organization in the dining hall.
  - Fewer complaints from parents in regard to the choice of food and service.
  - Improved knowledge of the children regarding the importance of eating a balanced meal and cooking skills.
  - Improved communications between the caterers and head teachers.
  - Less food wastage and packaging used.
- The *actual product*, the desired behavior, is for key stage 2 pupils to eat school meals. As with the core product, the actual product in phase 1 is also:
  - Dinner nannies to manage the dining hall environment and to talk to pupils about healthy and balanced meal choices.

- Children to eat a nutritionally balanced meal.
- Head teachers to promote school meals to parents and children and become engaged in the agenda.
- Head teachers to understand the nutritional standards, incorporating what can and cannot be served in foods since the new standards have come in.
- The *augmented product* includes:
  - A laminated myth-busting card and case study compendium that highlight local successful initiatives and overcome the misconceptions with the new school meal standards (saying what the children can still eat—e.g., chicken nuggets, etc.).
  - A new dining room experience, created by queue management, lunchtime rotation, and improved 1:1 management by the dinner nannies.
  - 1:1 meetings between head teachers and caterers to develop new menus for their individual schools based on their children's favorite meals.
  - Development of new menus for individual school meal tastes.
  - Puddings served in bowls and at the table so they are hot and do not run over into their savory main course.
  - A "healthy tuck shop," where the children help cook the healthy snack food (such as banana bread, etc.), thus learning about food and cooking skills.
  - Development of the single-choice menu.
  - Training for dinner nannies and kitchen assistants on customer service skills, presentation of food, first aid, nutrition standards, and positive behavioral management/motivational techniques. Due to a low average reading age and lack of formal educational qualification of the dinner nannies, the training is being developed with the health literacy team at the Department of Health in England and will also be accredited.

Price

The research showed that price is a major factor in school meal uptake. Recent increases in food costs are seen as a threat to current school meal pricing and could lead to detrimental, but unavoidable, price increases.

Monetary

Cost was also a factor for many of the families, who had more than one child but who did not satisfy the criteria for free school meals. Cost was also a factor for the caterers as they were experiencing rising food, fuel, and labor costs.

Therefore, they could not run any price-reduction offers. However, by piloting a one-choice menu scheme, many were able to freeze costs in this financially difficult time.

Nonmonetary

The following nonmonetary costs were identified through the research:

1. Children who are late into the dining hall often miss out on the most popular menu choices. By switching to a one-choice system, designed in partnership with the children, every school meal taker was given the same choices; the rotation system also ensured every class group was able to be served first once a week.
2. Food is poorly prepared, unappetizing, and carelessly presented. This is sometimes due to time constraints, which were addressed through the one-choice menu system, allowing cooks to devote enough time to prepare one high-quality meal. Training for school cooks was going to be delivered at the local level. However, just before the training was commissioned, the School Food Trust launched a national scheme to offer training for school cooks. To avoid duplication of resources, the steering group agreed to ensure all local cooks benefited from this existing scheme.
3. One repeated issue for school meal takers is that they have to remain in the dining hall eating while packed-lunchers can finish quickly and have longer playtime (or in summer can eat outside). Some schools are running a rotation system so that school meal takers can eat outside on special tables during sunny weather.

Place

Through this project, it has become clear that children should not be considered as passive recipients of a service. They are consumers and make choices based on their own experiences and judgment. Therefore, they cannot be expected to eat unappealing food in an unattractive environment. Many successful and creative approaches are already under way to encourage school meal uptake by improving the dining hall experience. The implementation of lunchtime rotations makes the dining hall a more relaxed, less noisy and bustling place so that it is more appealing. Children are able to sit outside in sunny weather and mix with packed-lunch friends. The training intervention developed for dinner nannies was delivered at the individual schools, because most of the dinner nannies did not have access to a car and were too scared to attend training delivered at a college.

Promotion

Communication between the catering services run by adjacent local authority and head teachers was inconsistent and reported to be poor. Strategies were put into place to improve communication.

Key Messages

Key messages were developed for each of the target audiences. The messages were clear, simple, and consistent and tried to address the barriers that were identified during the qualitative research.

The key messages that were communicated to head teachers were:

- A child who has a healthy meal is easier to teach and achieves more academically.
- Head teachers have a right to be involved in their kitchen: their school, their kitchen.
- Children can still eat their favorite foods (e.g., tomato ketchup and Yorkshire puddings).
- With the catering manager, head teachers can develop bespoke menus for their school so that the children can still eat the foods they like.

Messengers

The local area head teacher consortiums were vital in establishing the credibility of messages, as were the local health nutritionists and the head teacher unions. This local representation was supported by national evidence from the Nutrition Foundation and School Food Trust reporting links between good food and behavior.

Key Media Channels

To ensure effectiveness, the messages were conveyed through a variety of media channels, including printed materials, events, and social networks.

Print Materials

Fact sheets, booklets, newsletters, and posters were designed to be displayed in teachers' staff rooms and on school notice boards.

Special Events

Leading-edge head teachers and the area caterers went to speak at established head teacher consortium groups. These heads are respected and well networked.

One-on-One-Communications

Poor communications among caterers, school cooks, and head teachers came out strongly in the research. Meetings in the intervention schools were set up among the three parties to define roles and responsibilities, to help head teachers and school cooks understand what services were available from the caterers, and to look at developing bespoke menus for their schools.

Online Communications

Head teachers often report they are time poor and the amount of paperwork they receive is high, so the print materials were backed up with e-newsletters and new sections on the caterer's Web sites, designed specifically for head teachers, carrying some of the myth busters and case studies from the local area.

SUMMARY

Social marketing is about increasing long-term, sustainable behavioral change; therefore, evaluation is ongoing and pilot sites are being run on a long-term basis. Nevertheless, results from the initial pilots and pre-testing work are positive. In particular, adopting a multipronged approach is vital because school meal uptake is a complex issue.

This project's ultimate goal was to increase the number of children eating school meals. As with many social marketing projects, the interventions were not delivered in a controlled environment. School meals are high on the political agenda in England, and therefore, there are numerous local and national initiatives going on at the same time. This means that we cannot say for sure if the positive changes that were recorded were solely due to the interventions described in this chapter. The results presented here are also just from phase 1 of the project and from a small number of schools where the initial testing and piloting work was conducted. However, in the schools that received the intervention mix, school meal uptake increased. The increases ranged from 3.5% to 9%, depending on which intervention mix the schools received. During phase 2, the local team will investigate which intervention mix was the most effective, as it is currently unclear which intervention was the most effective.

Other measures were also used to evaluate the interventions. Other indicators included:

- Environmental factors, including packaging and food wastage.
- Head teachers' satisfaction with the communications between caterers and themselves.

- Dinner nannies' satisfaction with their work, their knowledge of nutritional guidelines, their belief in the importance of providing children with a balanced diet, and their self-reported confidence at managing the dining room (including speaking to children, organizing queues, etc.).
- The number of head teachers who downloaded the newsletter and the number who meet with their catering manager.

These other measures will be evaluated in Autumn 2009.

Due to financial difficulties, the one-choice menu, although implemented in some schools, was not evaluated. The training for dinner nannies has also been delayed, and will now be piloted in Autumn 2009.

QUESTIONS FOR DISCUSSION

1. What kind of health communication activities are suitable in a school setting for children aged 7 to 11?
2. What interventions would you develop for the *too busy* and *engaged and passionate* head teachers?
3. How important is stakeholder engagement in the development of a project such as the one described in this chapter? What objectives might the different stakeholders have, and how might they conflict?

REFERENCES

British Broadcasting Corporation (BBC). (2005, August 11). Health inequality gap widening. *BBC News*. Retrieved July 28, 2009, from http://news.bbc.co.uk/2/hi/health/4139440.stm

Department of Health. (2004). *Choosing health: Making healthy choices easier*. Retrieved July 28, 2009, from http://www.dh.gov.uk/en/Publicationsandstatistics/Publications/PublicationsPolicyAndGuidance/DH_4094550

Department of Health. (2009). *About us*. Retrieved July 28, 2009, from http://www.dh.gov.uk/en/Aboutus/HowDHworks/DH_074813

Jamie's School Dinners. (2005). Retrieved July 28, 2009, from http://www.jamieoliver.com/schooldinners/history

Nelson, M., Nicholas, J., Suleiman, S., Davies, O., Prior, G., Hall, L., et al. (2005). *School meals in primary schools in England*. Research Report RR753. London: Department for Education and Skills.

Office for National Statistics. (2001). *Population of Great Britain by religion*. Retrieved July 28, 2009, from http://www.statistics.gov.uk/cci/nugget.asp?id=954

Office for National Statistics. (2008a). *Local area labour markets: Statistical indicators*. Retrieved July 28, 2009, from http://www.statistics.gov.uk/downloads/theme_labour/LALM_statistical_indicators_Apr08.pdf

Office for National Statistics. (2008b). *North East: Selected key statistics.* Retrieved July 28, 2009, from http://www.statistics.gov.uk/cci/nugget.asp?id=1149

Ofsted. (2007, October). *Food in schools: Encouraging healthier eating.* Retrieved July 28, 2009, from http://www.warrington.gov.uk/Images/Food%20in%20Schools_tcm31-21448.pdf

School Meal Arrangements. (2006). *Schools census.* Retrieved July 28, 2009, from http://www.teachernet.gov.uk/management/ims/datacollections/scplasc2006/schoolcensus2006/

School Meals Review Panel. (2005). *Turning the tables: Transforming school food. A report on the development and implementation of nutritional standards for school lunches.* Retrieved July 28, 2009, from http://www.dcsf.gov.uk/consultations/index.cfm?action=conResults&consultationId=1319&external=no&menu=3

CHAPTER 7

Choose Health in Food Vending Machines

Obesity Prevention and Healthy Lifestyle Promotion in Italy

Giuseppe Fattori, Paola Artoni, and Marcello Tedeschi

ITALY: A COUNTRY OVERVIEW

General Information

Italy is a state in southern Europe. It is a peninsula in the central Mediterranean Sea, bordering France to the west, Switzerland and Austria to the north, and Slovenia to the east. Other neighboring countries are the Vatican City and the Republic of San Marino. On the whole, it covers an area of 30,133,601 hectares (301,336 square kilometers) with more than 59 million inhabitants (Istituto Nazionale di Statistica [ISTAT], 2007).

Since 1946, it has been a democratic republic, with Rome as its capital. The constitution, the fundamental law that runs the republic, has been in force since 1948. Italy is a member of the European Union and of the North Atlantic Treaty Organization (NATO). It is known worldwide for its natural beauties, its history, and its art.

Major Public Health Issues

The life expectancy at birth in Italy is one of the longest in the world: it reaches 78 years for males and 84 for females, while the healthy life expectancy (HALE) at birth[1] is, respectively, 71 years and 75 years. Furthermore, the infant mortality rate—data traditionally linked to socioeconomic and environmental conditions, and to performance of health services—suggests that the health of the Italian population has reached a good level. In fact, this rate in Italy is low (4 per 1,000 live births), as compared to that of other countries (WHO, 2007).

Italian Health Service is founded on the principles of equity and of universal healthcare coverage: it guarantees everyone access to appropriate services. The right to safeguarding health is defended by the constitution. Total expenditure on health is 8.7% of the gross domestic product; 75.1% is covered by the general government and 24.9% is private. In 2004, the per capita total expenditure on health at the international dollar rate was US$2,414. In comparison, the average value of the entire European region was US$1,564 (WHO, 2007).

As in other European countries, chronic diseases are one of the main public health issues. According to recent WHO statistics (2007), noncommunicable diseases cause 86% of years of life lost in Italy. It is also estimated that in 2004, tumors and cardiovascular illnesses caused almost 390,000 deaths, a total of 72% of overall deaths (ISTAT, 2007). It is widely recognized that unhealthy lifestyles are the major cause of chronic diseases. To reduce their spread, the WHO Regional Office for Europe (2006) launched *Gaining Health: The European Strategy for the Prevention and Control of Non-Communicable Diseases*. In coherence with European strategy, the Italian government (*Decreto del Presidente del Consiglio dei Ministri 4 maggio 2007* [Decree of the President of the Council of Ministries, May 4, 2007]) has approved the national *Gaining Health: Making Healthy Choices Easier* program (*Guadagnare salute: Rendere facili le scelte salutari*, in Italian), whose focus is on diet, physical activity, smoke, and alcohol. Through communication and environmental interventions, this national program aims to create favorable conditions in adopting healthy habits. Its strength is the promotion of activities that involve different subjects of the society, such as public institutions, private business (production, distribution, management, etc.), and scientific associations, with the purpose of health promotion.

---

[1]The World Health Organization (WHO) defines healthy life expectancy at birth as the "average number of years that a person can expect to live in 'full health' by taking into account years lived in less than full health due to disease and/or injury." This definition was retrieved February 10, 2009, from the WHO Web site at: www.who.int/whosis/indicators/compendium/2008/1hat/en/index.html.

Social Marketing and Health Communication in Italy

In 2000, a national law (*Legge No. 150 del 7 giugno 2000* [Law No. 150, June 7, 2000]) was approved that represents a milestone for the development of public communication in Italy because it regulates information and communication activities in public institutions and defines the educational training required of operators who work in these professional fields.

Since then, social marketing and communication have been acquiring importance and, in recent years, are becoming part of prevention and health promotion strategies, as was specified by recent national and regional planning documents discussed later.

The National Health Plan 2006–2008 (*Piano Sanitario Nazionale 2006–2008*, in Italian) states the importance "of developing strategies for coherent and effective communication, since this is a necessary and decisive instrument to reach the objectives of risk prevention and health promotion" (translation from the *Ministero della Salute* [Ministry of Health], 2006, p. 29). Coherently, the National Prevention Plan 2005–2007, *Piano Nazionale della Prevenzione 2005–2007*, in Italian (*Intesa Stato Regioni del 23 marzo 2005* [Regions State Agreement, March 23, 2005]), and the Italian *Gaining Health* program reaffirm the strategic and central role of communication for the development of prevention activities. In particular, the *Gaining Health* program states that it "favors health communication," defining communication as "an integrated component of the prevention interventions regarding the *Gaining Health* program" and "an important instrument for information and knowledge" (translation from the *Decreto del Presidente del Consiglio dei Ministri 4 maggio 2007*, p. 8).

The Social and Health Plan 2008–2010 (*Piano Sociale e Sanitario 2008–2010*, in Italian) of the Emilia-Romagna Region (*Deliberazione dell'Assemblea Legislativa della Regione Emilia-Romagna 22 maggio 2008, No. 175* [Deliberation of the Legislative Assembly of the Emilia-Romagna Region No. 175, May 22, 2008]), along with communication activities, focuses its attention on social marketing as a tool to create partnership for the purpose of empowering citizens. Meanwhile, in the Prevention Plan of the Veneto Region (*Delibera della Giunta Regionale del Veneto No. 188 del 31 gennaio 2006* [Deliberation of the Regional Council of Veneto No. 188, January 31, 2006]), among the interventions to reduce obesity, there exists a specific recommendation for the development of a social marketing project to promote health through food vending machines.

To support the diffusion of effective communication and social marketing strategies for health promotion, the Italian Association of Public and Institutional Communication has activated the research area, Social Marketing and Health Communication, and a National Social Marketing Work Group, which gather the contributions of Italian experts, professionals, and operators. The research area has developed two working tools—a Web site (www.marketingsociale.net) and a newsletter—and organizes periodical conventions, focusing on the following themes:

- Applying social marketing to health promotion activities.
- Enhancing public health communication.
- Organizational models.
- Impact of socioeconomic inequities on health status and the role of communication.
- Communication evaluation.
- Communication of social responsibility.
- Appropriate practices.

Moreover, to collect and enhance health promotion activities that use social marketing principles, the Italian Association of Public and Institutional Communication and the Local Health Unit of Modena organize an annual national competition, denominated "Health Marketing," which reached its fourth edition in 2007. Overall, more than 220 projects took part in that initiative to give proof of the increasing interest toward this innovative strategy.

CASE STUDY
Choose Health

This case study involves an experimental social marketing project, *Choose Health*, aimed at transforming vending machines into a tool for preventing obesity and promoting healthy lifestyles in schools, workplaces, and universities through the delivery of communication activities and the introduction of healthy products (see Figure 7-1).

CAMPAIGN BACKGROUND, PURPOSE, AND FOCUS

The WHO estimated that unhealthy habits—being overweight or underweight, not eating enough fruits and vegetables, physical inactivity, smoking, and drinking alcohol—account for almost 50% of all diseases in men and for 25% in women (measured as disability-adjusted life-years, or DALY) in developed European countries (WHO, 2002).

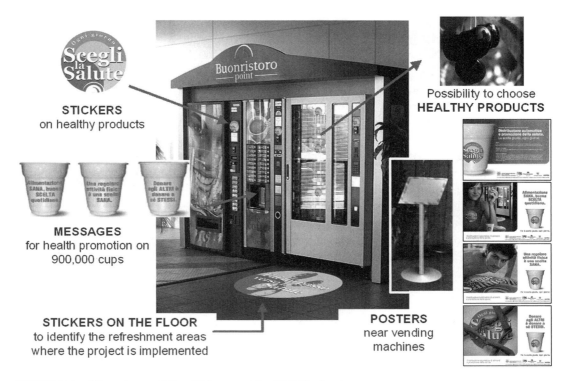

STICKERS
on healthy products

MESSAGES
for health promotion on
900,000 cups

STICKERS ON THE FLOOR
to identify the refreshment areas
where the project is implemented

Possibility to choose
HEALTHY PRODUCTS

POSTERS
near vending
machines

FIGURE 7-1   Structure of the "Choose Health" Project
Courtesy of Daem S.p.A.–Buonristoro Vending Group

The *Choose Health* project was implemented in the province of Modena (in the Emilia-Romagna Region, in the northeast of Italy) with approximately 670,000 inhabitants and 47 municipalities. In this territory, according to the national behavioral risk factor surveillance system called *Passi*, 35.3% of citizens surveyed were reported as not being sufficiently active, 21.4% were completely inactive, and 40% were obese or overweight (Centro Nazionale di Epidemiologia, Sorveglianza e Promozione della salute [National Center for Epidemiology, Surveillance, and Health Promotion], 2006).

To support the development of effective healthy lifestyle promotion activities in the province of Modena, the Local Health Unit (*Azienda USL di Modena*, in Italian) has activated the Health Promotion program that includes coordinated interventions in different settings, such as schools, workplaces, supermarkets and shopping centers, mass media, and fairs, in collaboration with several public and private partners in the context of the Local Health Plan. *Choose Health* was developed as a part of this program.

The project's purpose was to contribute to reducing the spread of obesity and of chronic diseases related to an unhealthy lifestyle. The focus was on accomplishing this through healthier and more appealing options at vending machines.

The rationale of the project was twofold. On the one hand, there was a growing request from citizens to improve the quality and the types of the products sold through vending machines. In fact, in Europe public opinions given believed that soft drinks, candies, and sweet snacks—often sold through vending machines—could be a cause of obesity. In recent years, this topic has become one of the priority actions affirmed by national and regional health planning documents. In particular, the *Gaining Health* program recommends the introduction of "fruit snacks, water, and low-calorie beverages with a good nutritional content" (translation from the *Decreto del Presidente del Consiglio dei Ministri 4 maggio 2007*, p. 22). The Prevention Plan of the Emilia-Romagna Region focuses its attention on schools and suggests increasing the use of "products that contain low simple carbohydrates, saturated fats, and additives," while sustaining the consumption of fruits and vegetables (translation from the *Delibera della Giunta Regionale dell'Emilia-Romagna n. 426* [Deliberation of the Regional Council of the Emilia-Romagna Region No. 426], 2006, p. 83).

On the other hand, vending machines were the place where nutritional choices occurred: using them for health promotion meant offering correct information regarding a proper lifestyle when an individual decided which products to buy and eat. Vending machines also provided opportunities to reinforce the effectiveness of the messages, because communication activities could be integrated with the offer of healthy foods. Vending machines were widely distributed, partly as a consequence of new ways of life and of work organizations that had reduced the possibility to have lunch at home. This trend has recently been confirmed by Confida, the Italian Vending Association, which estimates that there are about 1.68 million vending machines in Italy and about 6 billion (6 thousand million) products (to eat or drink) sold through these machines (Confida, 2007). These statistics suggest that a great number of people can potentially benefit from the use of vending machines, which promote healthy lifestyles.

The SWOT analysis of micro- and macro-environments specified the following aspects.

Micro-Environment

- Internal strengths:
  - The Buonristoro Vending Group (a group of vending firms) contacted the Local Health Unit of Modena and offered its willingness to develop

a project for preventing obesity and promoting health as part of its cause-related marketing activities.
- The Local Health Unit of Modena had a staff with expertise in communication and health promotion (Communication and Social Marketing Department) and in nutrition (Office of Food Hygiene and Nutrition). Moreover, health promotion was part of the mission of the Local Health Unit.
- Internal weaknesses:
  - Funding sources for development of the project were limited, and the budget was low.
  - The Local Health Unit of Modena had no experience in working with the vending machine sector.

Macro-Environment

- External opportunities:
  - Because of the concerns of citizens toward this topic, the development of a project that related to health and vending machines could be perceived as interesting and remarkable.
  - New technological and organizational solutions had been developed, which made it possible to insert healthy food in vending machines: for example, fresh fruit or fruit salads that had to be kept cold or cooked.
- External threats:
  - Most citizens were skeptical about vending machines and thought they only sold products with low nutritional profiles.
  - The vending machine sector was a private sector, so its economic interests may influence the products that it sold.

At international levels, there had been some cases of vending machines being banned because of the types of products sold (e.g., candies and soft drinks). *Choose Health* was among the first projects developed in Italy aimed at promoting health through vending machines; other projects are now under way, also due to the development of the national *Gaining Health* program. The project, and its most recent developments, have gathered information on past and similar efforts documented by scientific literature and by the Web (Food Standards Agency, 2004; Higgs & Styles, 2006; Indiana State Department of Health, n.d.; San Diego & Imperial Nutritional Network, n.d.; Welsh Assembly Government, 2005). As a guide for the definition of the social marketing approach, Kotler, Roberto, and Lee's book, *Social Marketing—Improving the Quality of Life* (2002), was consulted.

TARGET AUDIENCES

According to the International Obesity Taskforce (2007), at the end of the 1990s and in 2000 the prevalence of obesity and excess weight in adolescents (aged 14 to 17) in Italy was among the highest in Europe. This suggested that adolescents should be considered a privileged target for healthy lifestyle promotion activities. Moreover, several experiences were described in the international context regarding the development of healthy vending machines in schools (Food Standards Agency, 2004; Higgs & Styles, 2006; Welsh Assembly Government, 2005).

Furthermore, existing data referred to the province of Modena (Centro Nazionale di Epidemiologia, Sorveglianza e Promozione della salute 2006) demonstrated that physical inactivity and prevailing obesity/excess weight increased with age: sedentary individuals reached 14.8% between the ages of 18 and 34 and 17.6% between ages 35 and 49; the data for obesity/excess weight were 23.8% in the 18-to-24 age group, 22.5% in the 25-to-34 age group, and 34.3% in the 35-to-49 age group. Recent data also indicated that about 40% of 25- to 44-year-olds in Italy were more likely to eat away from home (ISTAT, 2007) and buy food from vending machines.

Given these data, the population groups that would enjoy the greatest advantages from a project that promoted health through vending machines were young and middle-aged adults, including students.

Choose Health was conceived as an experiment with the intention of defining an intervention strategy that promoted health through vending machines and that could be repeated in various settings by adapting the communication activities and the choice of products for different targets.

In conjunction with these remarks and considering the project's experimental approach, the main targets were:

- students aged 14 to 19.
- people who were studying or teaching in universities.
- those who were working in some firms in the province of Modena.

CAMPAIGN OBJECTIVES AND GOALS

The project's objectives were as follows:
- Behavior objectives:
  - To choose healthy products (foods and beverages) available at vending machines during breaks at school, university, and work.

- Knowledge objectives:
  - To know what a healthy lifestyle is and how to put it into practice.
  - To know the health advantages of having a good lifestyle.
- Belief objectives:
  - To believe that a balanced diet, regular physical activity, and, in general, a good lifestyle can aid in preventing diseases and in feeling well.
  - To believe that having a healthy lifestyle does not necessarily require a great effort and can be achieved through simple everyday actions.

Indirectly, the project also had affective objectives aiming to reinforce the trust of citizens toward the Local Health Unit of Modena and to improve the Unit's reputation and reliability.

The goal was that at least 25% of all products that target audiences purchased through the project's vending machines were healthy (considering that there were no healthy choices before the campaign, the vending machines were new, and they offered both traditional and healthy products).

TARGET AUDIENCE BARRIERS, MOTIVATORS (BENEFITS), AND COMPETITION

Two focus groups were run with samples of the target audiences in order to explore their points of view regarding the project and collect important information regarding how to develop customer-oriented marketing mix strategies. These groups were led by a trained psychologist; the first involved school students between the ages of 18 and 19, and the second involved university students and working people. Several subjects were discussed during the focus groups: how often the target audiences bought certain groups of products and their perception regarding these products, their proposals about how to increase healthy products consumption (instead of traditional consumption), and how to realize health communication activities through vending machines.

In addition, several meetings were held with representatives of the Local Health Unit and of the Buonristoro Vending Group to discuss the characteristics of the target audiences. Their consumption habits, for example, could be inferred from data regarding the products sold through traditional vending machines found in locations similar to the project settings.

In synthesis, the following aspects were highlighted:

- Perceived and real barriers related to eating healthy products from vending machines:
  - The cost of fruit snacks, which were often expensive.
  - The practical difficulties of consuming healthy foods, like yogurt and fruit salads, which require, for example, a spoon.

- Factors that could act as motivators or could be perceived as benefits:
  - The availability of fresh food instead of prepackaged food.
  - A correct and reliable communication regarding healthy lifestyles, with positive, appealing, and easy-to-read messages, instead of negative warnings.
  - A clear identification of healthy products.
- Competition:
  - Vending machines selling fatty and sweet foods and beverages.
  - Attractive pictures on vending machines aimed at promoting traditional product consumption.
  - Nearby snack bars that offered a wider variety of products.

POSITIONING STATEMENT

The positioning statement of the project can be summarized as follows: We wanted our target audiences to see consuming healthy foods and beverages from vending machines, instead of sweet and fatty products, as an important, motivational, and pleasant everyday life activity, which could positively influence their health.

CAMPAIGN STRATEGIES (4Ps)

Figure 7-2 synthesizes the 4P strategies developed for the project.

Product Strategies

- Core product (benefits of desired behavior): healthier life and reduction in the risk of becoming obese/overweight.
- Actual product (behavior, service, or program being promoted): eat and drink healthy foods and beverages during breaks at school, university, or work; have a balanced diet; practice regular physical activity; and think of the value of donating (blood, tissue, or organs to those in needy situations).
- Augmented product (ancillary goods and services): introduction of healthy products in vending machines, selected through the following steps:
  - Analysis of the products that the Buonristoro Vending Group could introduce in the vending machine distribution chain.

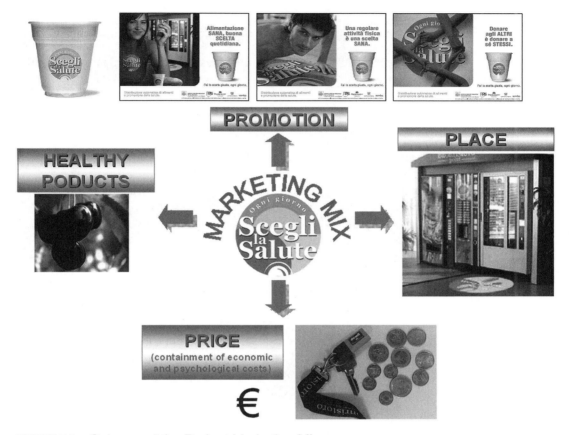

FIGURE 7-2   Scheme of the Project Marketing Mix
Courtesy of Daem S.p.A.–Buonristoro Vending Group

- Technical judgments expressed by nutritionists of the Local Health Unit of Modena, which took into account the nutritional contents and the portion sizes available for introduction in vending machines.
- Opinions and needs expressed by the target audiences during the focus groups.

As a result, the healthy products selected were:

- Fresh fruit salads.
- Fresh fruits and vegetables.
- Ham sandwiches (prepared each morning).
- Yogurt with active milk enzymes.

- Fruit juices with 70% fruit content.
- Snacks with crackers and Parmigiano Reggiano (a typical Italian cheese).

To guarantee free choices to target audiences, the vending machines, where the project was implemented, sold both traditional and healthy products.

Pricing Strategies

- The costs associated with the behavior being promoted were:
  - Monetary costs, which included the economic costs for buying healthy products.
  - Nonmonetary costs, which were mainly psychological and consisted of renouncing good-tasting foods and beverages; not feeling completely full; feeling guilty with oneself, or feeling annoyed, or bored, while reading health promoting advice.
- To manage costs, and counterbalance them, the following strategies were adopted:
  - The healthy products of the vending machines were priced less than those sold in the cafés and snack bars where workers and students often had their breaks and/or lunches.
  - Stickers with the slogan, "Choose Health," were used to signal healthy products in vending machines; they were a nonmonetary incentive since people were encouraged to prefer healthy products by the fact that they could see others choosing something with a healthy label.

Place Strategies

- As specified in the section regarding the project rationale, the same vending machines were the point of the decision-making process aimed at nutritional choices and where the target audiences carried out their behavior.
- To make the area convenient for the target groups, the vending machines were located inside some schools, firms, and in two locations in the university—in positions that were easy to reach and that the audiences already knew as places where they could have a break.
- The refreshment areas, where the vending machines with healthy foods and beverages were located, were made pleasant through the use of bright graphic presentations.
- To make the locations easy to identify, the project's vending machines stood out with a green sticker placed on the floor with images of footprints and the invitation to approach through the writing, "Welcome to health."

Promotion Strategies

- The key messages of the project were that "you can choose to have a healthy life" and "you can achieve it through a good diet, through practicing regular physical activity, and through active attention towards the value of donation."
- Based on the characteristics of the target groups (mainly young individuals), the message delivery strategy was developed through the use of an emotional style, which should solicit the association of positive feelings—such as wellness, joy, and happiness—to the concept of health. In coherence with the project's slogan, "Choose Health" (*Scegli la salute*, in Italian), three slogans were created: "Healthy diet, a good daily choice"; "Regular physical activity is a healthy choice"; and "Giving to others is giving to ourselves." Short and straightforward, these slogans were mainly based on two words—*health* and *choice*—repeated in each one. Pictures were key elements of the communication strategy, and they were coherent with the idea of choosing health in that they, respectively, represented the actions of healthy lifestyles being promoted: a smiling girl with an apple in her hand, a young boy exercising, or a hand chain for solidarity. Bright colors (such as yellow, green, and light blue) were largely employed both in the images and in the text of the slogans. Figure 7-3 illustrates the image used to present the project.
- Original, innovative, and appealing communication channels were used to give

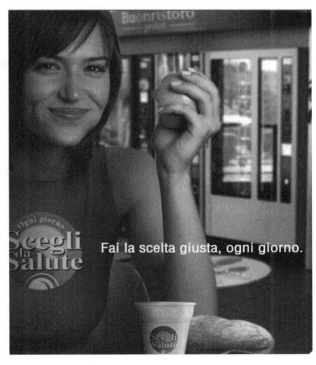

FIGURE 7-3   Image Used to Present the "Choose Health" Project

Courtesy of Daem S.p.A.–Buonristoro Vending Group

advice regarding healthy habits: the three slogans were written on 900,000 plastic cups and were repeated on posters (positioned near the vending machines), where they were associated with the images described earlier. Practically, the vending machines themselves became a communication channel.

Other Important Strategies

- *Partnership strategy:* The development of a collaboration between public and private partners was a key element of the project, because the contribution of each of them was fundamental for its realization and success. The partnership strategy could be specified as follows:
  - The Local Health Unit of Modena was responsible for the scientific validity of the health message contents and of the types of healthy foods chosen (but not of the specific brands).
  - The Buonristoro Vending Group found the technological solutions, which allowed the introduction of healthy products (in fact, they had to be kept at different temperatures).
  - Confida promoted the project in Italy and toward associated vending firms.
  - Confindustria–Modena contacted the firms where the project was implemented and collected their agreements.
- *Supporting strategy:* There were several additional activities carried out to support the project and to create favorable conditions for its future development. In this case, the strategy was aimed at increasing the community's interest and attention toward experimentation issues and at increasing the number of partners that could contribute to health promotion through vending machines.

To promote *Choose Health*:
- A folder was created to present the project, its activities, and its results.
- A specific area within the Modena Health Plan Web site was created to collect information and materials.
- Numerous articles were published in local and national newspapers and in specialized magazines.
- The project was presented during meetings, public conferences, and national exhibitions.

CAMPAIGN BUDGET

The total project budget amounted to approximately €50,000 (euro; about US$63,700 based on 2004 rate). Costs were divided into the following:

- Approximately €5,500 for the staff involved (including the psychologist heading the focus groups).
- Approximately €11,500 for the design and creation of the health communication and project promotion materials (e.g., posters, slogans on plastic cups, and stickers on floors and healthy foods).
- About €33,000 for the 13 vending machines (including a change-giver mechanism, a system that stopped fresh products delivery after their date of expiration, and the supports for the health-promoting posters).

The costs were covered by the project partners.

The strength of the *Choose Health* campaign was its capacity to autonomously finance its activities. This meant that it had the possibility of being long-lasting and of being extended to other locations, because it did not depend on the availability of external funds.

CAMPAIGN TIME FRAME

1. Plan and preparation of the project (beginning in November 2004):
   a. Definition of the target audiences, campaign objectives, goals, and strategy through meetings between representatives of the Local Health Unit of Modena, Buonristoro Vending Group, and Confindustria–Modena.
   b. Realization of two focus groups with samples of the target audiences.
2. Presentation and promotion of the project (beginning in November 2004).
3. Realization of the project (from May 2005 to November 2005), through the creation of the refreshment areas and its implementation for six months.
4. Evaluation (during the development of the experiment and after its end).

CAMPAIGN EVALUATION

From the 13 vending machines where the experiment was initially implemented, about 30% of all products sold were healthy ones: on the whole, 25,000 healthy foods/beverages were purchased during the six months of experimentation.

A survey about opinion, satisfaction, and intention to buy was implemented in collaboration with the Communication and Marketing degree course taught at the University of Modena and Reggio Emilia in order to evaluate the consumer attitude about healthy food consumption and purchasing from vending machines. Items and questions from the questionnaires were evaluated according to a seven-point Likert-type scale. The period selected was the first month, just at the beginning of the *Choose Health* campaign, and the assigned locations were university and firms. Respondents were 144 students and 75 workers.

In general, beliefs about healthy food from both students and workers were similar, even if their purchasing and consumption habits differed somewhat. Students used this alternative quite often, as a reasonable option to lunchtime, while workers chose vending machines mainly as an alternative to break time or during other moments, if strictly necessary, due to lack of time. Concerning the traditional products delivered through the vending machines, quality as well as taste and freshness were perceived to be just acceptable, prices not really moderate, and the variety of products offered not satisfactory. These opinions were tested both at the beginning of the experiment and at the end (as described later).

The "intention to buy" healthy products, measured during the first month, showed a moderately higher value for students (an average of 5.3) than for workers (an average of 4.8). Among students, 64.6% noticed the new healthy products, and 51.6% bought them at least once.

Among workers, a higher percentage (81.3%) noticed the healthy products. In this case, 54.7% of workers combined their purchase, buying both healthy and traditional products.

Both students and workers tested the new products, even if they did not necessarily notice the special sticker. They were satisfied with the healthy options but hoped to have a wider variety to select from. When choices were directed toward more conventional alternatives, brand names still played a relevant role. Because purchasing behavior at vending machines could be considered as a low-involvement action, the selection of known brands or categories of food resembled more the application of default choice heuristics instead of real preferences. Past behavior appeared to be a relevant reference point of how individuals tended to behave.

Six months later, a new survey to verify habit changes was conducted. Beliefs about the goodness of the *Choose Health* project reflected a different level of attention. First, beliefs about quality, taste, and freshness of healthy food were higher compared to the beliefs expressed toward products at the beginning of the experimentation. It was found that 41.7% of students, as compared to 62.9% of workers, said they were very familiar with the project and, moreover, that they were aware that colleagues bought healthy products, too. Information about healthy products was thought to be extensive, even if only a few believe this information could be a relevant strategy to change individual nutritional styles. Higher brand knowledge, awareness, loyalty, and a clearer product identity probably fostered a more traditional approach to product selection through vending machines.

The project could be considered successful because the results exceeded the initial goal (that at least 25% of the products that target audiences purchased through the campaign's vending machines were healthy). The project has been able to develop a great interest in its goal and its activities. In fact, interest has been lasting and continuous, even after the six-month trial period: the number of participating vending machines increased from the initial 13 to approximately 175 by the end of 2007, upon citizens' requests.

In 2007, a similar project was developed in some secondary schools in the city of Modena. In this case, vending machines offered children aged 11 to 13 only healthy products, together with information on healthy habits and health education activities in the classrooms. Health education and communication interventions have been studied according to the characteristics of the young targets.

Based on this experience, a proposal of healthy public procurement for vending machines has been realized by a national network composed of representatives of the Social Marketing National Work Group, Health Plan–Modena Local Health Unit, FARE (an association of public purchasers), the Institute of Nutritional Science–University of Rome "La Sapienza," Confida, the Italian Association of Local Agenda 21, and Federconsumatori (a national consumer association). The objective of the proposal was to spread health promotion values through public procurement for vending machines. In particular, the proposal supported the following activities:

- Increase the availability (and therefore the access) of fresh, local, biological, and fair trade products.
- Enhance local, typical, and traditional foods and beverages (fruits, vegetables, and water).
- Introduce guarantees for environmental protection among the selection criteria—for example, a short supply chain (to reduce distances from place of production to point of purchase).

By law, public administrations in Italy must develop public procurement if they want to purchase goods or services, and usually a point system is used to compare the different offers. One of the main strengths of the proposal was that it recommended paying more attention to the characteristics of the products. In fact, it recommended giving 50 points to the economic offer and 50 to the qualitative offer. Among these, 40 points should be attributed to the choice of the products. Table 7-1 summarizes the proposed score attribution.

TABLE 7-1 Proposal of Healthy Public Procurement for Vending Machines: Synthesis of Evaluation Criteria and Score Attribution

Criteria for Evaluation	Best Score
Economic Offer	
a.1 Annual fee	A.1*
a.2 Prices for consumers	A.2*
Total	**50**
Qualitative Offer	
b.1 Characteristics of the products	40
Fresh foods	
• Fruit salad	
• Fruits/vegetables	
• Sandwich with ham	
• Yogurt with active milk enzymes	
Fruit juices with 70% fruit content	
Local products (fruits, vegetables, and water)	
Biological products	
Fair trade foods	
b.2 Service utilities	6
b.3 Quality certifications	4
Total	**50**

*The proposal described earlier in this chapter was one of the first attempts to include in public procurements the quality of the products sold through vending machines between the criteria requested to the service. Note that a.1 refers to the amount of the rent that vending firms can pay to the public administration for the installation of vending machines; a.2 refers to the prices for the consumers of the products sold through the vending machines. The attribution of single scores to the a.1 and a.2 criteria (called A.1 and A.2 in the table) is decided by the public administration taking into account the economic and geographical characteristics of context.

Great efforts have been made to promote the proposal of healthy public procurement for vending machines: it has been presented in national conferences; published in a specialized national health magazine (mainly addressed to Italian Local Health Services and to health professionals); and sent to some ministries, the Emilia-Romagna regional administration, and some Italian provincial and municipal administrations.

SUMMARY

After two years, it can be said that the main success of the *Choose Health* project has been its capacity to increase the community's interest and attention, as demonstrated by its developments. An analysis of the experimentation specifies some aspects that must be taken into consideration when developing such a project:

- Creation of an easy-to-recognize healthy product identity is necessary, because customers are more attracted by brand-name foods.
- Choice of a healthy food portfolio is crucial to the success of the project. In fact, the traditional food portfolio appears too often to be a dominant alternative.
- Pricing strategies should lower healthy product costs: Because traditional brand-name foods have a great appeal to customers, economic advantages should be offered to favor healthy product purchases.
- Coherence of health communication activities is needed. Health messages should be specific and suitable to the vending machine context. In this case, nutrition and physical activity appear to be the best theme for the objective of the project.
- The position of healthy products, and of the stickers used to illustrate them, should be rigorously defined and should be the same in all vending machines, in order to make healthy foods easier to find.
- A good definition of habits and purchasing behavior for vending machines is requested in order to face the lack of information regarding behavioral patterns and contextual preferences.

For more information regarding the project, see www.ppsmodena.it/vending.

QUESTIONS FOR DISCUSSION

1. What kind of health communication activities are suitable for a setting such as vending machines? How would you use the refreshment area around the vending machines to develop health communication activities?
2. What kind of packaging would you develop for non-brand-name healthy foods? In your opinion, what is the value of a project such as *Choose Health*?
3. How important is partner involvement for the development of an experiment like *Choose Health*?

ACKNOWLEDGMENT

We thank Alex Gozzi (Demil S.p.A.—Buonristoro Vending Group) for his collaboration on the *Choose Health* project.

REFERENCES

Centro Nazionale di Epidemiologia, Sorveglianza e Promozione della salute—Profea & Azienda USL di Modena. (2006). *Studio Passi per l'Italia—Progressi nelle Aziende Sanitarie per la Salute in Italia, Azienda Unità Sanitaria Locale di Modena.* Retrieved July 28, 2009, from www.ausl.mo.it/dsp/epi/pdf/pubblicazioni/2006/rapporto_passi_mo_05/Passi_Modena_2005.pdf

Confida. (2007, September 21). *La distribuzione automatica aiuta a "Guadagnare Salute"* (press release). Retrieved July 28, 2009, from www.ausl.mo.it/pps/iniziative/buoris/2006/download/01_10/Comunicato%20confida.pdf

Decreto del Presidente del Consiglio dei Ministri 4 maggio 2007. (2007). Documento programmatico "Guadagnare salute." Published in *Gazzetta Ufficiale della Repubblica Italiana*, 22 maggio 2007, No. 117. Retrieved July 28, 2009, from www.ministerosalute.it/imgs/C_17_normativa_1435_allegato.pdf

Delibera della Giunta Regionale dell'Emilia-Romagna n. 426 del 27 marzo 2006. (2006). *Approvazione del Piano Regionale della Prevenzione 2006–2008 relativamente a: prevenzione dell'obesità, prevenzione delle recidive nei soggetti che già hanno avuto accidenti cardiovascolari, prevenzione degli incidenti nei luoghi di lavoro, stradali e domestici.* Retrieved July 28, 2009, from www.saluter.it/wcm/saluter/sanitaer/ssr/assistenza_territoriale/Dipartimento_sanita_pubblica/documentazione/lk_prevenzione/page/p_prevenzione/pagina_piano_prevenzione/allegati_parte2/prev_2.pdf

Delibera della Giunta Regionale del Veneto No. 188 del 31 gennaio 2006. (2006). *Piano nazionale per la prevenzione 2005–2007—Integrazione DGR 2031 del 26 luglio 2005. Approvazione progetti regionali.* Retrieved July 28, 2009, from www.ccm-network.it/Pnp_Prp_Veneto

Deliberazione dell'Assemblea Legislativa della Regione Emilia-Romagna 22 maggio 2008, No. 175. (2008). *Piano Sociale e Sanitario 2008–2010.* Published in *Bollettino Ufficiale della Regione Emilia-Romagna*, 3 giugno 2008, No. 71. Retrieved July 28, 2009, from http://www.saluter.it/wcm/saluter/news/notiziedallaRegione/2008_maggio_agosto/017pubblicato_PSSR.htm

Food Standards Agency, the Dairy Council, & the Health Education Trust. (2004, October 7). *Vending healthy drinks. A guide for schools.* Retrieved July 28, 2009, from www.food.gov.uk/multimedia/pdfs/vendingmachinebooklet.pdf

Higgs, J., & Styles, K. (2006). Principles and practical aspects of healthful school vending. *Nutrition Bulletin* 31(3), 225–232.

Indiana State Department of Health. (n.d.). *Healthy vending.* Retrieved July 28, 2009, from www.in.gov/isdh/20062.htm

International Obesity Taskforce. (2007, December 10). *Childhood and adolescent overweight in Europe.* Retrieved July 28, 2009, from www.iotf.org/database/Childhoodandadolescentoverweightineurope.htm

Intesa Stato Regioni del 23 marzo 2005. (2005). *Il Piano Nazionale della Prevenzione 2005–2007* (allegato 2). Retrieved July 28, 2009, from www.ccm-network.it/documenti_Ccm/normativa/Intesa_23-3-2005.pdf

Istituto Nazionale di Statistica (ISTAT). (2007). *Annuario statistico italiano 2007.* Roma (Italy): C.S.R. Centro stampa e riproduzione S.r.l. Retrieved July 28, 2009, from www.istat.it/dati/catalogo/20071212_00/contenuti.html

Kotler, P., Roberto, N., & Lee, N. (2002). *Social marketing—Improving the quality of life.* Thousand Oaks, CA: Sage Publications.

Legge No. 150 del 7 giugno 2000. (2000). Disciplina delle attività di informazione e di comunicazione delle pubbliche amministrazioni. Published in *Gazzetta Ufficiale della Repubblica Italiana*, 13 giugno 2000, No. 136. Retrieved July 28, 2009, from www.senato.it/parlam/leggi/00150l.htm

Ministero della Salute. (2006). *Piano Sanitario Nazionale 2006–2008.* Retrieved July 28, 2009, from www.ministerosalute.it/resources/static/primopiano/316/PSN_2006_08_28_marzo.pdf

San Diego & Imperial Nutritional Network. (n.d.). *San Diego and Imperial/Bay Area regional nutrition network vending machine toolkit.* Retrieved July 28, 2009, from www.sdnnonline.org/tools_vending_machine_toolkit.htm

Welsh Assembly Government. (2005, May). *Think healthy vending. Guidance on vending machines in schools.* Retrieved July 28, 2009, from http://new.wales.gov.uk/topics/health/improvement/food/publications/vending/;jsessionid=bnqzJpzDTtrns5sZJ1NS1yRpsnyQ0QNQvBkvKGjy3BjcdNsGGHLR!-1414164158?lang=en&ts=1

World Health Organization (WHO). (2002). *The World Health Report 2002.* Retrieved July 28, 2009, from www.who.int/whr/2002/en/index.html

World Health Organization (WHO). (2007). *World Health Statistics 2007.* Retrieved July 28, 2009, from www.who.int/whosis/whostat2007/en/index.html

World Health Organization (WHO), Regional Office for Europe. (2006). *Gaining health: The European strategy for the prevention and control of non-communicable diseases.* Retrieved July 28, 2009, from www.euro.who.int/document/E89306.pdf

CHAPTER 8

Establishing a Healthy Drinking Culture

Systembolaget—Alcohol Monopoly and Public Health in Sweden

Karin M. Ekström and Lena Hansson

The European Union (EU) has lately recognized that alcohol consumption is a major social problem causing health problems, crime, and deaths. Alcohol is considered the fifth leading risk factor for death and disability in the world (WHO, 2008). Sweden has had a restricted view on alcohol policy for a long time, with high taxes on alcohol, an alcohol retail monopoly to limit accessibility, and harsh drunk driving laws. The Swedish alcohol retail monopoly, Systembolaget, is discussed in this chapter with a focus on two campaigns aiming to increase the number of Swedes who support it, as part of an integrated communication assignment.

SWEDEN: A COUNTRY OVERVIEW

Sweden is the third largest country in western Europe, a country with long distances (longest north–south distance 978 miles or 1,574 km) and a comparatively small population (9 million inhabitants; Sweden.se, 2008). The language is Swedish, and all Swedes start to learn English as a second language in third grade. The literacy rate is 99% (CIA, 2009). At the end of 2007, 14% of the Swedish population was immigrants (Immigrant Institute, 2008). The major religion is the Evangelical Lutheran Church of Sweden, to which 80% of the population belongs (Sweden.se, 2008).

Since 1995, Sweden has been a member of the EU. Sweden has a market economy and, during the twentieth century, built up a substantial tax-financed social welfare system. The Swedish welfare state idea—"the Swedish model"—has inspired other countries. Even though there are structural and financial problems related to the economic security system today, the main features of the Swedish welfare state still remain intact (Sweden.se, 2008). Sweden is a constitutional monarchy based on a parliamentary democracy. Social democratic governments have been in power for most of the twentieth and twenty-first centuries. Presently, there is a collaboration government, representing conservative and liberal parties. Swedes have one of the world's largest average life expectancies: 83 years for women and 79 years for men (Sweden.se, 2008). Swedish people have an active lifestyle and are open to trends and new patterns of behavior. Therefore, Sweden is used as a test market by major multinational corporations when launching new products and services (Sweden.se, 2008). New culinary trends have been noticeable during the past decades, and Sweden has become internationally famous for its gastronomy (Landes, 2008). A reason for an increased interest in new food trends could be increased immigration, but also the fact that Swedish people are extremely well traveled.

Alcohol Consumption in Sweden

Historically, Sweden has had high alcohol consumption, but today it is among the lowest in Europe (Anderson & Baumberg, 2006). However, alcohol consumption in Sweden has increased dramatically since the middle of the 1990s when Sweden joined the EU. The yearly consumption was 7.8 liters of pure (100%) alcohol per inhabitant (aged 15 years and older; including unrecorded estimated consumption) in 1995, and it increased to 10.2 liters in 2005. Since then, consumption has decreased marginally—with the exception of 2007, when consumption remained virtually unchanged (Centre for Social Research on Alcohol and Drugs [SoRAD], 2008). Statistics for 2008 show that consumption decreased to 9.5 liters (SoRAD, 2009). Reasons for the increase since 1995 are changes in lifestyle and drinking occasions

(Swedish National Institute of Public Health [SNIPH], 2008a), increased disposable income, and accessibility. Since 2004, it is possible to bring in larger quantities of alcohol across borders within the EU due to lifted import restrictions. Persons who are 20 years old can bring in 10 liters of liquor, 20 liters of strong wine, 90 liters of regular wine, and 110 liters of beer from another EU country to Sweden every time they travel, without paying custom (Swedish Customs, 2009). It is relatively common for many Swedes to travel regularly to purchase alcohol at a lower cost in countries like Denmark and Germany; this practice is particularly common among people living in the south of Sweden. The introduction of bags in boxes might also have had an effect on increased alcohol consumption. People drink in particular on weekends. Seasonal variations are noticeable in that people drink more during the summer and bigger holidays. Over time, drinking habits have changed from a focus on snaps and hard liquor to strong beer and wine, the latter being the most consumed drink (SNIPH, 2008a). In Sweden, men drink twice as much as women, but over time women have also increased their alcohol consumption, in particular women who are between 50 and 75 years old (SNIPH, 2008a). The reasons for the decrease in consumption is explained by fewer imports and less smuggling (SoRAD, 2009).

Swedish Alcohol Policy

Sweden has historically faced societal problems caused by alcohol consumption. Excessive drinking can result in health problems and substantial social costs related to hospital care, violence, and crime. Problems related to alcohol have been tackled by political goals and by introducing restrictions regarding alcohol consumption. The overall aim of Swedish alcohol policy is to reduce total alcohol consumption at all levels of society (Government Offices of Sweden, 2008). The Swedish government has established different goals regarding alcohol policy in order to reduce medical and social damage of alcohol: (1) promote an alcohol-free childhood; (2) postpone the age of first experiences with alcohol; (3) provide more alcohol-free environments; (4) prevent drinking among drivers, in working life, and during pregnancy; and (5) combat illegal alcohol trading (Government Offices of Sweden, 2008). There are also a number of governmental instances that work to implement the alcohol policies. Established in 1992, the Swedish National Institute of Public Health (SNIPH) is responsible for monitoring and coordinating implementation of national public health policy—exercising supervision in the areas of alcohol and developing regulations and general recommendations (SNIPH, 2008b). Most of the practical public health work in Sweden is carried out by local authorities and county councils. The National Board of Health and Welfare (NBHW) is the supervisory authority for social services and health and medical services (NBHW, 2008).

Alcohol consumption is affected by accessibility, price, and marketing. Alcohol accessibility has been restricted by attempts to limit sales through an alcohol retail monopoly and municipal control over licensed premises for restaurants. Also, the high level of taxes on alcohol in Sweden has resulted in high alcohol prices. Lower alcohol taxes have lately been proposed in Sweden in order to reduce private imports from neighboring countries with cheaper alcohol, but at the moment, there are no such discussions. Recently, a European court decision to overturn the Swedish law that bans Internet sales of alcohol has made it possible to purchase alcohol via the Internet.

CASE STUDY
The Swedish Alcohol Retail Monopoly—Systembolaget

Systembolaget, the Swedish alcohol retail monopoly, is a state-owned corporation for off-premise retail sale of all alcoholic beverages containing more than 2.25% alcohol by volume. Systembolaget has 411 stores, of which 310 are self-service outlets. The first self-service store opened in 1991. By December 2010, all stores will be self-service. Also, Systembolaget has 520 agents in smaller communities where there is a lack of a sufficient customer base to establish stores.[1]

Systembolaget is a Swedish innovation established in the mid-1800s. Similar monopolies exist in Norway, Finland, Iceland, Faeroes, Canada (except Alberta), and several states in the United States. Systembolaget is based on a nonprofit idea because a lack of profit is expected to limit consumption and thus keep alcohol-related problems down. By limiting availability to specific shops with restricted opening hours on weekdays and Saturday, consumption levels are also kept low. The legal age limit for selling alcoholic beverages in Systembolaget's stores is 20 years. In grocery stores where soft beer is sold, as well as on-premise sale (restaurants) of different types of alcohol, the legal age limit is 18 years, the age for Swedish suffrage.

Systembolaget has approximately 4,000 employees who receive ongoing training, making them expert advisers in the field of food and drink (Systembolaget, 2008a). The company monitors employee satisfaction regularly by an employee satisfaction index (ESI; Systembolaget, 2007a). Systembolaget has also developed a customer satisfaction index (CSI) based on a yearly survey

[1]Information from former marketing director Per Bergkrantz, Systembolaget, November 6, 2008.

distributed to 60,000 customers representing all stores. CSI has increased slightly since 2003 (Systembolaget, 2007a). Competent personnel are expected to contribute to customer satisfaction.

Historically, alcohol advertising has been prohibited in Sweden. Since 2003, advertising for products below 15% alcohol by volume is allowed, but it is regulated in the Swedish alcohol law; for example, warning texts regarding the damage of alcohol must be visibly included (STS, 1994). Even though there is no Swedish law forbidding Systembolaget to advertise its products, promoting alcohol would contradict its vision to establish a healthy drinking culture and its mandate to avoid promoting additional sales and being brand-neutral.[2] However, distributors do advertise alcoholic products in Sweden.

CAMPAIGN BACKGROUND, PURPOSE, AND STRATEGY[3]

Since 1995, when Sweden joined the EU, Systembolaget can no longer be taken for granted. There has been pressure over time from the EU to eliminate aspects of the national alcohol policy since the EU wants to encourage free trade between its member states. Although Systembolaget has no competitors in the Swedish market, it faces competition from travelers' import and online purchases. There is also a black market for alcohol and home-distilled strong liquor, even if it is an illegal activity in Sweden.

An alternative to Systembolaget is either a private licensing system or sales in grocery stores. The debate about the alcohol monopoly's continued existence was rather heated around the turn of the millennium, both in the EU and among politicians in Sweden. Systembolaget needed to reinforce its position in order to stay on the market. A new strategic plan was, therefore, implemented in 2000 in order to maintain Systembolaget's role in Swedish alcohol policy. The aim was "to make Systembolaget into a modern retail organization, without compromising the organization's social responsibilities" (Systembolaget, 2001).

Forsman and Bodenfors (F&B), a well-known Swedish advertising agency, was in 2002 given the assignment to help increase the public's positive attitude toward Systembolaget. It was argued that the alcohol monopoly can only survive if it is supported by a majority of the Swedish population. Advertising campaigns to reinforce Systembolaget's position as an alcohol monopoly promoting the benefits of the monopoly were developed, as well as strategies for increasing

[2]The information is based on information from Forsman and Bodenfors (F&B), along with interviews at F&B.

[3]The campaign material is based on internal information from Systembolaget and F&B, along with interviews at F&B.

customer orientation in order to continue and further customer satisfaction. A change of people's attitudes requires continuous campaigns over a long period of time.

In this chapter, we focus on two alcohol monopoly campaigns, one from 2002 and another from 2007, in order to study the effects over time. The purpose of all the campaigns has been to increase the number of Swedish people who understand and hence support the existence of Systembolaget. In total, 13 campaigns have been carried out since 2002, each including one to five ads:

- 2002: one alcohol monopoly campaign.
- 2003: three alcohol monopoly campaigns.
- 2004: two alcohol monopoly campaigns.
- 2005: two alcohol monopoly campaigns.
- 2006: three alcohol monopoly campaigns.
- 2007: two alcohol monopoly campaigns.

The first campaign in 2002 represents a breakthrough in terms of communicating the benefits of the alcohol monopoly. It was carried out at a time when Systembolaget was questioned in Sweden, as discussed earlier. Currently, the discussion in the EU is not focusing on the existence of the Swedish alcohol monopoly, but rather on alcohol politics involving health issues and costs related to alcohol consumption. The second campaign in 2007 was developed with these perspectives in mind, also referring to health implications if Systembolaget was abolished and the alcohol market set free.

In addition to the campaigns, the F&B assignment included a remake of Systembolaget's store communication (store functionality and design) and graphic profile (such as an updated logotype, a special font, and a graphic manual for all printed material used within Systembolaget). Systembolaget's communication strategy distinguishes between inside and outside communication. The "inside" represents the store and includes the physical area before, but not beyond, the cashiers. It is the area where the customers are expected to make decisions regarding purchases. The "inside" also includes the Web site, the customer magazine, and the product catalog. The "outside" includes the area beyond the cashier, the area the customers pass just before leaving the store. The "outside" also includes advertisements such as in print media, outdoors, on the radio, and at PR events. The intention with the distinction between "inside" and "outside" is to separate different communication strategies. While the outside targets the Swedish public (both customers and noncustomers), the inside targets only customers. The outside is the focus of the alcohol monopoly campaigns where the advantages of Systembolaget are emphasized by communicating the downside of a free alcohol market. The inside communication is expected to show the advantages with Systembolaget in practice—for example, a wide product assortment and quality customer service. To maintain Systembolaget, it is necessary to increase the understanding of the benefits of the monopoly and to increase customer satisfaction. Therefore, both outside and inside communication arenas are required.

TARGET AUDIENCES AND OVERALL CAMPAIGN OBJECTIVES

The target audiences for the campaigns are Swedish citizens over the age of 18, customers as well as noncustomers (those who are too young to buy alcohol at Systembolaget and those who do not drink at all or others). The young should like the idea of the alcohol monopoly, and the nondrinkers and others should believe that the alcohol monopoly is better than a free alcohol market.

The overall goal for the alcohol monopoly campaigns is to show the advantages with Systembolaget, thus arguing for its continued existence. Because Systembolaget is owned by the government, it is not allowed to serve as an opinion leader and to propagate for the alcohol monopoly. Instead, it focuses on facts and the consequences of a free alcohol market, believing that given the full picture, more Swedish citizens (including customers) will support the idea of an alcohol monopoly. Systembolaget is continuously interested in measuring the public attitude and has investigated this since 2001, as will be discussed later for the individual campaigns. The attitude toward Systembolaget is also affected by customers' satisfaction, and this has been emphasized since 2001.

POSITIONING STATEMENT

Systembolaget wants the target audience to believe that the alcohol monopoly is a better alternative than a free alcohol market. In addition to an increase in the number of people feeling positive toward Systembolaget, there is a need to make Systembolaget more customer oriented in order to ensure continuing and growing customer satisfaction.

THE 2002 ALCOHOL MONOPOLY CAMPAIGN

Campaign Objectives and Audience Barriers

In 2002, the alcohol monopoly campaign objective was to increase the proportion of those who are positive about Systembolaget from 49% to 54% in three years. It represents the attitude objective—that is, to increase the number of Swedish people who support the existence of the monopoly. The knowledge objective was to make the public more aware of the advantages of an alcohol monopoly and Systembolaget. The campaign focused on changing attitudes in order to maintain the monopoly. Even though no behavioral objective was expressed for the campaign, Systembolaget is still interested in that it wants people who are going to consume alcohol to purchase it at Systembolaget. This requires a positive attitude toward Systembolaget. To communicate the advantages of an alcohol monopoly is a difficult task. The consequences of a free alcohol market also have to be highlighted. The message, therefore, becomes rather complicated and requires a lot of copy. This puts more demands on the readers and could be seen as an audience barrier. The audience must have the time to read the serious messages in the ads.

Campaign Communication Strategies

Message

The traditional image of Systembolaget is that it is a typical governmental institution, which should not promote alcohol, but should control and restrict alcohol consumption, due to concerns over alcohol-related health and social problems. Systembolaget's mandate is to help limit the medical and social damage caused by alcohol and thereby improve public health. Systembolaget's vision is to promote a "healthy drinking culture, whereby we can enjoy Systembolaget's drinks without harming either ourselves or other people" (Systembolaget, 2009a) but it does not dictate if it is right or wrong to drink. Rather, people should be inspired to become interested in what they drink and to focus on quality, not quantity, of drinking (Systembolaget, 2009b).

In 2002, when Systembolaget started to advertise its advantages, there was a risk that the public would react negatively if they thought it was inappropriate to advertise a governmental alcohol monopoly. Also, the employees needed to be informed about the new communication approach. A campaign kit was, therefore, developed in order to explain why Systembolaget started to advertise. It was first distributed to the employees to keep them informed and prepare them for questions from customers. The kit was also distributed to journalists, and Systembolaget's chief executive Anitra Steen discussed the needs and advantages of an alcohol monopoly in morning TV shows and on radio. The kit was available in all Systembolaget's stores when the campaign was launched.

Advertisements

The core message of the 2002 campaign was to argue for the Swedish alcohol monopoly or what would happen if Systembolaget was abolished. Every ad in this campaign presented advantages of Systembolaget and was frank in tone, and each headline was followed by a large section of text. In total, there were five ads, two of which are shown in Figures 8-1 and 8-2.

Media

Newspapers were used as the prime media group to disseminate the campaign message in 2002. Morning press was considered the most appropriate for the campaign because the ad would then be surrounded by social and news reports. The intention was to catch the readers at the most convenient moment when they read the daily news. A large share of the Swedish population reads the morning press (74% in 2002), especially people between 30 and 49 years old (70%) and between 50 and 85 years old (84%; Westlund, 2007).

For the first campaign, five ads were placed in both national and local morning press, in a total of 90 newspapers. The reach was at least 70%. The ads ran on five occasions, mainly during weekdays, during two weeks in November 2002. A new ad was used each time. In addition to this, ads were placed in the subway in Stockholm, the capital of Sweden, to increase the reach. The total official gross media cost for the campaign was SEK10.7 million (approximately US$1.16 million). The total production time was six weeks carried out in late 2002.

Evaluation

The campaign has been thoroughly evaluated by different marketing research companies using two different types of measurements. One focused on the effects of the ads (outputs), and the other focused on the attitude to the alcohol monopoly (outcome).

The Campaign Outputs

The evaluation of the 2002 campaign was made toward the end of the year. A telephone survey was conducted among a national random sample of 1,018 individuals from age 16 and older. The reason for monitoring consumers from age 16 is that they are becoming customers in a few years, and their attitudes are, therefore, of interest for Systembolaget. The purpose was to evaluate how the

Sweden is dead last in the EU. That's what happens when you don't adapt.

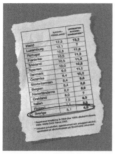

An honourable 15th place.

It may be hard to believe, especially at 11pm this evening, but we Swedes actually drink less than other EU citizens.

And because we drink less alcohol, we have fewer alcohol-related problems. Cirrhosis of the liver, for example, is three times more prevalent in our neighbour, Denmark, than it is in Sweden.

The most important reason is a Swedish invention called "alcohol monopoly".

The idea is based on alcohol being sold without the private profit motive. Because if you have no incentive for financial gain, you do not need to maximise sales.

And, of course, there are other factors that influence the amount we drink. Recently, such things as lower tax on wine and more continental drinking habits have caused Swedish consumption to increase considerably.

But we would drink much more if there were no monopoly.

Nevertheless, that is not self evident any longer.

The EU does not like monopolies in principle. And the trend in our world is, of course, that the private profit motive is getting increasingly dominant.

The monopoly (and Systembolaget) will only exist as long as a majority of Swedes want it.

Therefore, we at Systembolaget will do everything we can to ensure that those who visit us will be more and more satisfied.

And therefore we have put together a series of advertisements in which we tell you things you perhaps did not know about the alcohol monopoly.

The next advertisement will appear on Wednesday.

SYSTEM BOLAGET

FIGURE 8-1   Advertisement from the 2002 Campaign, Translated into English. The Picture Shows a List of Alcohol Consumption in the EU Countries. Sweden Ranks Last, with the Lowest Consumption.

Courtesy of Forsman & Bodenfors and Systembolaget

Do you like Systembolaget without really knowing why?
Here are some good reasons:

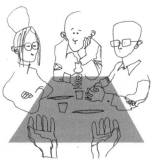

One day you may have to explain yourself.

* "It's a Swedish invention. And an export commodity! The idea, which was born 152 years ago, has decreased the consumption of alcohol and alcohol-related problems in Sweden, Norway, Finland, Canada and several states of the USA, among other places."
* "During the early 1800s, that is before Systembolaget had been invented, we Swedes drank roughly four times as much as we do now, and Swedish consumption was one of the highest in Europe. Today, it is the lowest in the EU."
* "Systembolaget has perhaps the world's largest range of beer, wine and spirits, with about 2,500 brands. And everyone in Sweden has access to it, not only people who live in Stockholm. Small stores, such as the one in Vansbro, have perhaps 600 in stock, but the other 1,900 can be ordered and be in the store the next day."
* "If Systembolaget happens to make a profit (in excess of the required yield of 9%, this money goes to causes such as alcohol research), margins come down. What other chain of stores does this?"
* "The advice that Systembolaget gives can be relied upon. They do not try to force more on you than you want. And they have no sales bonuses."
* "Because the monopoly will only exist as long as people support it, Systembolaget does its utmost to ensure that its customers are satisfied."

If those who disagree with you are still sceptical, ask them to visit www.systembolaget.se

FIGURE 8-2   Advertisement from the 2002 Campaign, Translated into English. Courtesy of Forsman & Bodenfors and Systembolaget

message was perceived by the target group, the entire population, and how the message influenced the attitude to Systembolaget. The evaluation shows the following results:

Recognition

Twenty-one percent of Swedes over 16 years of age noticed the campaign. The attention was higher in big cities, among customers who frequently visited the store, among men, older people (age 45 and above), and people in the south of Sweden. The reason for the high recognition in big cities might be that full-page ads were used, which was not the case for rural newspapers. A possible explanation for the higher recognition in southern Sweden might be that comparisons are made with Denmark, a country where alcohol is cheaper and more easily accessed.

Recall

Among people who had recognized the campaign, three-fourths had read the entire text or part of it. In particular, younger people (16- to 44-year-olds) had read the entire text. Again, it was mostly men and people in big cities who had read the text. People in the northern part of Sweden and noncustomers showed less recall.

Comprehension

Among the people who had recognized the campaign, 58% remembered the message of the ad. Among the people who remembered the message, 9 out of 10 mentioned the advantages of the alcohol monopoly: fewer alcohol problems, less alcohol consumption, or a larger assortment. However, one-tenth remembered the wrong message. Again, noncustomers, older customers (age 60 and above), and people in northern Sweden showed less comprehension in comparison to people living in big cities.

Acceptance

Among the people who had recognized the campaign, 18% answered that their attitude had become more positive to Systembolaget as a result of the campaign. In particular, the attitude was more positive among people who had read part of or the entire text and among the youngest respondents (16- to 29-year-olds). In total, 76% of the respondents had not changed their attitude as a result of the campaign.

Attitude to Advertisement

One-third of the respondents answered that it is good that Systembolaget advertises the benefits of the alcohol monopoly, one-third disliked the idea, and one-third had no opinion. The attitude was more positive among the respondents who had seen the campaign: 54% were positive, 20% were negative, and 26% were neutral.

Satisfaction with Systembolaget

In total, 40% of the respondents were satisfied with Systembolaget overall (not only concerning the attitude to the alcohol monopoly), 4% were dissatisfied, and 56% were neutral. The most satisfied were frequent customers, respondents living in big cities, and persons being 30 to 59 years old. The least satisfied were younger respondents (ages 16 to 29) and persons living in rural areas. The non-customers were the most dissatisfied.

The Campaign Outcomes

A marketing research company has regularly conducted public opinion surveys over the years with a national random sample of 1,500 individuals. In the end of 2001, before the first monopoly campaign was launched in November 2002, the OPI (public opinion index) was 49% (people positive toward maintaining the alcohol monopoly). A public opinion survey was performed in December 2002, right after the first campaign (see Figure 8-3). The question asked when determining the attitude to Systembolaget was whether they would vote for keeping the alcohol monopoly if a referendum was carried out.[4] The initial goal to increase the OPI from 49% to an average of 54% in three years had already been reached at the end of 2002, when the OPI was 57%. The increase in OPI could be due to the campaign, but it could also be explained by the overall change of Systembolaget into a modern retail organization with a new store concept and graphic profile.

The results show that 57% of the public wanted to keep the alcohol monopoly. The customers were less positive (53% of the customers wanted to keep the alcohol monopoly) than the general public. More women than men were in favor of keeping the alcohol monopoly.

---

[4]The exact question asked was, "Do you think one should keep Systembolaget and the alcohol monopoly for sales of strong beer, wine, and strong liquor, or do you want strong beer, wine, and strong liquor to be sold in other stores?"

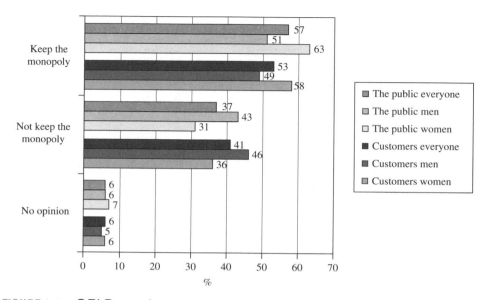

FIGURE 8-3 OPI December 2002, the Public and Customers

Data from SIFO Research International, Opinion measurement December 2002 for Systembolaget

THE 2007 ALCOHOL MONOPOLY CAMPAIGN

Campaign Objectives and Audience Barriers

Since 2002, the public opinion of keeping Systembolaget has been strength-ened. The 2007 campaign had the same objective as the first one in 2002—that is, to increase the positive attitude toward keeping the alcohol monopoly to 57% (the 2002 campaign objective was 54%). The audience barriers were the same as for the 2002 campaign. Also the objectives remained the same. The at-titude objective was to increase the number of Swedish people who support the existence of the monopoly. The knowledge objective was to make the public more aware of the advantages of an alcohol monopoly and Systembolaget. Even though no behavioral objective was expressed for the campaign, Systembolaget was still interested in that people who are going to consume alcohol purchase it at its stores.

Campaign Communication Strategies

Messages

The 2007 campaign message was based on the Holder report (2007) published by the National Institute of Public Health. The report examines two scenarios focusing on health and social consequences if the Swedish alcohol retail monopoly is abolished. In the first scenario, the alcohol monopoly was replaced with privately licensed alcohol stores, which specialize in alcohol sales. As a consequence, (1) there would be an increase in the number of stores from the current 400 Systembolaget stores to more than 1,000 private outlets; (2) total alcohol assortment in Sweden would be greater, but the assortment in each store smaller; (3) there would be no price change if current Swedish alcohol excise taxes were maintained; (4) the promotion effect is expected to increase consumption by 5% in addition to other price promotions; (5) opening hours would be longer; and (6) it seems very likely that privatization would increase availability for underaged buyers.

In the second scenario, all alcohol would be available in grocery stores. The consequences could be that (1) all alcohol beverages would be sold in up to 8,000 grocery stores; (2) total alcohol assortment in an average grocery store would be much smaller than in a Systembolaget store; (3) opening hours would mirror grocery store hours; (4) grocery stores would offer low-priced alcoholic beverages, with lower quality than the cheapest wines and spirits currently at Systembolaget; (5) there would be no price change if current Swedish alcohol excise taxes were maintained; (6) grocery stores would subsidize the price of selected alcoholic beverages with profit on other products in order to generate store traffic; (7) point-of-sale promotions and advertising are expected to increase total consumption by 8%; and (8) it seems very likely that privatization would increase availability for underaged buyers.

Current estimates of alcohol consumption are 9.5 liters per capita (100% alcohol content; SoRAD, 2009). The Holder report shows that privatization of all retail sales of alcohol in Sweden would raise consumption by 14% (approximately 1.4 liters per capita) if sales were restricted to specialty stores or by 29% (approximately 2.8 liters per capita) if alcohol were available in grocery stores. Holder (2007) claims that these estimates are conservative; the actual increase would likely be higher. A forecasting model was used in the Holder report to estimate the health and social effects on alcohol consumption if Systembolaget were replaced by specialty stores only or grocery stores. Alcohol sales in privately licensed specialty shops would annually result in an estimated 700 deaths (alcohol-related illness deaths, fatal accidents, suicides, homicides), 6,700 non-fatal assaults, and 7.3 million sickness absence days. With alcohol sales in grocery stores, the estimated additional annual toll would be 1,580 deaths (alcohol-related illness deaths, fatal accidents, suicides, homicides), 14,200 nonfatal assaults, and 16.1 million sickness absence days.

Advertisements

The 2007 campaign featured three newspaper ads and one Web ad, all based on the Holder report. Every ad in this campaign presented consequences if Systembolaget were abolished. Each ad was frank in tone, and each headline was followed by a lot of copy. Two print ads from this campaign are presented in Figures 8-4 and 8-5.

Media

For the 2007 campaign, print media was also used in order to communicate a more complex message. However, fewer local morning papers were used due to budget limits. Instead, evening press and free newspapers were used to obtain 70% reach. In addition, a Web ad was developed. Home Internet coverage is very high in Sweden (83%), and 64% of Swedes use the Internet daily. Among those using the Internet daily, younger consumers rank highest (86% for ages 15 to 24), but usage is also relatively high among older consumers (29% for ages 65 to 79; Nordicom, 2008). The Web strategy was to cover the sites with the highest reach for the target group, as well as major national newspapers' Web sites. The three print ads were placed during three weekdays between November 16 and November 26, and the Web ad ran for three weeks. The total official gross media cost for the campaign was SEK13.5 million (approximately US$2.09 million), exclusive of the Internet cost. The total production time was six weeks carried out in late 2007.

Evaluation

The 2007 campaign was evaluated in a similar way as the 2002 campaign by two different marketing research companies for Systembolaget.

The Campaign Outputs

The evaluation of the campaign was made toward the end of the year. A telephone survey was conducted among a national random sample of 1,033 individuals (16 years and above). The purpose was to evaluate how the message was perceived by the target group and the entire population and how the message influenced the attitude toward Systembolaget. The results are discussed next.

A happy story about sickness, violence and death.

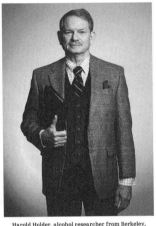

Harold Holder, alcohol researcher from Berkeley, led an investigation which shows that the Swedish alcohol monopoly saves a lot of lives each year.

It's not in vain that you put up with the alcohol monopoly.

An international research group has just investigated what would happen if it was abolished, and they found that alcohol-related problems would be much worse.

Many other studies have shown this previously, but this is the first one carried out since the import regulations for alcohol were changed. Today, you can bring an almost unlimited quantity back with you when you have been abroad.

Nevertheless, the group of researchers believe that Swedes would increase their consumption by almost 30 per cent if strong beer, wine and spirits were sold in food stores. And that would bring about the following consequences:

About 1 600 more deaths each year.

About 14 000 more cases of assault.

And about 16 million more sick days.

But the alcohol monopoly will only last as long as people want it. So we will continue to do everything we can to ensure that you are more and more satisfied with our stores, our range and our service.

(If you want to know how the researchers arrived at their conclusions, you can see the entire report on folkhalsoinstitutet.se)

FIGURE 8-4 Advertisement from the 2007 Campaign, Translated into English
Courtesy of Forsman & Bodenfors and Systembolaget and photographer
Emmet Malmström

What would the price of alcohol be if it was sold in food stores?

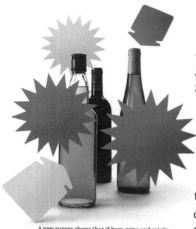

A new survey shows that if beer, wine and spirits were sold freely, alcohol-related problems would be much greater. And cost a great deal more.

An international group of researchers has just investigated what would happen if the Swedish alcohol monopoly was abolished.

They concluded that consumption would increase by almost 30 per cent if strong beer, wine and spirits were sold in food stores. Which would cause a considerable increase in alcohol-related problems. And those kinds of problem cost society a great deal of money.

Exactly how much is difficult to say, it depends how you calculate it. Some people think that the current social costs are 20 billion per year, others that they are 70 billion.

If the monopoly was abolished, it is estimated that costs would increase to the same extent as drinking. Which would mean additional costs of between 6 and 21 billion each year.

But the alcohol monopoly will only remain as long as people want it. So we will continue to do everything we can to ensure that you are more and more satisfied with our stores, our range and our service.

(If you want to know how the researchers arrived at their conclusions, you can see the entire report on folkhalsoinstitutet.se)

FIGURE 8-5 Advertisement from the 2007 Campaign, Translated into English
Courtesy of Forsman & Bodenfors and Systembolaget

Spontaneous Recall (Both Print and Web)

About 17% of the respondents could spontaneously remember the ad campaign. More men (24%) than women (11%) remembered the ads spontaneously. Also, frequent customers (24%) could spontaneously recall the ads to a greater extent than noncustomers (13%). Furthermore, older people (age 45 and above) scored higher than younger respondents.

Aided Recall (Print)

"Aided recall" means that the respondents are given a short description of the message of the campaign ads. The result shows that 32% of the respondents had either read or seen the ads—more men (40%) than women (25%) and more customers (39%) than noncustomers (26%). More specifically, 24% of the respondents had read the ads—again, more men (31%) than women (19%) and more customers (30%) than noncustomers (19%). Among the ads, the first one, with the expert male researcher, scored highest regarding reading (19%), as well as either reading or seeing the ad (25%). The other ad (the bottles) scored 9% on reading and 15% on either reading or seeing the ad.

Aided Recall (Web)

For the Web advertisement, the aided recall was 7%. It scored highest among the youngest group, 16- to 29-year-olds (15%) and higher among men (11%) than women (4%).

Acceptance (Both Print and Web)

Among the people who had read and seen the campaign, 22% answered that their attitude had become more positive toward Systembolaget as a result of the campaign. The youngest respondents (16- to 29-year-olds) were both the most positive and the most negative, indicating that the effect of the campaign was the strongest for this group. The older (age 60 and above) were the least positive. People in small cities (24%) and rural areas (26%) were more positive than people in big cities (17%). There were no major differences between men and women; 24% of frequent customers and 13% of noncustomers had become more positive. In total, 66% of the respondents answered that they had not changed their attitude as a result of the campaign.

Attitude to Advertisement

About 60% of the respondents answered that it was good that Systembolaget advertises its business, 21% disliked it, and 15% were indifferent. More men (67%) than women (54%) were positive, as well as more frequent customers (64%)

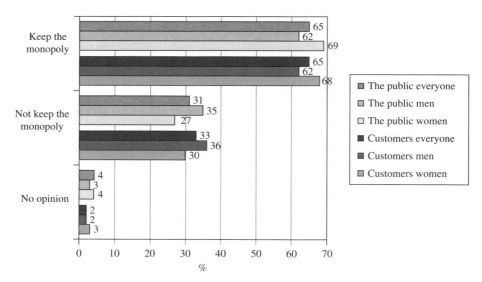

FIGURE 8-6   OPI November 2007, the Public and Customers

Data from SIFO Research International, Opinion measurement November 2007 for Systembolaget

than noncustomers (45%). The older (age 60 and above) were more negative (26%) in comparison to other age groups.

The Campaign Outcomes

In October 2007, the OPI (public opinion index) was 58% (people positive about maintaining the alcohol monopoly).[5] After the campaign a public opinion survey was made with a national random sample of 1,500 individuals. The results are presented in Figure 8-6.

The results show that both 65% of the public and 65% of the customers wanted to keep the alcohol monopoly. Again, female customers appear to be more positive than the male customers. The number of people positive to the alcohol monopoly has increased from 57% in December 2002 to 65% in November 2007. In other words, the campaign goals have been exceeded. The number of people negative toward Systembolaget has decreased from 37% to

[5]The exact question asked was, "Do you think one should keep Systembolaget and the alcohol monopoly for sales of strong beer, wine, and strong liquor, or do you want strong beer, wine, and strong liquor to be sold in other stores?"

33% during the same time. The number of people having neither positive nor negative opinions about Systembolaget has decreased from 6% to 2%.

AN INTEGRATED MARKETING MIX

The preceding discussion has primarily dealt with promotion in the marketing mix. For Swedes to be interested in keeping Systembolaget and become loyal customers, however, the campaigns are not enough. The other components in the marketing mix must also be considered: place, product, and price.

Place: A Modern Retail Outlet

Many changes have been made in Systembolaget's stores to become a more modern retail outlet. Historically, sales have been made over the counter and created a feeling of supervision. Customers could not pick up alcohol bottles themselves, but had to ask cashiers for specific brands or recommendations. This old-fashioned way of organizing Systembolaget's stores has now changed. Since 2001, many stores have been made into self-service stores, where customers can look around and pick out whatever they want themselves. The store layout has also become more appealing and consumer-friendly.

Customer service has also improved over the years. Systembolaget has a customer service department that answers questions regarding food and drink, in addition to anything that has to do with Systembolaget's operations. Systembolaget organizes in-store tastings in 32 locations led by the store staff. The employees are offered training by taking courses, attending tasting sessions, and taking study trips.

Product: A High-Quality Assortment

Systembolaget's product range is one of the biggest in the world and consists of high-quality products. It carries almost 7,000 items, including beer (with 400 strong beers from 37 countries), wine, hard liquor, and nonalcoholic beverages stocked by Systembolaget or its suppliers (Systembolaget, 2008b). Approximately 1,000 new products are launched every year. The product assortment is continuously revised in order to consider trends and changes in consumers' tastes (Systembolaget, 2009c). Quality control is rigorous, and both new and old products are tested in a laboratory (Systembolaget, 2009d). The products are described in a product catalog. Before the F&B assignment, it was mainly a price list but has now been developed to include flavor charts and food symbols recommending suitable food and drink combinations. Books containing Systembolaget's expertise on food and drink are published and sold in the stores.

Drink auctions are held twice a year when valuable collectors' items are offered for sale. All this has likely increased customer satisfaction, in addition to the wide assortment and high-quality products. In addition, Systembolaget has a customer magazine that describes different products more in-depth, as well as offering food recipes. However, these positive aspects of alcohol consumption are mitigated by discussing the downside of alcohol consumption in the magazine (Systembolaget, 2009e). This is in line with Systembolaget's mission to educate people about the downside of alcohol, including information on its home page, in the stores, and in different campaigns about bootlegging. Difficulties to communicate disadvantages with alcohol should, however, be recognized. In particular, excessive drinkers may be difficult to reach due to selective perception.

Price: A Noncompetitive Factor

An alcohol monopoly by definition eliminates competition, although Systembolaget faces competition from travelers' imports, online purchases, and the black market for alcohol. Still, Systembolaget does not use price as a competitive factor. High taxes make this impossible. The advantages promoted are instead the wide assortment and high-quality products.

CONSUMPTION AND MARKET SHARE

Alcohol consumption has increased since Sweden joined the EU in 1995 but shows a decrease during more recent years. Still, consumption is considerably higher than before Sweden joined the EU. Systembolaget's sales have increased over time, from 33.6 million liters in 2001 to 40.5 million liters in 2007 (Systembolaget, 2007a). Also, the number of customer visits in the stores has increased during the past few years (Systembolaget, 2007b). The question is whether this increase is due to an increased number of new customers or an increase in consumption among existing customers. One possible explanation could be the increase in disposable income among Swedes during the recent years. It is noticeable that Systembolaget has increased its market share of the total alcohol consumption since 2004 (SoRAD, 2008). Because private imports of alcohol have decreased (Systembolaget, 2006, 2007a), it is likely that Systembolaget has taken shares from this market. The campaigns, a stronger focus on customer orientation, and an integrated marketing mix may have contributed to a decrease in private imports. Rather than importing alcohol, Swedes may rather choose to support Systembolaget.

CONCLUSION AND IMPLICATIONS

The purpose of the alcohol monopoly campaigns was to increase people's under-standing and positive attitude toward Systembolaget. Campaign results show that the number of people positive to Systembolaget has increased from 49% before the 2002 campaign to 65% after the 2007 campaign. The campaigns have been success-ful. The impact of the alcohol monopoly campaigns has been an increase of citi-zens who are in favor of an alcohol monopoly in Sweden. As long as public opinion is strong, Systembolaget is not threatened at a national level. It is interesting to no-tice that among customers, the number of persons who are uncertain about whether they think Systembolaget is good or bad has been 11%,[6] and this has been a relatively constant share throughout the campaign years. The changes in attitudes over time are believed to have occurred in steps from negative to uncertain and from uncertain to positive; in other words, not directly from negative to positive. The number of negative customers has decreased, but there are still uncertain cus-tomers to convince about the benefits of Systembolaget.

Systembolaget's efforts to improve store atmosphere, quality assortment, and customer service may also have contributed to the customers' positive attitude to-ward it. The 2007 campaign result shows that the numbers of frequent customers (24%) who have become more positive toward Systembolaget are greater than the noncustomers (13%). Systembolaget was aware of the importance of customer ori-entation before the monopoly campaigns. Customer orientation has thus been highlighted over the past years and has resulted in increased customer satisfaction since 2003. The campaigns may have also contributed to increased customer satis-faction and that people have become more interested in Systembolaget and visiting its stores.

Another reason for the increase in positive attitude toward Systembolaget could be the change in political climate during the past several years. Resistance to the al-cohol monopoly has decreased both among the public and politicians. Health and social problems related to alcohol have received more attention lately both in Sweden and in the EU. In the EU, the cost of alcohol-related harms (e.g., mortality and absenteeism from work) was estimated to be €125 billion (approximately US$156 billion) for 2003, equivalent to 1.3% of gross domestic product (European Commission, 2006). The spending on alcohol-related problems (e.g., crime, health, and traffic accidents) was estimated to be €66 billion (approximately US$82 billion;

---

[6]The number of customers who are uncertain is calculated based on the number of answers ranked 5 and 6 on a 10-point rating scale. The answers ranged from "Not at all certain" (1) to "Very certain" (10). The exact question asked was, "How certain is it that you would vote for keeping the alcohol monopoly of Systembolaget?"

European Commission, 2006). The EU is also realizing the benefits of alcohol control. Alcohol monopolies are one way of keeping the societal costs of alcohol-related harm down. An alcohol monopoly keeps alcohol consumption down by 30% compared to a free market where alcohol can be bought in any retail store (Holder, 2007). This is also likely to be of interest in the EU where a free market is advocated. A restriction of alcohol accessibility and alcohol taxes keeps the societal costs down. In May 2008, the World Health Organization adopted a resolution requesting a development of a draft global strategy to reduce harmful use of alcohol (WHO, 2008).

From a global perspective, Sweden's alcohol monopoly may provide some interesting and helpful experience to other countries. Systembolaget's campaigns shed new light on the applications of social marketing principles in a new sociocultural context. The 2002 campaign was the first advertisement campaign that was launched by Systembolaget advocating the advantages of an alcohol monopoly. The campaign created interest but also required preparations in the form of an information kit explaining the reasons for the campaign to external as well as internal stakeholders. The complexity of the issue required extensive copy, which is unusual in today's image-focused, advertising-intense society. This kind of copy also required an appropriate choice of media. Morning newspapers were used to a large extent in order to create a trustworthy setting. The advertisements stuck out and created attention. The timing was right in that the political opinion for deregulating the Swedish alcohol monopoly had weakened at the time of the campaign launch. Furthermore, the importance of recognizing the link between attitudes and behavior needs to be noticed in social marketing. The campaigns have resulted in a higher number of Swedes with a positive attitude toward Systembolaget, but this is not sufficient. The integrated marketing mix has succeeded in making shoppers more satisfied at Systembolaget. Moreover, changing attitudes and, even more so, changing behavior takes time and requires continuity. The collaboration between F&B and Systembolaget has, from the beginning, been a long-term relationship, which is expected to have positive effects on the results.

Finally, it may be perceived as a paradox that Systembolaget promotes restricted consumption of alcohol by limited accessibility (number of outlets and opening hours) and campaigns focusing on health consequences of alcohol and bootlegging, while at the same time emphasizing customer orientation (a wide product assortment, customer service) in order to increase its market share. However, we believe a nonprofit alcohol monopoly needs to focus on customer satisfaction in order to be attractive in a global marketplace. The idea to limit consumption—and thus, alcohol-related problems—by an alcohol monopoly such as Systembolaget and its focus on customer satisfaction could, from an international perspective, be considered a smart solution to a global public health problem.

QUESTIONS FOR DISCUSSION

1. What are the advantages and disadvantages of keeping the Swedish alcohol retail monopoly from the perspective of the consumer and from the perspective of the Swedish state?
2. Describe the alcohol policy defined by the government in your own country, and explain if and how regulation is carried out by your government.
3. Apart from governmental regulations, how are alcohol-related problems handled in your own country? Please give also suggestions for preventive actions.
4. Underage and young consumers are a group at risk when it comes to alcohol consumption. Systembolaget has developed bootlegging campaigns to put a stop to consumption in this group. Please suggest other strategies that may help prevent underage and young consumers from consuming alcohol.

ACKNOWLEDGMENTS

The authors wish to thank Per Bergkrantz, former marketing director at Systembolaget; Fredrik Thor, brand manager at Systembolaget; Maria Hallenborg, project leader; and Hans Andersson, account manager at Forsman & Bodenfors for information and accessibility to material for this case.

REFERENCES

Anderson, P., & Baumberg, B. (2006). *Alcohol in Europe.* UK: Institute of Alcohol Studies). Retrieved July 28, 2009, from http://ec.europa.eu//health-eu/news_alcoholineurope_en.htm

Central Intelligence Agency (CIA). (2009). *The World Factbook—Sweden.* Retrieved July 28, 2009, from https://www.cia.gov/library/publications/the-world-factbook /geos/sw.html

Centre for Social Research on Alcohol and Drugs (SoRAD). (2008). *Alcohol statistics* [Fact sheet]. Retrieved July 28, 2009, from http://www.sorad.su.se/alcohol_statistics.php

Centre for Social Research on Alcohol and Drugs (SoRAD). (2009). *News, the total alcohol consumption in Sweden during 2008* [Fact sheet]. Retrieved July 28, 2009, from http://www .sorad.su.se/pub/jsp/polopoly.jsp?d=11320&a=57064

European Commission. (2006). *Alcohol-related harm in Europe—Key data, October 2006* [Fact sheet]. European Commission, Health & Consumer Protection, Directorate-General. Retrieved July 28, 2009, from http://ec.europa.eu/health/ph_determinants/life_style/alcohol/ documents/alcohol_factsheet_en.pdf

Government Offices of Sweden. (2008). *Swedish national alcohol policy.* Retrieved July 28, 2009, from http://www.sweden.gov.se/sb/d/2901/a/16516

Holder, H. (Ed). (2007). *If retail alcohol sales in Sweden were privatized, what would be the consequences?* Swedish National Institute of Public Health. Retrieved July 28, 2009, from hppt://www.fhi.se

Immigrant Institute. (2008). *Immigrants in Sweden 2000 and 2007—statistics by continent/ region in the world and country* [Fact sheet]. Retrieved July 28, 2009, from http://www.immi .se/migration/

Landes, D. (2008, March 11). New Swedish restaurants added to Guide Michelin. *The Local, Sweden's News in English*. Retrieved July 28, 2008, from http://www.thelocal.se/10410/ 20080311/

National Board of Health and Welfare (NBHW). (2008). *Fact sheet.* Retrieved July 28, 2009, from http://www.socialstyrelsen.se/en/about/

Nordicom. (2008). *Nordicom—Sveriges Mediabarometer 2007* [Nordicom—Sweden's Media Barometer 2007]. Report MedieNotiser Nr. 1, 2008. Göteborgs Universitet: Author.

STS. (1994). *Alkohollag* [Alcohol law], SFS 1994:1738 [Fact sheet]. Socialdepartementet [Ministry of Social Affairs]. Svensk författningssamling. Retrieved July 28, 2009, from http://www.riksdagen.se/webbnav/index.aspx?nid=3911&bet=1994:1738

Sweden.se. (2008). *Sweden in brief* [Fact sheet]. The official gateway to Sweden. Retrieved May 28, 2008, from http://www.sweden.se/templates/cs/CommonPage____2707.aspx

Swedish Customs. (2009). *Riktlinjer och referensnivåer* [Guidelines and reference levels] [Fact sheet]. Tullverket. Retrieved July 28, 2009, from http://www.tullverket.se/en/startpage.4.4ab 1598c11632f3ba9280002814.html

Swedish National Institute of Public Health (SNIPH). (2008a). *Alcohol—Alcohol consumption Fact sheet.* Retrieved July 28, 2009, from http://www.fhi.se/templates/Page____141.aspx

Swedish National Institute of Public Health (SNIPH). (2008b). *Fact sheet.* Retrieved July 28, 2009, from http://www.fhi.se/default____1417.aspx

Systembolaget. (2001). *Annual report 2001.* Retrieved July 28, 2009, from http://www.system bolaget.se/Applikationer/Knappar/OmSystembolaget/Ekonomi/Ekonomiskinfo.htm

Systembolaget. (2006). *Annual report 2006.* Retrieved July 28, 2009, from http://www.system bolaget.se/Applikationer/Knappar/OmSystembolaget/Ekonomi/Ekonomiskinfo.htm

Systembolaget. (2007a). *Annual report 2007.* Retrieved July 28, 2009, from http://www.system bolaget.se/Applikationer/Knappar/OmSystembolaget/Ekonomi/Ekonomiskinfo.htm

Systembolaget. (2007b). *Bokslutskommuniké 2007.* Retrieved July 28, 2009, from http://www.system bolaget.se/Applikationer/Knappar/OmSystembolaget/Ekonomi/Ekonomiskinfo.htm

Systembolaget. (2008a). *Why does Systembolaget exist?* [Fact sheet]. Retrieved July 28, 2009, from http://www.systembolaget.se/Applikationer/Knappar/InEnglish/History.htm

Systembolaget. (2008b). *For suppliers and producers* [Fact sheet]. Retrieved July 28, 2009, from http://www.systembolaget.se/Applikationer/Knappar/InEnglish/suppliers.htm

Systembolaget. (2009a). *Our vision* [Fact sheet]. Retrieved July 28, 2009, from http://www.system bolaget.se/Applikationer/Knappar/InEnglish/ourvision.htm

Systembolaget. (2009b). *Systembolaget's mandate* [Fact sheet]. Retrieved July 28, 2009, from http://www.systembolaget.se/Applikationer/Knappar/InEnglish/systembolagetsmandate.htm

Systembolaget. (2009c). *This is Systembolaget* [Fact sheet]. Retrieved July 28, 2009, from http://www .systembolaget.se/Applikationer/Knappar/InEnglish

Systembolaget. (2009d). *About Systembolaget. A presentation of Systembolaget, our history and our aims* [Fact sheet]. Retrieved July 28, 2009, from http://www.systembolaget.se/NR/rdonlyres/8C39020E-492A-47A1-B578-021AF5833CD6/0/foretagspres_03_eng.pdf

Systembolaget. (2009e). *The company—a magazine from Systembolaget* [Fact sheet]. Retrieved July 28, 2009, from http://www.systembolaget.se/Bolaget/Artiklar.htm

Westlund, O. (2007). Svenskarnas Dagstidningsläsning ur ett förändringsperspektiv [Swedish people's reading of daily newspapers from a transformation perspective]. In S. Holmberg & L. Weibull (Eds.), *Det nya Sverige [The New Sweden]* (p. 323). Göteborgs Universitet: SOM-Institutet.

World Health Organization (WHO). (2008, May 28). *Strategies to reduce the harmful use of alcohol. 61st World Health Assembly adopts resolution on developing a global strategy* [Press release]. Retrieved July 28, 2009, from http://www.who.int/mediacentre/events/2008/wha61/issues_paper3/en/print.html

CHAPTER 9

Creating a Commercial Market for Insecticide-Treated Mosquito Nets in Nigeria

Willard D. Shaw

The best-laid schemes of mice and men often go awry.
—Robert Burns

Malaria is one of the greatest health scourges on the planet, infecting 300 to 500 million people every year and causing at least 1 million deaths—mostly among pregnant women and children under 5 years of age in Africa. Malaria costs Africa $12 billion in lost gross domestic product (GDP), reducing economic development by 1.3% annually. Many poor families spend a significant portion of their income on the prevention and treatment of multiple cases of malaria each year. It is Africa's leading cause of under-5 mortality (20%) and constitutes 10% of the continent's overall disease burden. It accounts for 40% of public health expenditure, 30% to 50% of inpatient admissions, and up to 50% of outpatient visits in areas with high malaria transmission (Roll Back Malaria [RBM], 2008).

The international health community has launched a variety of initiatives to reduce the impact of malaria, including the Roll Back Malaria (RBM) Partnership in 1998; the Global Fund for AIDS, Tuberculosis, and Malaria (2001); and the $2 billion

U.S. President's Malaria Initiative (2001). All of these efforts have focused primarily on the public sector. In 1999, the U.S. Agency for International Development (USAID) created the NetMark Project—the first program focused entirely on harnessing the skills, investment, and infrastructure of the commercial sector to combat malaria through the creation of commercially sustainable markets for insecticide-treated nets (ITNs) in five to seven sub-Saharan African countries.

In Africa, malaria is carried by the night-biting anopheles mosquito; more than 97% of infective bites occur between the hours of 10 p.m. and 6 a.m. Sleeping under an ITN, therefore, is one of the best ways to prevent malaria. The insecticide is deadly for the anopheles but poses little human health risk. NetMark was issued for competitive bidding by USAID in 1999 and awarded in September 1999 to AED, a nonprofit social development organization. It was signed as a "cooperative agreement" instead of a "contract" because it was seen as an experimental effort to determine if and how commercially viable markets for ITNs could be established in multiple African countries and how far down the economic scale commercial products could reach. There was no certainty it would be successful.

At the start of NetMark, ITNs were available in African countries mainly through donor and government programs. In most countries, they were not available in commercial markets; thus, families seeking the protection provided by ITNs were not able to buy them. NetMark sought to change this situation by partnering with international net and insecticide manufacturers to create retail markets for ITNs in partnership with African distributors and retailers. For a variety of reasons (e.g., prohibitive cost of educating consumers about ITNs, lack of market data, competition from free and subsidized products, etc.), no ITN producers invested in building retail markets but focused instead on the institutional market with its large tenders from governments and donors. It was safe, clients were likely to pay on time, orders were large, and it involved a simple response to an invitation to bid. NetMark offered these commercial firms an opportunity to create retail markets through its Joint Risk—Joint Investment Strategy. NetMark would carry out market research, cover the heavy costs of educating the populace and creating consumer demand for ITNs, help companies enter into the retail market, and serve as a link with national malaria control programs and other public sector efforts to establish a supportive environment for the commercial marketing of ITNs. AED's Full Market Impact (FMI™) approach to public health social marketing addressed all elements of the marketing mix in close collaboration with the public and private sectors. FMI™ provided the framework for engaging the commercial sector, nongovernmental organizations (NGOs), and the public sector in comprehensive efforts to increase the practice of healthy behaviors and generate and fulfill demand for an affordable and accessible range of public health products and services with three outcome goals: equity, commercial viability, and sustainable public health impact.

NetMark established a regional office in Johannesburg, South Africa, where many of the multinational insecticide and advertising companies had their sub-Saharan headquarters. The regional office established, supported, and supervised the country programs with backstopping from AED headquarters in Washington, DC. NetMark started as a $15.2 million project scheduled to run from September 1999 through September 2004. Its mandate was later expanded and the end date extended to September 2007 and then to September 2009, with its budget ceiling increased to $65.2 million. Country programs started based on USAID country missions "buying into" NetMark by providing funding. NetMark eventually worked in seven countries: Zambia, Ghana, Nigeria, Mali, Senegal, Uganda, and Ethiopia.

Nigeria is presented here as a case study, not because it was NetMark's most successful country program, but because of the many challenges that were navigated, the variety of issues that were addressed, and the wide range of activities created to respond to changes in the country situation. NetMark started with a process and a plan and then found it had to adapt that plan periodically so it could move forward and achieve its goals.

NIGERIA: A COUNTRY OVERVIEW

With an estimated population in 2008 of 146,255,000, Nigeria is the most populous country in Africa, comprising 18% of the total population of sub-Saharan Africa. The median age is 19 years, and life expectancy is under 46 years. Nigeria is a multiethnic and multilingual society. It has more than 250 ethnic groups, with the largest and most influential being the Hausa and Fulani (29%), Yoruba (21%), Igbo (18%), and Ijaw (10%). Half the population is Muslim, while 40% are Christians and 10% follow indigenous beliefs. The main languages are English (official), Hausa, Yoruba, Igbo, and Fulani (Central Intelligence Agency [CIA], 2008). There is ongoing tension between the largely Muslim north (mainly Hausas and Fulanis) and the Christian south (mainly Yorubas and Igbos; CIA, 2009).

Since emerging from British colonialism in 1960, Nigeria has had a troubled history replete with periodic ethnic conflicts, a civil war with a breakaway region (Biafra, 1967–1970) that caused a million deaths, long periods of military rule, and an oil-driven economy that has seen US$300 billion in oil pumped since independence. Oil provides 20% of GDP, 95% of foreign exchange earnings, and about 80% of budgetary revenues. Transparency International has consistently ranked Nigeria as one of the world's more corrupt countries. The GDP per capita is US$2,100 while the literacy rate is 68% (CIA, 2009).

Nigeria is a nation of great promise with an energetic and creative citizenry and natural resources, but sociopolitical instability continues to hinder its progress. It is a federal republic composed of 36 states and the Federal Capital Territory of Abuja. The state governors generally have significant autonomy. The Federal Ministry of Health (MOH) and National Malaria Control Program set policies and guidelines, but each state has its own health minister and malaria director and often acts independently.

CASE STUDY
Insecticide-Treated Mosquito Nets

CAMPAIGN BACKGROUND AND ENVIRONMENT

Malaria in Nigeria

Malaria is endemic throughout much of Nigeria, with more than 90% of the population at risk. Malaria accounts for 25% of infant mortality and 30% of childhood mortality with up to 200,000 child deaths occurring every year. Malaria is the most common cause of hospital outpatient attendance in all age groups. It is estimated that 50% of the population has at least one episode of malaria each year. In the southern half of Nigeria, malaria is perennial (7 to 12 months a year), while in the northern regions it is seasonal (4 to 6 months a year; NetMark, 2000).

The National Malaria Control Program made ITN use a key strategy for malaria prevention. In 2000, NetMark's survey of households with a child under 5 years of age found that only 10% of households had at least one mosquito net, and none was a treated net. Only 6% had ever heard of an ITN. For a long time, the importation of ready-made nets was prohibited. The few Nigerian net manufacturers made nets only part of the year and manufactured other products like mattress covers the rest of the time. Local production was not adequate to meet the needs of the Nigerian market. The four main insecticide treatments are imported from multinational companies with some brands packaged in the country.

ITN Activities before NetMark

Before NetMark started in Nigeria, no major efforts had been undertaken to expand the availability and use of ITNs. Untreated nets were sold in most parts of the country. A small number of net manufacturers produced nets as a sideline, and other nets were made by local stitchers from a variety of materials—but insecticide-treated nets were a rarity and unknown to the general public. A 1999 UNICEF project sold ITNs for US$4.50 in 10 states; a second project had NGOs sell ITNs for $5 in four communities to test the possibility of full-cost recovery. Although there was strong support in the Ministry of Health for the involvement of the local net manufacturers in NetMark, there was not broad support for the commercial sector in general. When the tariff on imported nets was increased to 75% in 2002, the Ministry of Health did not back the efforts of NetMark and other RBM partners to get it reduced.

TARGET AUDIENCES

There were three main target audiences for NetMark's efforts to build a commercial ITN market:

1. *Consumers.* This group includes families with women of reproductive age and/or children under 5 who are most likely to die from malaria. A secondary group is everyone else likely to get malaria—which constitutes 90% of Nigeria's population.
2. *Public sector policy makers.* These are the decision makers who can create a facilitating environment for the commercial sector by targeting free and subsidized ITNs to the poorest segments of the population, lowering taxes and tariffs on ITNs, and enabling a vibrant commercial market to develop to meet the needs of those who can afford a commercial product.
3. *Commercial distributors and retailers.* While NetMark had collaborative agreements with multinational insecticide and net suppliers, they had to identify and appoint national distributors that could jumpstart a retail ITN market for their brands.

PROGRAM GOALS AND OBJECTIVES

NetMark's goals fell into four categories (see Table 9-1). Its projected outputs changed over time as its end date was extended from September 2004 to September 2007 and then to September 2009; however, funding for Nigeria was decided annually.

TABLE 9-1 NetMark Goals and Objectives

Goals	Objectives and Strategies	Projected Outputs
Availability Increase ITN availability and number of brands in the market.	Have multiple "formal" brand partners and informal "collaborating" partners competing. Link to major textile traders and stitcher associations. Involve community-based distributors and open markets.	Increase net sales to 5 million by 2007, including conical and long-lasting ITNs (LLINs). Make ITNs available in all five major open markets to supply the other open markets.
Supply and Quality Increase Nigerian net and ITN production capacity, quality, and variety.	Improve quality control. Provide data on consumer preferences (e.g., size, shape, colors, price, etc.). Introduce conical nets. Develop local LLIN production capacity. Get stitcher associations to package their nets with ITN kits.	Raise net production to 5 million by 2007 and transfer LLIN technology to at least one company.
Demand and Use Increase consumer demand and appropriate ITN use.	Increase demand and use for all ITNs in the market. Increase use and demand for partner brands. Increase use by high-risk groups. Use behavioral research to understand barriers and motivators for ITN use.	Have an additional 19 million Nigerians sleeping under an ITN by 2007 (1.5 people per 1 ITN).
Equity Demonstrate models for targeted subsidies.	Provide subsidies for high-risk groups. Provide commercial discount voucher. Obtain corporate sponsorships. Help with free ITN distributions using local partners.	Allow for 120,000 pregnant women to buy an ITN with vouchers. Distribute 120,000 ITNs for free using local partners.

NetMark's goal was to try to create a sustainable commercial market for ITNs with Nigerian companies procuring, packaging, distributing, and marketing a variety of ITN brands at competitive prices through ever-expanding sales networks, thus increasing the availability of ITNs throughout the country. To do this, the commercial firms needed a ready supply of quality ITNs, retail networks that reached a wide swath of the public, and strong consumer demand that could grow and sustain the market. NetMark and its commercial and communication partners would have to achieve major changes in the knowledge, attitudes, and behaviors of the three key target audiences.

1. Families with children under 5 and pregnant women would have to:
   - Understand that malaria is solely caused by mosquitoes.
   - Understand that ITNs can prevent malaria by repelling or killing malaria-carrying mosquitoes.
   - Understand that pregnant women and children under 5 are most likely to get life-threatening cases of malaria and, therefore, need to be protected.
   - Believe that ITNs are safe and effective.
   - Believe that purchasing an ITN is a good investment.
2. Public sector policy makers would have to:
   - Recognize that having the commercial sector invest in the ITN market would be an important addition to the public health effort to reduce malaria.
   - Believe that a facilitating environment is needed to encourage companies to invest in the marketing of ITNs (e.g., removing tax and tariffs on imported ITNs so they can be sold at affordable prices; segment markets for commercial, subsidized, and free ITNs; open up tender market to local companies).
   - Recognize that programs based on free and subsidized ITNs should be coordinated with commercial sector activities to prevent undermining them.
   - Prevent leakage of subsidized product into commercial markets.
   - Recognize that the public sector does not have the ability to make the commercial sector successful—but it does have the power to kill it.
3. Distributors/retailers would have to:
   - Believe that ITNs could be marketed profitably.
   - Invest in procurement, distribution, and marketing of ITNs.
   - Expand current distribution and retail networks to reach increasing numbers of the high-risk population, particularly in peri-urban and rural areas.

TARGET AUDIENCE BARRIERS, MOTIVATORS (BENEFITS), AND COMPETITION

Barriers for Consumers

Affordability

Were ITNs priced in a range that made sense to consumers (US$4.00 to US$6.00)? Before NetMark started, there was anecdotal information that untreated nets were sometimes selling for more than US$30 in some parts of the country. NetMark's pricing study that showed photos of potential products to consumers revealed that people thought US$4.40 was a reasonable price for a "theoretical product" consisting of a net with an insecticide treatment. Consumers were already spending a considerable portion of their income on malaria prevention and treatment. They had to be convinced that an ITN would prevent malaria and save them money.

Availability

Were ITNs available for sale in the markets where these consumers shopped? ITNs were not available before NetMark started. In addition, market research showed that most people purchased their nets in open markets—not in shops or pharmacies. Therefore, NetMark undertook a study of the open market network to see how it could be penetrated.

Safety

Was the insecticide safe, particularly for babies who might suck on the netting? Research showed that public education using credible voices could overcome this concern.

Heat

Did the net make it hotter and therefore more difficult to sleep? Some people felt that sleeping under a net made them feel warmer. This was particularly seen as a problem in the hot season when mosquitoes were in abundance. Most locally stitched nets were made from textiles like curtain material and not from actual mosquito netting. NetMark's research showed that Nigerians were more likely to cite heat as a barrier compared to consumers in the four other countries surveyed.

Modern Product

Weren't nets an old way of dealing with mosquitoes while aerosols and coils are the modern way? This feeling was much more prevalent in Nigeria than in other

NetMark countries. The education emphasized that ITNs were "new" products with a special insecticide designed to kill mosquitoes (the feature of aerosols that consumers liked best).

Insect Control

Will it kill mosquitoes so there are fewer in my house to deal with? NetMark's research showed that killing power was the prime feature that consumers sought in an insect control device—and the main reason they purchased aerosols. Therefore, a main campaign theme was "Mosquitoes Kill—Kill Mosquitoes."

Barriers for Public Sector

Among some policy makers, there was an innate distrust of the commercial sector and a strong feeling that public health goods should be free to people—particularly the poorest people. There was reluctance to have people pay for a life-saving product and an uneasy feeling that businesses would be profiting. There was also a lack of understanding of the pricing structure and the cost of bringing an ITN into a local shop. Many public sector people only saw the price of an ITN in official bids for tens of thousands of nets delivered to Lagos port; they did not understand the heavy costs of moving nets from port to shop shelf (e.g., storage, transport, credit costs, and distributor and retailer margins). Some desired to keep large procurements in government hands.

Barriers for Distributors/Retailers/Manufacturers

Businesspeople had to be convinced that a retail market did exist for ITNs and that people would buy them in enough quantities to create a sustainable market. There was concern about the turnaround time from procurement to consumer sale so that they could pay off the 90- to 100-day letters of credit used to purchase imported ITNs. Many retailers were reluctant to pay up-front for an unproven product and asked for a small stock of ITNs on consignment (payment following sale). Retailers' reluctance worried distributors who could not afford to put a large number of ITNs into shops without some prepayment. Distributors also felt pressure from NetMark's constant push to expand their sales networks into new shops. NetMark helped the distributors and suppliers arrange longer and larger terms of credit.

Motivators and Perceived Benefits

For consumers, the motivations for purchasing an ITN ranged from getting a good night's sleep to protecting themselves against malaria to avoiding the cost of treating malaria cases and the number of days lost by illness.

For policy makers, the motivators were to improve the public health of their citizenry, decrease the number of malaria cases, and reduce the amount of health funding that was being spent on malaria treatment.

For distributors and retailers, the motivators were to add another product line that would increase income and profit. For some, there was also the pride of being involved in selling a life-saving product. Everyone knew someone who had been ill or died from malaria. Once the sales of ITNs picked up, some retailers felt that the ITN campaign brought more consumers into their shops—who then bought other products.

Competition

In the marketplace, the main competitors in the insect-control category were aerosols and coils, seen by many as modern products. They also were cheaper per unit. Aerosols were plentiful and cost between US$2.25 and US$3.00 per can (sufficient for two weeks), and a pack of 10 mosquito coils was US$0.75. Some street vendors even sold single coils. For low-income families, the cost of an ITN for US$4.50 to US$7.00 was a considerable expense that required time for thought and saving before purchase. In 2001, the insect control market was dominated by aerosols, with 60% of households claiming to buy an aerosol product as their most common anti-mosquito product and 36% buying mosquito coils. Coil usage was higher in rural areas while aerosol usage was biased toward urban areas (Research International, 2001).

The main competition to commercial ITNs, however, was really the free and subsidized ITNs provided by donor and government programs. If not well managed and targeted, these ITNs would undermine commercial sales. In some cases, ITNs purchased with public sector funds "leaked" into the commercial market and were sold at very low prices. The threat of massive free distributions made distributors very wary of building up a large inventory of ITNs in their warehouses and retail networks and made retailers reluctant to put the product in their shops and see demand disappear if free or highly subsidized ITNS entered their area.

POSITIONING STATEMENT

As the host of the African Summit on Roll Back Malaria in April 2000, Nigeria fully adopted the Abuja Declaration goal of having:

> at least 60% of those at risk of malaria, particularly pregnant women and children under five years of age, benefit from the most suitable combination of

personal and community protective measures such as insecticide treated mosquito nets and other interventions which are accessible and affordable to prevent infection and suffering.

Few countries met this goal by 2005; however, funding for millions of free long-lasting insecticide-treated nets has since been flowing to many countries. RBM's Global Malaria Action Plan now establishes a target of 80% coverage by 2010.

CAMPAIGN STRATEGIES (4Ps), IMPLEMENTATION, AND EVALUATION

Product Strategies and Implementation

NetMark's first year was spent on conducting quantitative and qualitative consumer research in its first set of countries and building relationships with the USAID missions, ministries of health, national malaria control programs, commercial firms, and donor organizations involved in ITNs.

Insecticide-treated nets (ITNs) consist of a mosquito net packaged with an insecticide treatment kit. Consumers purchase the ITN and treat it at home by mixing the insecticide with 500 milliliters of water in a bucket and dipping the net until it absorbs almost all of the mixture. The insecticide is effective in repelling or killing the anopheles mosquito for 6 to 12 months (depending on the insecticide product) or three washes. Each wash depletes the insecticide until it no longer meets the World Health Organization (WHO) standard of 90% mortality for anopheles mosquitoes landing on it. An untreated net provides an effective barrier to mosquitoes, although they may bite an arm pressed against the netting or find their way inside a net through a small hole. A treated net is twice as effective in preventing malaria because it kills mosquitoes that land on it and repels others. Over the course of NetMark, ITN technology has evolved: (1) factory-made, long-lasting insecticide-treated nets (LLINs) have been introduced that maintain their killing power for at least 20 washes; (2) LLIN treatment kits became available to convert an untreated net into an LLIN; and (3) production of polyethylene LLINs with the insecticide incorporated into the yarn has greatly increased. In this chapter, ITNs will also refer to LLINs, and the marketing of insecticide kits will not be covered.

Pricing Strategies and Implementation

ITN prices were set by the supplier, distributor, and retailer. NetMark's only restrictions were that there had to be a range of products (varying in size, color, and shape) with most pricing within the range likely to attract Nigerian consumers

(US$5 to US$7); it discouraged any ITNs/LLINs priced over US$10. At least once a year, NetMark reviewed the pricing strategies for each brand with the brand owner and its distributors. Distributors and retailers were generally very price-sensitive and tried to keep their profit margin low, so they could build a market. During the 2002–2008 period, the ITNs sold by NetMark's commercial partners ranged from a single "student size" bundled ITN for US$4 to an extra-large family LLIN for US$12.

To achieve the goal of equity, NetMark replicated its model of targeted subsidies. This model was developed in Zambia when NetMark saw that public-sector subsidy programs spent a large portion of their scarce funds on procuring, storing, and distributing ITNs through the health clinics—thus using scarce funds for the logistics of the program and lessening the amount available for ITNs. To some extent, these programs also undermined the growth of a commercial market by taking potential customers away. NetMark devised a strategy of giving discount vouchers to specific target audiences through the public health system for redemption at commercial shops, thereby putting the logistics burden on the commercial sector that already possessed the skills and infrastructure to distribute large amounts of ITNs and manage the voucher redemption process. The public sector focused on what it did best—identifying those at risk and providing them with malaria counseling and a voucher, while the logistics of the ITNs was left to the private sector. Voucher recipients went to local shops prestocked with a variety of ITNs by NetMark partners and selected the size, shape, color, and price range of ITN they wanted. Almost always, families purchased the largest ITN they could afford—not the cheapest one. The Zambia pilot provided vouchers and counseling to pregnant women attending antenatal clinics and achieved a 70% redemption rate. It was replicated in other countries, including Nigeria, where funding was obtained from ExxonMobil to support two voucher programs. These programs distributed more than 180,000 vouchers to pregnant women and families with children under age 5, and 161,000 (89%) were redeemed for ITNs. The voucher program was well received by all involved. Parents were able to purchase an ITN at a 50% discount; health staff were able to provide their clients with a tangible benefit that immediately started to reduce the number of malaria cases in their clinics; retailers were more willing to stock ITNs, knowing that there was a nearby customer base and soon found that voucher customers bought other items in their stores; and distributors found that vouchers made it easier to recruit local retailers and provided a reliable level of sales if they were active in stocking shops near the clinics and promoting their brand.

NetMark was also asked by USAID and other agencies to distribute free ITNs to very poor rural populations. Working with the commercial partners,

NetMark helped set up four major distribution programs that provided 885,000 ITNs and LLINs in very poor districts. These free ITNs provided immediate relief from malaria while also serving as "free samples" to stimulate the market and increase appreciation for the ITN product line.

Place Strategies and Implementation

The Nigerian distributors represented a range of distribution networks, including agro-chemical shops, pharmaceutical outlets, textile stores, and food markets. NetMark continually pushed the distributors to expand these networks and to find new ones. One distributor signed agreements with several states to place a small kiosk on the grounds of their main health clinics to sell its ITNs. When research showed that the majority of Nigerians purchased their current nets in the open markets, NetMark studied the open-market system and identified five giant open markets that supplied most of the open markets throughout the country. NetMark and its partners recruited retailers in these open markets and tracked down the stitcher associations (one with 200 members) that supplied these markets with nets. The stitchers produced more nets per year (5 to 6 million) than the formal manufacturers (1 to 1.5 million). Seeing this potential, NetMark linked the largest stitcher associations to a supply of WHO-standard netting, arranged for insecticide kits at a special introductory discount, and gave them heat-sealing machines, so their nets and insecticide kits could be bundled in plastic bags. In the first year of this effort, the stitcher associations sent more than 648,000 ITNs into the open markets, where NetMark's demand creation efforts were causing shoppers to ask for ITNs. In 2008, they produced 2.1 million.

Promotion Strategies and Implementation

When NetMark's baseline survey was conducted from September to November 2000, public awareness of ITNs among households with children under age 5 was only 6%. Many people knew of mosquito nets and malaria, but many also thought that nets were an old way of mosquito control and that aerosols and mosquito controls were the modern means. The NetMark demand creation effort ran on two tracks: (1) a NetMark-run "generic" communication campaign that utilized integrated media channels (such as TV, radio, billboards, posters, and point-of-purchase materials such as the store poster shown in Figure 9-1) and interpersonal communication (such as road shows, clinic counseling, "town storming" to recruit retailers, and "cash vans" selling directly to shops) to deliver messages derived from NetMark's extensive market research; and (2) brand promotion carried out by each of the brand owners/distributors. The generic campaign carried key messages such as the night-biting mosquito is the sole carrier

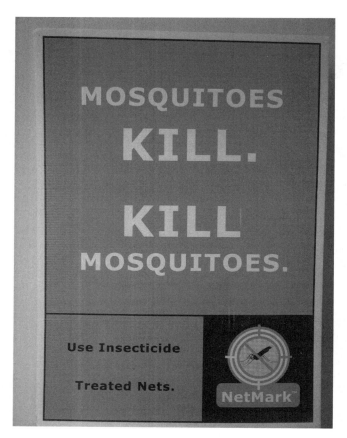

FIGURE 9-1   Generic Point-of-Sale Poster

of malaria and the importance of ITNs for preventing malaria, especially for pregnant women and children under 5. This campaign was meant to generate demand for the entire ITN product category—not just for partner brands—and increase the sales of all ITNs. A link to the partner brands was made by the use of the NetMark logo (called a "seal of quality") on the packaging of partner ITNs and on point-of-sale materials developed by NetMark for its partners. Brand promotion strategies and materials were usually developed by the brand owners (e.g., Bayer, Vestergaard) and provided directly to their distributors. Because brand marketing budgets are generally derived from a percentage of sales, NetMark knew there would be limited funds for brand marketing in the early years when sales and revenue were low. To stimulate a rapid roll-out of the brands, NetMark created a "matching funds" process for the support of brand promotion. Each year, NetMark helped the brand owner and national distributors finalize their annual country marketing plans. Based on their plans for expanding distribution beyond its current network, NetMark agreed to reimburse specific costs up to a ceiling of US$20,000 to US$50,000. The brand owners and distributors paid for such costs as additional sales staff to recruit and supply new outlets, radio spots, point-of-sale materials, and in-store promotions; they were reimbursed by NetMark for half of the cost up to the ceiling amount.

NetMark worked closely with a regional advertising agency to develop a core set of high-quality communications materials (e.g., two TV commercials, four radio spots, newspaper ads, and numerous point-of-sale materials) to launch ITN campaigns in all countries. Staff from the agency's affiliates in

NetMark countries were involved in the development of these materials and pretested them in their countries. While the TV commercials (in English and French) were fixed, the radio spots were meant to be translated into local languages and adapted to suit local situations. Affiliates produced additional radio spots in local languages. Point-of-sale materials were common across countries; however, generic materials were gradually replaced by brand materials. Signs for shops selling NetMark ITNs were sized according to local standards. A large pricing chart for group discussions was used to illustrate the annual cost of using coils, aerosols, and ITNs. For voucher programs, malaria counseling cards were produced for clinic staff to educate women about malaria, ITNs, and the voucher process.

Other Strategies and Implementation

Policy

NetMark did not initiate commercial activities in Nigeria until April 2002, mainly because the tariff on imported nets was more than 25%. In 2000, Nigerian President Obasanjo convened an Africa Summit on Roll Back Malaria attended by 17 heads of state from the 49 malaria-affected countries and territories in Africa. High-ranking officials from 26 other countries attended, along with representatives from the major donor agencies. The summit endorsed RBM's goals for reducing malaria and most countries signed the Abuja Declaration with its resolution to "reduce or waive taxes and tariffs for mosquito nets and materials, insecticides, anti-malarial drugs and other recommended goods and services that are needed for malaria control strategies" (RBM, 2000). Some countries like Tanzania and Zambia immediately acted on this commitment, but Nigeria was slower to do so. It finally cut its tariff from 25% to 5% in 2002, thereby paving the way for NetMark's commercial partners to launch activities.

Partners

In Nigeria, NetMark started with Bayer, Aventis, Vestergaard Frandsen, Siamdutch, and A-Z Textiles as the multinational suppliers, which then recruited national distributors. As the program grew and adapted to changes in the environment, other distributors and brand owners were added. They varied in size and type of core business (including pharmaceuticals, foodstuffs, agrochemicals, and textiles). One of the smaller distributors ultimately outsold all the others because it focused much of its energy and investment on its ITN business while the larger companies divided their time and attention among a number of product lines that brought in larger profits than ITNs.

For demand creation, NetMark used competitive bidding to select the Africa division of Foote, Cone, & Belding (FCB), a multinational advertising agency. FCB had a broad network of African-owned affiliates in more than 20 sub-Saharan countries and a history of helping those affiliates improve their skills and capabilities through periodic training activities. Group Africa, a company specializing in product promotion and market development through consumer education and mobilization, was already a member of the AED team that won the NetMark contract. It had its own offices in more than 25 countries, including a range of vehicles and promotional staff skilled in carrying out road shows, educational programs in schools and health facilities, and other product promotion activities. In Nigeria, NetMark worked closely with Centrespead FCB, an advertising and public relations firm, and with Group Africa's Nigeria office. Both worked together with NetMark staff and commercial partners on the marketing plans.

Production

One of the major issues affecting the Nigeria program was the source of the ITNs to be sold by the commercial sector. The MOH strongly pushed for the exclusive use of locally produced nets because Nigeria had the only net-production capacity in West Africa and a large textile industry under siege by Chinese imports. NetMark favored using local nets, but found their quality was poor and that local net manufacturers were very passive about developing the net market and improving quality. When asked to show their nets to NetMark's commercial partners, only a few showed up—and one sample net had holes in it. The commercial partners could not launch a new product under their brand name with a poor-quality net and decided to start with high-quality imported nets to break into the market.

There was also a sensitive issue of production capacity. The MOH presented a three-page listing of "net manufacturers" that claimed a total annual production of millions of nets. This capacity was not real. Most production projections were based on a theoretical capacity and not a realistic assessment. The list of "manufacturers" also contained a number of companies that had no production capacity. After a British aid employee reported that many of those companies were importers and that actual net production was only about 1 million nets per year, the MOH finally admitted that there was an important role for imports. NetMark brought two textile experts to Nigeria to visit the factories of the six largest manufacturers and to provide them with confidential assessments on how they could improve net quality. Some problems were fixed as the experts moved through the factory; other changes were made after the report; but no manufacturer made an intensive effort to improve quality by addressing all recommendations made in the assessment.

The ITN campaign was formally launched in April 2002, with imported nets bundled with insecticide kits and one pretreated ITN; however, this strategy was upended when President Obasanjo and his cabinet surprisingly voted in July to increase the tariff on textiles (including nets) to 75%. This virtually ended imports as a source of quality nets. One distributor (one of the largest companies in the country) was awaiting a shipment of 50,000 ITNs and canceled his order when the ship was three days from Lagos port—and the manufacturer diverted the shipment to Togo. That distributor then halted his plans to sell ITNs because he wanted to market a premium-quality product and did not want to rely on locally produced nets. Thus, NetMark and Vestergaard Frandsen lost a distributor with a national distribution network and more than 1,500 delivery vehicles.

To facilitate the use of local nets, NetMark convened a meeting of 24 net manufacturers, insecticide suppliers, and distributors to foster partnerships and challenge net manufacturers to increase the quality, quantity, and variety of their nets. NetMark also presented multicountry data showing the popularity of conical nets, which were not produced in Nigeria. The distributors noted that their imported conical nets sold very quickly. NetMark offered to teach the manufacturers how to make conical nets; two distributors offered to buy them if a local company could produce a quality product. Two manufacturers agreed to produce some prototypes if they were provided with samples. Within six weeks, both manufacturers sent the distributors conical nets. Within a year, four manufacturers were producing conical nets for the first time ever in Nigeria. In 2005 and 2007, NetMark involved Nigerian net manufacturers in workshops on LLIN production, and in 2008, the largest net manufacturer decided to install an LLIN treatment process developed by NetMark and started producing LLINs in 2009.

CAMPAIGN BUDGET AND TIME FRAME

NetMark received approximately US$1 million per year from USAID/Nigeria with supplemental support coming from the NetMark core budget for regional staff time and the design and production of the initial campaign materials—radio and TV spots, newspaper ads, and point-of-sale materials. The time frame for the project changed twice. NetMark was originally timed to run through September 2004. USAID/Nigeria put funds into NetMark one year at a time, with verbal commitments to maintain that funding until 2004. When NetMark was extended to September 2007 and then September 2009, USAID Nigeria agreed to continue funding its activities. From 2001 to 2008 NetMark received a total of $9,993,250 from USAID/Nigeria (see Table 9-2

TABLE 9-2   NetMark/Nigeria Funding 2001–2008

Project Component	Expenditures (US$)	Percentage of Budget
Management and administration	$2,114,795	21.16
Advertising/promotions/distribution	3,095,222	30.97
Research/evaluation	766,379	7.67
Market impact studies	570,841	5.71
Program development	598,510	5.99
Policy/advocacy	73,025	0.73
Vouchers/free ITNs	2,609,728	26.11
Technical assistance manufacturing	164,264	1.64
Total	**$9,992,764**	

for details). In addition, ExxonMobil contributed US$400,000 to fund two discount voucher programs for pregnant women. The commercial partners invested approximately $10 million over the same period in product, staff, and the marketing of their own brands. None of those funds went through NetMark.

RESULTS

NetMark conducted a baseline survey of 1,000 households with children under 5 in five states in 2000; because of the government delay in reducing the tariff from 25% to 5%, it did not launch the ITN products and communications until May 2002. During that period, no major ITN activities were carried out in Nigeria by the government or donors, and only very limited demand activities occurred. A second survey that encompassed 2,000 households was conducted in 2004, and a final survey was conducted in late 2008. All three surveys were conducted during the rainy season (September–October). Some of the key findings from those studies (with preliminary results from 2008) are presented in Table 9-3 (NetMark, 2001, 2005).

As anticipated, there was a great increase in public awareness of ITNs rising from 6% at baseline in 2000 to virtually 100% in late 2008. NetMark was by far

TABLE 9-3   NetMark Household Survey Results

Household Indicators	2000	2004	2008
Awareness of ITNs	6%	59%	100%
Households owning any bed net (treated or untreated)	10	26	29
Households owning an ITN	0	7	20
Urban households owning an ITN	0	5	23
Rural households owning an ITN	0	8	18
Pregnant women sleeping under a net the previous night	6	15	14
Pregnant women sleeping under an ITN the previous night	0	4	10
Child under 5 sleeping under a net the previous night	8	10	13
Child under 5 sleeping under an ITN the previous night	0	2	9

the largest investor in ITN promotion in Nigeria over that period, starting with its media launch in 2002. During this time, the commercial partners increased their brand marketing each year, and other organizations occasionally promoted ITN use. As usual, the actual use of nets and ITNs lagged behind awareness; however, ITN use steadily increased over this period. While the use of ITNs by pregnant women and children has registered significant increases, overall net use has not increased at the same pace, indicating that many of the ITN users are those who used to sleep under an untreated net. NetMark's baseline research had shown that Nigerians were more negative about using nets compared to people in other NetMark countries. Given the size of Nigeria's population and the fact that it has grown by 23 million since 2000, more resources need to be applied to ITN promotion. NetMark's resources were very modest compared to the target population.

REACH OF THE COMMERCIAL SECTOR

The data did show that the commercial sector played a powerful role in making nets available to consumers: in 2004, 80% of respondents reported that they got their nets or ITNs from a commercial outlet. Obviously, the commercial sector was the main source of the nets owned by households in every economic quintile (see Figure 9-2).

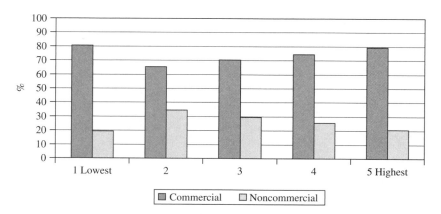

FIGURE 9-2   Sources of Nets for all Socioeconomic Quintiles

The data, however, also showed that net and ITN ownership increased in every economic quintile. In some countries where public sector distribution of ITNs dominates, the richer quintiles sometimes obtain more ITNs than the poorer segments (see Figure 9-3).

A survey of the five largest open markets—the ones that provide most of the nets to the entire open-market system—showed that ITNs were now available in all of them as opposed to one of five in 2002 when NetMark first began studying the open-market system.

Sales of ITNs were tracked by NetMark's formal partners (those holding a signed agreement with NetMark and receiving direct marketing support) and

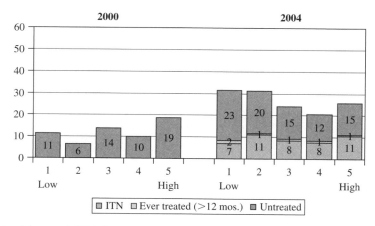

FIGURE 9-3   Net and ITN Ownership among all Socioeconomic Quintiles

TABLE 9-4   Number of ITNs Sold by NetMark Formal Partners

2002	2003	2004	2005	2006	2007	2008
167,914	270,210	648,452	1,312,040	2,611,227	3,479,283	6,055,846

informal partners (those who benefited from the generic advertising and other NetMark activities but were willing to report their sales to NetMark even though they had no signed agreement; see Table 9-4).

SUMMARY

There are many lessons to be learned from NetMark's Nigeria experience. One of the welcome surprises was discovering how well the commercial sector was already reaching the poorest segments of the population. NetMark began with the premise that it would see how far down the economic spectrum the commercial sector could reach; it was pleasantly surprised to see that in most countries, the commercial sector was already getting nets to all economic levels. It was on the ground before the public sector took on the challenge of malaria and hopefully will continue to serve those markets when the current wave of donor funding inevitably shifts away from ITNs to other emerging health problems or solutions (e.g., an HIV/AIDS or malaria vaccine). One of the major limitations of local businesses, however, is finding the capital and credit to serve a large and growing national market.

The Nigeria project once again reaffirmed the necessity of paying attention to all components of the marketing mix: the 4Ps and beyond. Changes are bound to happen and surprises are bound to occur—particularly in projects in developing countries. Although a plan may be thorough, well reasoned, and optimal (at least at launch time), program implementers need to be flexible and creative in responding to changing conditions. These changes may be subtle ones detected by a good monitoring system generating accurate data. Others may hit you in the face as when a tariff increases from 5% to 75% overnight.

In developing public–private partnerships, there is an important need for a catalyst that can bring the two sectors together and help them create a win–win situation in which both sides can achieve their goals. Oftentimes, there is a need for a party that understands the motivations and capabilities of both sides and the inherent tensions of these relationships. The public sector is eager to move ahead to address an urgent health problem where lives may be at stake. In a life-or-death situation, public officials are willing to take risks and not worry so much about cost versus benefit. The commercial sector, however, plays with its own money—not public funds. It needs to slowly build its business while continually watching the bottom line. If a public sector program fails, another program is created to take its place. If a commercial venture fails, people lose their jobs and the company may go bankrupt. This difference gives rise to very different perspectives.

Nigeria also points out the need for a close relationship between implementer and client. The best situation is when the client and implementer function as a team, both focusing on the overall goals with ongoing and frank discussions about the steps ahead. When the inevitable problems occur, the "team" is more likely to surmount them.

In designing and implementing projects in developing countries, in particular, there are only two things to worry about: the things you can control and the things you cannot. Keeping an eye on both with regular monitoring and adapting to changing circumstances is the only way to achieve success.

The NetMark Nigeria project resulted in 14 million ITNs getting into households and protecting at least 21 million people from malaria. Even more important was that this was accomplished through educating consumers and building a commercial infrastructure and investment pattern that will keep supplying the fight against malaria for as long as the fight needs to be waged.

QUESTIONS FOR DISCUSSION

1. What are some of the inherent tensions in creating and maintaining public–private partnerships for the marketing of a health product? How can you find a win–win situation as the basis for a public–private partnership?
2. What are the pros and cons of balancing sustainability (e.g., systematically building a viable market for ITNs) and achieving quick public health impact (e.g., distributing millions of free ITNs)? What can be done to balance cost recovery and equity?
3. NetMark decided it had to go far beyond the 4Ps in order to succeed in Nigeria. Under what conditions should a social marketing program go beyond the 4Ps? What are the risks, rewards, and other factors to consider?

REFERENCES

Central Intelligence Agency (CIA). (2008). *The World Factbook*. Nigeria. Retrieved January 3, 2009, from www.cia.gov/library/publications/the-world-factbook/

Central Intelligence Agency (CIA). (2009). *The World Factbook*. Retrieved July 28, 2009, from www.cia.gov/library/publications/the-world-factbook/

NetMark. (2000). *NetMark regional Africa program briefing book: Insecticide-treated materials in Nigeria* (internal document).

NetMark. (2001). *Baseline survey on insecticide-treated materials.* Retrieved July 28, 2009, from www.netmarkafrica.org

NetMark. (2005). *2004 survey on insecticide-treated nets (ITNs).* Retrieved July 28, 2009, from www.netmarkafrica.org

Research International. (2001). *Microtest research report.* NetMark (internal document).

Roll Back Malaria (RBM). (2000). *The Abuja declaration and plan of action.* Retrieved July 28, 2009, from http://rbm.who.int/docs/abuja_declaration.pdf

Roll Back Malaria (RBM). (2008). *Economic costs of malaria.* Retrieved July 28, 2009, from www.rbm.who.int/cmc_upload

CHAPTER 10

"Safe Water Saves Lives"

Clean Drinking Water Reduces Diarrhea-Related Mortality in Madagascar

Steven W. Honeyman

MADAGASCAR: A COUNTRY OVERVIEW

Madagascar is a lush island nation in the Indian Ocean, east of Mozambique, with a wealth of biodiversity. Situated off the southeastern coast of Africa, nearly 60% of the island's 300 bird species, about 90% of its 13,000 plant species, and 96% of its nearly 400 reptile species are found nowhere else in the world (Conservation International, 2009). Madagascar has a diverse history as well. Formerly an independent kingdom, Madagascar became a French colony in 1896 and regained independence in 1960. With National Assembly and presidential elections in 1997, 17 years of single-party rule ended.

Madagascar is the fourth largest island in the world at 587,040 square kilometers, almost twice the size of Arizona, with a population of 19.4 million people (World Bank, 2008). There are more than 18 different ethnic groups; the official languages are Malagasy, French, and English. The major religions are indigenous beliefs (52%), Christianity (41%), and Islam (7%; Central Intelligence Agency [CIA], 2009).

Health and Social Indicators

More than 85% of the population of Madagascar lives on less than US$2.00 per day (Government of Madagascar, 2007) with half of the population falling below the poverty line. Strikingly, 88% of the rural population lack access to safe drinking water and only 36% of children age 12–23 months have been fully immunized—factors that contribute to the deaths of an estimated 100,000 children each year (UNICEF, 2005). Literacy rates are low, and only 68.9% of the population are able to read (UNICEF, 2005). Leading causes of death and disability include malaria, sexually transmitted infections (STIs), diarrheal diseases, and adverse conditions arising from pregnancy and birth (USAID, 2005). Despite these challenges, rates of infant and child mortality have declined by more than 40% between 1997 and 2004 (USAID, 2005). These successes can be attributed to highly effective public health interventions by the government of Madagascar, donors, and nongovernmental organization (NGO) development partners. During the same time period, there was a 50% decrease in the prevalence of diarrhea and a doubling of the percentage of those with diarrhea who received either oral rehydration salts (ORS) or a homemade diarrhea treatment solution. In spite of this notable progress, diarrheal disease morbidity and mortality, especially in young children, remains a leading public health issue across Madagascar.

UNSAFE WATER-RELATED GLOBAL DIARRHEAL DISEASE BURDEN

Today, more than a billion people worldwide lack access to improved water sources. It is estimated that 1.9 million children worldwide die every year due to diarrhea (Bryce, Boschi-Pinto, Shibuya, Black, WHO Child Health Epidemiology Reference Group, 2005). High levels of child mortality continue to burden many countries around the world, with diarrheal disease as the second leading cause of death among children under age 5. Each day, nearly 5,000 children die from dehydration due to infectious diarrhea.

Unsafe drinking water contaminated by microbiological pathogens is a major contributor to diarrheal disease. About 88% of diarrheal disease is attributed to unsafe water supply, inadequate sanitation, and poor hygiene practices (WHO, 2005). This not only leads to negative health effects, but also carries significant other human and economic costs. A total of 443 million school days are lost each year from water-related illnesses (UN Development Program, 2006). Sub-Saharan Africa loses about 5% of gross domestic product (GDP; some US$28.4 billion annually) from costs related to diarrheal disease.

GLOBAL TRENDS IN HOUSEHOLD WATER TREATMENT

Since 1996, a growing body of research has examined the health impact of interventions to improve household water treatment and safe storage (HWTS; Fewtrell, Kaufman, Kay, Enanoria, Haller, et al., 2005). The results of these studies, including several randomized controlled intervention trials, have highlighted the public health implications of post-source contamination of drinking water during collection, transport, and storage and the health value of effective HWTS (Luby, et al., 2004). A recent meta-analysis found that hygiene education and water quality interventions were effective in reducing diarrheal disease by 42% and 39%, respectively (Fewtrell & Colford, 2004).

In 2003, as the evidence base for the health benefits of HWTS methods accumulated, academic and government institutions, NGOs, and private sector organizations engaged in research and implementation of HWTS approaches formed the International Network to Promote Household Water Treatment and Safe Storage, with a secretariat hosted by the World Health Organization (WHO). Its stated goal is "to contribute to a significant reduction in waterborne disease, especially among vulnerable populations, by promoting household water treatment and safe storage as a key component of water, sanitation and hygiene programmes" (WHO, 2003). The network serves as a forum for professional collaboration and a technical resource for starting and implementing water treatment programs.

The four proven household water treatment options are chlorination, ceramic filtration, solar disinfection, and combined filtration/disinfection (Centers for Disease Control and Prevention [CDC], 2009). Chlorination was first used for disinfection of public water supplies in the early 1900s, contributing to dramatic reductions in waterborne disease in cities in the developed world.

Although small trials of point-of-use chlorination had been implemented, larger-scale trials only began in the 1990s as part of the Pan-American Health Organization and the CDC's response to epidemic cholera in Latin America. The CDC developed the Safe Water System (SWS), which included three elements:

1. A water treatment product consisting of a diluted sodium hypochlorite (chlorine) solution.
2. Storage of water in a safe container.
3. Education to improve hygiene and water use practices.

Although the chlorination treatment left a slight aftertaste, the process made water safe to drink in 30 minutes. In randomized controlled trials, use of the SWS resulted in a 44% to 84% reduction in the risk of diarrheal disease (Lantagne, 2006).

THE CDC-PSI PARTNERSHIP

In 1996, the CDC and the international nongovernmental organization Population Services International (PSI) began a strategic partnership to introduce the Safe Water System globally (see Box 10-1). The two organizations designed, piloted, and evaluated the first Safe Water System field project in Bolivia; CDC developed and tested the prototype, while PSI fielded the first commercial application. Controlled trials found that use of the SWS significantly reduced the incidence of diarrhea under field conditions. The field trial led to 44% fewer diarrhea episodes in intervention versus control households (Quick, Venczel, Mintz, Soleto, Aparicio, et al., 1999). PSI, with continuing technical support from the CDC, has since applied the lessons learned from the Bolivia pilot program to expand social marketing of the SWS throughout much of the developing world.

BOX 10-1   Population Services International

PSI is a nonprofit organization that harnesses the vitality of the private sector to address the health problems of low-income and vulnerable populations in more than 60 developing countries. It promotes products, services, and healthy behavior in its malaria, reproductive health, child survival, HIV/AIDS, and tuberculosis programs that enable people to lead healthier lives. It engages private sector resources and uses private sector techniques to encourage healthy behavior and make markets work for the poor.

Core Values

1. The power of markets and market mechanisms to contribute to sustained improvements in the lives of the poor.
2. Results and a strong focus on measurement.
3. Speed and efficiency, with a predisposition to action and an aversion to bureaucracy.
4. Decentralization, empowering staff at the local level.
5. A long-term commitment to those served.

"Safe Water Saves Lives" Campaign

CAMPAIGN BACKGROUND AND RATIONALE

In 2000, following a cholera outbreak after one of the most devastating series of cyclones in more than 50 years, the government of Madagascar, PSI, CARE, and CDC partnered to introduce a Safe Water System (SWS) emergency response. Together, the partners recognized SWS as an essential tool to prepare communities against future cyclones, flooding, and other natural disasters.

In addition, the need for safe drinking water extended beyond natural calamities because the majority of Madagascar residents do not have access to improved drinking water. A Madagascar Ministry of Health survey in 2000 showed that some 75% of the population—up to 88% in rural areas—lacked access to an improved source of drinking water, placing them at significant risk of diarrheal disease (USAID, 2004). There are an estimated 119 deaths per year for every 1,000 children under the age of 5 in Madagascar (UNICEF, 2007), and approximately 20,000 under-5 deaths per year are related to diarrhea (Institut National de la Statistique and ORC Macro, 2005; Parashar, Hummelman, Bresee, Miller, & Glass, 2003). Large geographic and socioeconomic disparities exist. Under-5 mortality is 64% higher in rural as compared to urban areas; among the poorest 20% of the population, children are twice as likely to experience diarrhea and are nearly three times more likely to die before their fifth birthday than children from the wealthiest families (USAID, 2005).

The overall situation, emergency and nonemergency, led to the introduction of a low-cost and easy-to-use chlorination (sodium hypochlorite) product, expanding the program over the next nine years with UNICEF and USAID financial support.

CAMPAIGN PURPOSE AND FOCUS

The Madagascar national SWS program was launched to improve the health and nutritional status of Malagasy children by reducing the incidence and prevalence of diarrheal disease related to unsafe drinking water. The program was a public–private partnership among the government of Madagascar (Ministry of Mines and Water and the Ministry of Health and Family Planning), UNICEF, USAID, PSI, CARE International, Madagascar NGOs, and the private commercial sector. As a focus, the partners developed and promoted a home water treatment product and related health messages using social marketing techniques.

SWOT ANALYSIS

Since 1998, PSI has worked in partnership with the government of Madagascar to develop social marketing components in their national health programs. Registered as a local NGO, it implements a comprehensive social marketing program to address major public health issues such as family planning, HIV/AIDS, malaria, and diarrheal disease as identified by the government of Madagascar. Diverse financial support from government, multilateral, and private foundation donors has resulted in a nationwide program that reaches all 22 regions throughout the country, with more than 200 employees trained in public health, marketing, research, and communications. PSI Madagascar designs and manages large-scale behavior change programs that include the provision of a wide range of high-quality reproductive and maternal and child health products and services at affordable prices through commercial and community-based distribution channels.

PAST AND SIMILAR EFFORTS

In early 2000, PSI launched its first two large-scale safe water programs in Madagascar and Zambia in the midst of public health emergencies—cholera epidemics in both countries followed by cyclone emergencies in Madagascar. Due to ongoing demand for safe water programs in both countries after the emergencies were addressed, SWS initiatives were scaled up into successful national programs—still vibrant and growing today—promoting safe drinking water for everyday use.

PSI saw the early success of the two SWS programs in Madagascar and Zambia as an exciting new opportunity to apply social marketing techniques to a global public health challenge: morbidity and mortality related to diarrheal disease. At that time, it had offices in more than 50 countries and, in partnership with the CDC, embarked on a global initiative to launch the SWS in countries where social marketing techniques could potentially create large-scale behavior change related to improved home water treatment. PSI's expertise and experience had previously resided in the intervention areas of HIV/AIDS, family planning, and malaria. In the absence of donor funding and presented with the opportunity to create significant new health impact with a global SWS program, PSI decided to invest substantial levels of its funds to launch and scale up household water treatment programs. It hoped that in doing so, successful programs would subsequently attract long-term donor funding. By 2008, PSI was leading SWS programs in 25 developing countries using its unique style of social marketing. That style includes designing a brand name and logo for a health product or service; selling those products at subsidized or affordable prices through local commercial channels and other networks; and generating demand for the products and practices through large-scale, targeted, behavior change communications (BCC).

TARGET AUDIENCES

When the national SWS program was launched in 2000, there were two types of target audiences.

Primary Target Audience

The primary target audience was 15- to 49-year-old mothers/caregivers of children under the age of 5. The primary target audience was the intended purchasers and users of SWS in the home. PSI Madagascar's experience with other maternal and child health interventions such as insecticide-treated mosquito nets for malaria prevention indicated that mothers or caregivers of young children were the most likely consumers of a new child health product. Caregivers were added to the target audience in order to include grandmothers, aunts, and sisters, who, in traditional Malagasy culture, often become temporary or permanent caregivers for young children.

Secondary Target Audience

Government employees and policy makers were the secondary target audience. Government employees and policy makers were also targeted with communication messages to create knowledge of and support for the national SWS program.

CAMPAIGN BEHAVIORAL OBJECTIVE

The program had the behavioral objective of increasing correct and consistent use of a SWS product. The program intended to achieve this objective on a national scale and to measure the performance of the program against national health indicators.

PSI's Research and Metrics Department developed a social marketing project framework in 2004. The framework, called PERForM, describes the social marketing process, identifies key concepts important for designing, monitoring, and evaluating social marketing interventions, and mirrors the four levels and concepts of the logical framework (see Figure 10-1). The aim of PERFoRM is to summarize known determinants of behavior and the relationship between behavior and health in order to provide social marketers with timely, actionable information for decision making. PERFoRM can be categorized into four levels, which incrementally help to better understand and explain behavior change and health status:

1. Goal (i.e., health status and quality of life).
2. Purpose (i.e., use, risk-reducing behavior, and need).
3. Outputs (i.e., opportunity, ability, motivation, and population characteristics).
4. Activities (social marketing intervention and the 4Ps).

PSI uses the PERFoRM framework in a five-step, iterative process to guide the development, implementation, and evaluation of its social marketing efforts

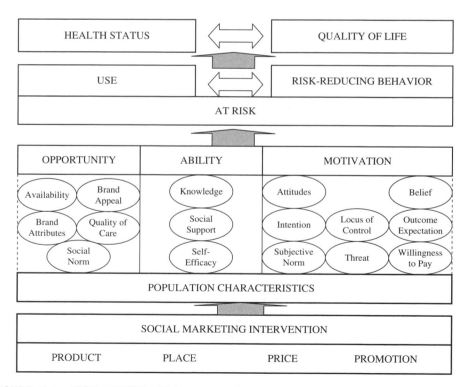

FIGURE 10-1 PSI's PERFoRM Framework

with the overall goal of changing behavior of target populations (Patel & Chapman, 2005).

PSI uses several PERForM research tools to plan, monitor, and evaluate its programs. One such tool is the Tracking Results Continuously (TRaC) survey, which informs programmers by routinely collecting data from cross-sections of populations at risk of adverse health outcomes. The data from these surveys provide information from populations about their behaviors, determinants of behaviors, risks, sources of supply of product or service delivery, and exposure to social marketing communication activities.

TARGET AUDIENCE BARRIERS, COMPETITION, AND MOTIVATORS (BENEFITS)

Barriers

There were many barriers for women, caregivers, and their families in treating water in their home. These barriers included lack of knowledge about diarrheal disease transmission, perceptions that the clarity of water indicated its safety, government sensitivity to criticism, and traditional forms of water gathering and use. At least one-third of Malagasy did not know that contaminated water causes diarrhea. Many believed that their water source was only unsafe during the rainy season and during cyclones, floods, and cholera episodes or that their water source has never been contaminated and therefore did not need treatment (PSI, 2007).

Other barriers to adopting home water treatment were the perceived costs. It was thought that significant time was needed to learn how to treat water. Materials were also needed, such as a vessel in which to treat and store clean water. Such additional financial costs deterred many from adopting a new practice.

In addition, a baseline TRaC survey was undertaken in 2004 and a follow-up survey in 2006 that found that self-efficacy, social norms, and availability were significant in determining the use of an SWS product by mothers and caregivers of children under 5. Self-efficacy represents the confidence an individual has in his or her ability to perform a promoted behavior effectively. Those who believe they can use SWS correctly were more likely to treat their water. Social norms are perceived standards for behavior that people follow. In other words, those who believe that others in their community use water treatment products are more likely to use them themselves. Finally, the product needed to be made widely available. A marketing intervention was designed to impact only those behavioral determinants known to positively influence use.

Competition

Competition from other behaviors and other water treatment options existed. Boiling had long remained a predominant home treatment for water. However, research had shown that on average water is not boiled long enough and re-contamination related to lack of residual protection and unsafe storage render the practice less effective than other water treatment methods (Clasen, McLaughlin, Nayaar, Boison, Gupta, et al., 2008). Solar disinfection (SODIS) and filtering are also used to treat water; however, the seasonality of the monsoon rains and longer treatment times (six hours or more), along with the added expense of a special container or filter, tend to make these types of treatment choices unpopular. The cost of one liter of bottled mineral water is half a day's wages for many workers, putting this form of safe drinking water out of the financial reach of most of the population.

Motivators

The Madagascar Action Plan calls for potable water to be made available to all citizens. Such commendable and ambitious policies and infrastructure plans often take decades to finance and construct. In the meantime, research indicated that the Malagasy population was open to trying a new home water treatment solution.

Research also indicated that many people knew contaminated water was causing family members to suffer from diarrhea, especially young children, yet still did not treat their water. The program team needed to find ways to motivate individuals in each community to begin changing their own behavior, which would eventually lead to communitywide changes.

A new and inexpensive water treatment system would find a significant consumer market if it met the needs of the consumer by (1) reducing the threat of diarrhea in the home, (2) being widely adopted as a new community behavioral norm, and (3) being an easily adoptable practice.

POSITIONING STATEMENT

The program developed the brand name Sûr'Eau and a positioning statement to clearly define how the product would be marketed to consumers. This would allow the marketing team to focus its efforts and resources on a common understanding of the consumer and the benefits offered by the Sûr'Eau brand. The positioning statement developed for Sûr'Eau is:

For conscientious mothers and caregivers wanting healthy children under age 5, Sûr'Eau is the easy-to-use and inexpensive home water treatment solution that gives safe water to whole the family. (PSI/Madagascar, 2006)

CAMPAIGN STRATEGIES (4Ps), IMPLEMENTATION, AND EVALUATION

In 2000, the team developed a plan to launch and scale up the new SWS product. They began by undertaking audience research to understand the target consumer and by creating product, pricing, packaging, and promotional strategies. As pioneers of household water treatment promotion and marketing, PSI had to depend on its own market research and expected to adjust the various program components—the marketing mix (4Ps)—as the program matured and valuable implementation, consumer research findings, and evaluation evidence came to light.

Product Strategies

Initially, following consumer research, the product strategy was to create a consumer good for home use in an economical "family size" and with attractive packaging. The packaging would include easy-to-use pictorial instructions to enable low-literate rural Malagasy to use the product. In 2000, PSI developed a product brand name, logo, and packaging for Sûr'Eau (pronounced "Syr-O" and meaning "safe water") water treatment. A 500-milliliter bottle with a cap that could be used for measuring out the chlorine solution was developed. A local private sector manufacturer was located and production of Sûr'Eau began. The only additional materials needed were a mixing pail and cloth, two inexpensive items that were locally available and normally found around the home (see Box 10-2).

The product was designed for ease of use and required three simple steps to correctly make water safe to drink (see Figure 10-2):

1. Add one cap of Sûr'Eau to one bucket of water.
2. Stir the mixture with a clean utensil.
3. Cover with a clean cloth and wait 30 minutes before using.

The product was designed to address one of the key behavioral determinants of use found through research—self-efficacy. By designing the product with self-efficacy in mind, the marketing team believed it would encourage use

BOX 10-2 **Getting the Product "P" Right in Uganda**

In contrast to Madagascar, PSI Uganda found developing the right product strategy a complex challenge. Selecting the right home water treatment and safe storage (HWTS) product for social marketing programs in developing countries often provides a difficult challenge. This is especially true in countries where the local context, differing health conditions, viability of the commercial marketplace, limited donor support, inadequate local marketing expertise, and other factors make product selection complex. HWTS has several competing proven treatment methods that all provide clean drinking water if used properly. These include chlorination (SWS), ceramic filtration, solar disinfection, and a combined flocculent/disinfectant (CDC, 2009).

PSI Uganda launched PUR (combined flocculent/disinfectant) in partnership with Procter & Gamble in November 2004. While the product was ideally fitted to the turbid water in rural areas of Uganda, it required simple but additional mixing equipment. This added cost to the product for transport and for communication on its use. In February 2005, a sodium hypochlorite solution (chlorine)—branded WaterGuard—was launched and targeted to those living with HIV/AIDS as a low-cost, easy-to-use, alternative water treatment method. WaterGuard solution was also easy to make but heavy to transport and, therefore, also more expensive. Finally, in December 2006, WaterGuard tablets were added to the marketing portfolio because they had less chlorine taste and because of the ease of use and lower cost of distribution and promotion. However, tabs still left some chlorine aftertaste and could not take the turbidity out of water.

Each of the HWTS products offers unique advantages and disadvantages. There is no one product that meets all the product needs of the Uganda water treatment marketplace. While on the surface it may seem that multiple product offerings in the same marketplace may be an inefficient use of public health resources, it is clear from the example of Uganda that public health interests might be best served by having multiple products available for different consumer segments or geographic areas of the marketplace. In this way, consumers are provided with options that they select given their personal situation and their own consumer preferences.

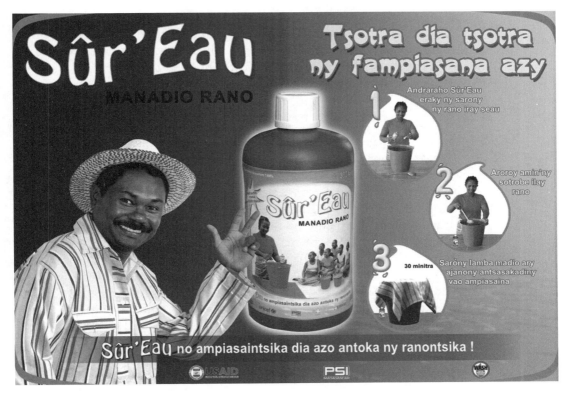

FIGURE 10-2   Sûr'Eau Demand Creation Poster on Self-Efficacy (It's as Easy as 1, 2, 3!)

of the product and make it easier for product use to become a societal norm—a second key behavioral determinant of use.

Pricing Strategies

Some social marketing research has provided evidence that the act of paying induces increased use of health products among households (Ashraf, Berry, & Shapiro, 2007). In a developing country like Madagascar, it is essential to establish a balance between product value and affordability to those who need it the most, especially low-income rural communities. Research was conducted in 2000 to determine the target audience's "willingness to pay." The determined pricing level required a substantial subsidy on the cost of manufacturing, distributing, and promoting the product to avoid a financial barrier to Sûr'Eau purchase and use. A key component of the pricing strategy was to select a price that was within the willingness of the consumer to pay while at the same time maximizing "cost recovery" to sustain the program. Too little subsidy would make the product unaffordable to the target audience, while too much subsidy would unnecessarily deplete program resources needed for other critical areas such as behavior change promotion (see Box 10-3).

Change in Product and Pricing Strategy 2004

Sûr'Eau sales averaged approximately 400,000 units per year from 2000 through 2003. However, the sales trend was flat, and program partners decided to reanalyze the price of Sûr'Eau as a potential barrier to use despite earlier willingness to pay research among target consumers.

PSI, CARE, and the CDC, under the guidance of the Ministry of Energy and Mines, and with financial and technical support from USAID, embarked on an eight-month project to increase the purchase and use of Sûr'Eau. The team conducted research that led to a major change in the product, its pricing, and its packaging. A smaller bottle prototype (150 milliliters versus the original 500 milliliters) was developed and went through two rounds of qualitative acceptability testing with consumers. Consumers indicated that the new bottle was more convenient and more affordable.

After a competitive bidding process, the selected private sector partner imported the customized injection mold from Germany and began production. The new bottle also required a higher concentration of sodium hypochlorite,

---

BOX 10-3   Making a Better Life for Her Community

Rahavana is a community-based sales agent in Madagascar associated with a faith-based organization called SALFA, in the commune of Shambavy. She received five days of training on key health issues and on the promotion of health products and healthier behaviors. She also received a starter stock of PSI's social marketed products: 5 bottles of Sûr'Eau, 5 insecticide-treated mosquito nets, 10 packets of birth control pills, and 48 condoms, all of which could be replenished at a subsidized price. Four weeks after she returned to her village, she had made a profit of more than 90,000 Aviary (US$50) for her family. This amount of money is a substantial addition to her family's income and provides motivation for her to work on improving the health of those in her community.

and the CDC provided technical assistance to the local manufacturer to ensure the correct concentration was produced and that quality controls were in place for its manufacture. The new bottle also meant that new packaging, promotional materials, and a relaunch media campaign were needed. Significantly, the new product format greatly reduced the price of the product, with the new consumer price of Sûr'Eau (now approximately US$0.17 per bottle) dropping by almost 60%. In August 2004, the new Sûr'Eau 150-milliliter product was launched. To further enhance the reach of Sûr'Eau, CARE piloted and scaled up new community-based promotional and distribution strategies.

The results of the changes were rapid and dramatic. Sales jumped immediately, and more than 600,000 units per year were sold in each of the following two years and more than 1 million units the subsequent two years.

Place Strategies

A key to program success was to ensure wide availability of Sûr'Eau across the country. Because Sûr'Eau was designed to be used in the home, it needed to be readily available in tens of thousands of rural villages as well as in densely populated urban centers. It was hoped that a community-based distribution model, in addition to a private sector distribution mechanism, would help in reaching rural populations not well served by local commercial networks. The team planned to leverage its existing national network of private sector retailers that were already distributing its other lifesaving social marketing products. In addition, the government of Madagascar and other NGO partners would assist with rural community–based distribution to both seed the launch of the new product and sustain availability of Sûr'Eau over the long term.

The marketing team contracted wholesalers, which made Sûr'Eau available in more than 20,000 retail outlets across the country. It managed the system similar to the methods used by fast-moving consumer goods companies. About 60% of national sales were achieved through this distribution mechanism.

Equally important was the task of designing and managing a community-based rural distribution network. Three innovative community-based distribution channels were developed:

1. *Rural distribution.* A network of community-based rural sales agents known as AVBCs ("Agent de Vente à Base Communautaire") was set up to reach remote villages. These agents, typically women, lived in the communities where they worked. The AVBCs were trusted community members available for follow-up questions. By using Sûr'Eau themselves, they began to change societal norms in their communities. The team also launched a network of women's associations, branded Ranoray ("Together for Water"), in five of the highest diarrheal disease

burden regions. Fifty women's associations were established with some 5,000 members trained in the importance of treated water and good hygiene, as well as in interpersonal communications (IPC) techniques. Sûr'Eau messages were integrated into other maternal and child health communications as part of a comprehensive approach to improve overall health in rural areas.

2. *School distribution.* The Sekoly Sûr'Eau (Sûr'Eau at schools) initiative was aimed at reaching schoolchildren with sanitation and hygiene messages as well as providing them with clean drinking water while they were at school. School-based programs have been found to effectively influence health behaviors with results such as children bringing messages of safe water home to their mothers. Working with NGOs such as Aide et Action, the team launched this distribution and promotion channel in 160 schools with a target of reaching more than 300 schools (see Box 10-4).

BOX 10-4 **Student Promotional Agents Change Behavior in Kenya**

Designing and implementing behavior change programs in rural areas provides unique challenges to social marketing programs. Traditional mass media (television and radio) are often not accessible to rural populations, while outdoor media such as billboards are only accessible along major roadways, and printed materials often end up in the hands of illiterate villagers.

This was the case when PSI Kenya launched PUR (flocculent/disinfectant) in 2005. To reach rural populations where drinking water was both turbid and unsafe, PSI partnered with the Ministry of Education and two local agencies to implement a school-based PUR promotion program. The idea of the initiative was to use schoolchildren to promote behavior change in their own households. One local NGO partner experienced in school-based program development designed and printed behavior change materials and acquired government approval for distribution. A second private sector communications partner conducted educational sessions at schools that included demonstrations of product use and gave three sample sachets of PUR to each student.

Evaluation of the behavior change intervention found that 95% of students could recall all of the steps necessary to correctly treat drinking water. In its first year, the school program reached almost 88,000 students in 446 schools at a cost of just over US$1.00 per student.

3. *Restaurant distribution.* To promote safe drinking and food preparation practices in small restaurants, the Hotely Sûr'Eau (Sûr'Eau in restaurants) initiative was developed in which restaurant owners signed an agreement to consistently use Sûr'Eau for all water and food preparation and to promote and sell Sûr'Eau to their clients. More than 300 small restaurants have become Hotely Sûr'Eau members with plans for an additional 350 members.

These community-based distribution channels achieved approximately 40% of Sûr'Eau's sales volume annually.

Promotion Strategies

Campaign Messages

The marketing team created a communications strategy that would affect two key behavioral determinants of Sûr'Eau use (self-efficacy and societal norms) by conveying critical messages to the target audience (see Table 10-1).

The communication messages were included in promotional materials including posters, pamphlets, T-shirts, pens, cups, banners, and packaging materials. The same messages were reinforced in radio and television spots. Campaign messages were integrated into government and other campaigns on hygiene and sanitation, while conversely, other hygiene and sanitation messages were integrated into Sûr'Eau communications efforts.

TABLE 10-1   Sample Communication Messages for Prevention of Diarrheal Disease

Target Audiences	Behavioral Determinant	Sample Communications Messages
Caregivers of children under 5, with a special focus on rural areas	Self-efficacy	• Sûr'Eau use is as simple as 1-2-3! (1) Add one cap of Sûr'Eau for one water bucket; (2) stir with a clean utensil; (3) cover with a clean fabric and wait 30 minutes before use (see Figure 10-3). • It takes 30 minutes to treat water with Sûr'Eau (it's the equivalent amount of time necessary to sweep a courtyard or cook rice).
Caregivers of children under 5, with a special focus on rural areas	Social norms	• Most people you know use a water treatment product. • Most Malagasy women use Sûr'Eau to treat their family's water. • Children whose mothers treat water with Sûr'Eau rarely get diarrhea.

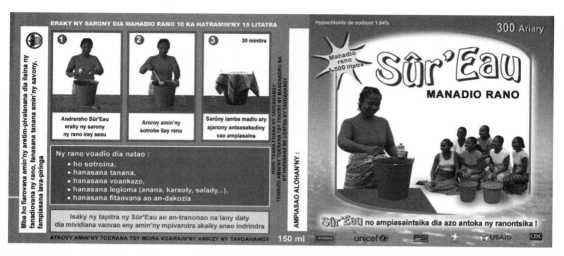

FIGURE 10-3   New Sûr'Eau Packaging Showing the Target Consumer Promoting Self-Efficacy While Creating a New Social Norm of Home Water Treatment

Communication Channels

Sûr'Eau promotion was achieved through multiple communication channels. These included interpersonal communications (either one-on-one in small group discussions or team-to-group), behavior change materials and promotional items used at special events or at point-of-sale and through mass media channels.

Analysis of the local mass media market determined that with high national listenership, radio was the most effective means to reach women and caregivers across the country. A radio edutainment series was developed that featured Sûr'Eau as a key component of the storyline. The show included a contest that became extremely popular. Radio commercials for Sûr'Eau were produced and played nationally. A limited number of TV commercials were also developed to link the brand and campaign visuals with the radio campaign, IPC, and other small media activities.

Behavior change communication (BCC) materials were used to ensure multiple exposures to the same messages through different channels. More than 5,000 posters were produced and placed in small shops, restaurants, and medical halls across the country. New BCC materials addressing self-efficacy, social norms, and the threat of diarrhea were developed approximately every three months to ensure the campaign remained fresh and "top of mind" with consumers (see Figure 10-4).

Sûr'Eau was highlighted at special promotional events such as the Government of Madagascar Maternal and Child Health Weeks (Semaine de la Santé Maternelle et Enfant), where branded T-shirts, caps, and brochures were given away. In April 2008, President Marc Ravalomanana attended and was captured in a national press photograph both drinking and distributing Sûr'Eau.

A wide variety of IPC activities provided additional exposure to campaign messages. In addition to the Ranoray women's associations initiative, Sekoly school-based program, and Hotely restaurant scheme, a Peace Corps volunteer training-of-trainers program edu-

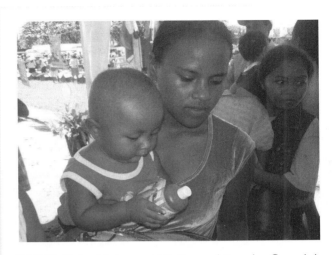

FIGURE 10-4   Malagasy Mothers Attend a Special Sûr'Eau Promotional Event to Learn How to Protect their Young Children from the Threat of Diarrhea

cated community individuals in hygiene, sanitation, and Sûr'Eau use. These activities were targeted to areas of the country most affected by unsafe water and diarrhea and were matched by additional distribution efforts to ensure the product would be available.

As part of the national health system, more than 12,000 government volunteer community healthcare workers were trained in hygiene, sanitation, and home water treatment and complemented the Sûr'Eau community-based sales agents and the other volunteers. The public sector volunteers were trained by the government, as well as local and international NGOs. The PSI marketing team trained the NGOs working with the volunteers and provided them with Sûr'Eau "starter kits" (see Box 10-5).

Mobile video units run on generators and capable of playing media in rural communities were developed to carry the communication messages into remote villages. The mobile units were built into trucks that hauled the equipment into places where television is rarely seen. Entertaining videos were projected onto a large outdoor screen, while Sûr'Eau commercials and health information were broadcast in between videos to crowds of villagers gathered around the screens. Sûr'Eau "animators" gave product demonstrations and sold bottles during the event.

BOX 10-5   **Union de Femmes FRAM du District Ambanja**

Suzette is a mother of two children who attend the primary public school of Ambanja in northern Madagascar. Since 2006, this school has collaborated with the NGO Aide et Action and PSI to implement a Sekoly Sûr'Eau project that promotes the use of safe drinking water and good hygiene practices at school and in the household.

The method was appreciated by the students and their families—so much so that Suzette took the initiative to create an association of the mothers of students (known as "Union de Femmes FRAM du District Ambanja") that partners with PSI for community-based education and distribution. The association began activities in March 2006 and had 12 active members. In the 15-month period through June 2007, they sold more than 23,000 bottles of Sûr'Eau. Thanks to Suzette, to the success of her association, and to the Sekoly Sûr'Eau program, it is estimated that more than 1,500 families now have regular access to safe drinking water in Ambanja.

CAMPAIGN TIME FRAME AND BUDGET

The Sûr'Eau program began in 2000 and continues to expand in 2009. Long-term additional funding has been acquired for national expansion of the program over the coming five years. To date, US$4.7 million has been spent over the nine-year life of the project.

CAMPAIGN OUTCOMES

The Sûr'Eau program in Madagascar has achieved remarkable success. Provision of Sûr'Eau is estimated to have led to more than 441,000 cases of diarrhea averted through September 2008.

The program has achieved 110,000 disability-adjusted life-years (DALYs) of health impact. Sales of Sûr'Eau over the last nine years have totaled more than 5.5 million units (see Figure 10-5). They continue to trend upward with an average of more than a million units now being sold annually. Research measuring access and performance (MAP) was conducted in 2005 to assess product coverage and quality of coverage. Coverage of outlets in urban settings averaged 66% while 21% coverage was achieved in rural areas. About 44% of urban consumers

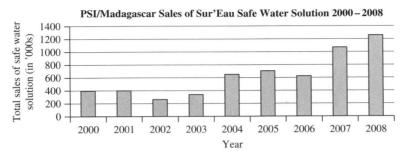

FIGURE 10-5   Sales of Sûr'Eau 2000–2008

and 8% of rural consumers reported that promotional materials were visible. The percentage of outlets that respected the expiry date by not carrying expired product was 66% in urban settings and 20% in rural settings (PSI MAP, 2005).

Research conducted in 2006 indicated that behavioral determinants had been positively affected by the program (PSI, 2007). Significant increases in perceived self-efficacy and the social norm of using Sûr'Eau were seen as well as for product availability and the belief that the product works.

Exposure to program communications showed positive trends; for example, 60.4% of respondents reported hearing the radio spots in 2006 versus 29.6% of respondents in 2004. Similarly, 52% of respondents saw or received BCC materials in 2006 versus 27.6% in 2004 (PSI, 2007).

The results indicate that intensified national-scale programming needs to be sustained over many years in order to effectively increase the purchase and consistent use of Sûr'Eau. In addition, more work needs to be done to better reach rural areas of Madagascar.

SUMMARY AND LESSONS LEARNED

The Sûr'Eau social marketing program in Madagascar has been a success. Today, all across the country, water is being treated in hundreds of thousands of homes, many in rural and poor areas. From its modest beginnings in 2000 until today, many lessons have been learned and many changes made to the program. These lessons have also informed and improved PSI's 25 other safe water programs around the world. In 2007, the U.S. Agency for International Development funded the Point of Use and Zinc (POUZN) Project, led by Abt Associates Inc., to undertake a review of 20 of PSI's international SWS programs around the world. The key lessons learned that were detailed in the report that apply to the Madagascar Sûr'Eau program include:

- *Project design.* The identification of appropriate target groups, technical expertise, and long-term funding are essential to the design of safe water programs.
- *Production of safe water product components.* Local production, product chlorine dosage and shelf life, and quality monitoring present challenges but are critical to cost-effectiveness and sustainability.
- *Regulatory environment.* Early government involvement and immediate response to concerns strengthen government support.
- *Marketing and communications.* Marketing communications should specifically address behavioral constructs and be positive and aspirational, complementary to existing efforts, highly context specific, and sustained long term to be successful.
- *Creating partnerships.* Successful partnerships with government, NGOs, and the private sector strengthen the program and increase the likelihood of success. They also provide unique opportunities to reach rural and high-risk populations.
- *Sales and distribution.* The commercial sector can be an efficient distribution channel for home water treatment products while encouraging entry of other commercial parties. To ensure access to the target audience, additional channels, including NGO networks, can improve rural reach.
- *Product costs, pricing, and cost recovery.* Product costs may be recovered, but prices must be affordable to target consumers.
- *Integrating safe water into HIV/AIDS programming.* SWS for People Living with HIV\AIDS (PLWHAs) in partnership with local NGOs is a successful model to reach this vulnerable population.

The report concluded:

> Household-level point-of-use water treatment has been shown to significantly reduce diarrheal diseases in vulnerable populations and should become an essential intervention within child survival, HIV/AIDS, and water supply programs. While challenges remain, such as ensuring consistent product use and program financial sustainability, the key elements in implementing household water treatment programs using safe water solutions are now quite well understood. These and other evidence-based POU [point-of-use] water treatment programs should be scaled up and expanded throughout the developing world, filling a critical public health gap in drinking water quality. (POUZN, 2007)

Last but by no means the least, the design, implementation, monitoring, and evaluation of social marketing projects in developing countries pose unique challenges to program teams. The execution of these social marketing programs can be challenging due to a lack of evidence for decision making or lack of solid research methodologies to collect it, weak private sector markets, limited infrastructure, weak governance, and inefficient systems. In addition, lack of transparency, divergent donor interests, limited viable partners, expensive media channels, limited professional capacity, and difficult social and political issues related to poverty compound the problem. Program teams that are creative, committed, flexible, dynamic, and willing to continuously learn and adapt will more likely be successful.

QUESTIONS FOR DISCUSSION

1. PSI Madagascar's program research found that while sales of Sûr'Eau continued to make impressive gains each year, the behavioral determinants of use (self-efficacy and societal norms) did not change between 2004 and 2006. Discuss why this might have happened and make recommendations as to what marketers could have done when these data came to light.
2. Social marketing programmers sometimes design national programs that utilize the public, private, and NGO sectors, simultaneously designing components of programs differently for each sector—also known as the total market approach. Discuss the advantages and disadvantages of such an approach, and cite examples where this approach would be useful.
3. Social marketing programs often sell products at highly subsidized rates targeting the poor in developing countries. Some say health products for the poor should be given away for free. Discuss the pros and cons of each approach.
4. Social marketing programs sometimes overlook the use of data or evidence in decision making. Give three reasons why this may happen and three disadvantages when it does.

ACKNOWLEDGMENTS

The author would like to kindly acknowledge Cecilia Kwak and Meg Galas for their generous contributions and give thanks to Nicole Andriamampianina, Megan Wilson, Ashima Khanna, Annalise Blum, and David Alt. All photographs, charts, tables, and sidebars used in this chapter were provided by Population Services International.

REFERENCES

Ashraf, N., Berry, J., & Shapiro, J. M. (2007). *Can higher prices stimulate product use? Evidence from a field experiment in Zambia.* Harvard Business School Working Paper 07-034. Retrieved July 28, 2009, from http://www.hbs.edu/research/pdf/07-034.pdf

Bryce, J., Boschi-Pinto, C., Shibuya, R., Black, R. E., & WHO Child Health Epidemiology Reference Group. (2005). WHO estimates of the causes of death in children. *The Lancet* 365(9465), 1114–11146.

Centers for Disease Control and Prevention (CDC). (2009). *Safe water systems (SWS) publications–other HWTS options.* Retrieved July 28, 2009, from http://www.cdc.gov/safe water/publications_pages/pubs_other_hwts.htm

Central Intelligence Agency (CIA). (2009). *The World Factbook*, Madagascar. Retrieved July 28, 2009, from https://www.cia.gov/library/publications/the-worldfactbook

Clasen, T., McLaughlin, C., Nayaar, N., Boisson, S., Gupta, R., Desai, D., et al. (2008). Microbiological effectiveness and cost of disinfecting water by boiling in semi-urban India. *American Journal of Tropical Medicine and Hygiene* 79(3), 407–413.

Conservation International. (2009). *Madagascar and the Indian Ocean Islands—Biodiversity hotspots.* Retrieved July 28, 2009, from http://www.biodiversityhotspots.org/xp/Hotspots/madagascar/Pages/biodiversity.aspx

Fewtrell, L., & Colford, J. (2004). *Water, sanitation and hygiene: Interventions and diarrhoea: A systemic review and meta-analysis.* Health, Nutrition, and Population Discussion Paper. Washington DC: World Bank.

Fewtrell, L., Kaufmann, R. B., Kay, D., Enanoria, W., Haller, L., & Colford, J. M. (2005). Water, sanitation, and hygiene interventions to reduce diarrhoea in less developed countries: A systematic review and meta-analysis. *Lancet Infectious Diseases* 5, 42–52.

Government of Madagascar. (2007). *Madagascar Action Plan 2007–2012.* Retrieved July 28, 2009, from http://www.imf.org/external/pubs/ft/scr/2007/cr0759.pdf

Institut National de la Statistique and ORC Macro. (2005). *Enquere Demographique et de Sante de Madagascar 2003–2004.* Calverton, MD: INSTAT and ORC Macro.

Lantagne. (2006). Engineering inputs to the CDC safe water system program. In *Frontiers of Engineering: Reports on Leading-Edge Engineering from the 2005 Symposium*, 46.

Luby, S., Agboatwalla, M., Hoekstra, R., Rahbar, M., Billhimer, W., & Keswick, B. (2004). Delayed effectiveness of home-based interventions in reducing childhood diarrhea, Karachi, Pakistan. *American Journal of Tropical Medicine and Hygiene* 71(4), 420–427.

Parashar, U. D., Hummelman, E. G., Bresee, J. S., Miller, M. A., & Glass, R. I. (2003). Global illness and deaths caused by rotavirus disease in children. *Emerging Infectious Diseases* 9(5). Retrieved July 28, 2009, from http://www.cdc.gov/ncidod/EID/vol9no5/02-0562.htm

Patel, D. S., & Chapman, S. (2005). *The dashboard: A tool for social marketing decision making.* Population Services International Concept Paper. Retrieved July 28, 2009, from http://www.psi.org/research/documents/dashboard2005.pdf

POUZN. (2007). Best practices in social marketing safe water solution for household water treatment: Lessons learned from Population Services International field programs. In *Social marketing plus for diarrheal disease control: Point-of-use water disinfection and zinc treatment (POUZN) Project.* Bethesda, MD: Abt Associates Inc.

PSI. (2007). *Madagascar (2006): Maternal and child health TRaC study evaluating the use of Sûr'Eau safe water solution among children younger than five years.* Social Marketing Research Series. Retrieved July 28, 2009, from http://www.psi.org/research/smr/627 madagascar_sureau_SMRS.pdf

PSI/Madagascar. (2006). *Sûr'Eau positioning statement.* Madagascar: Population Services International, Diarrhea Prevention Program.

PSI MAP. (2005). *Madagascar (2005): Enquête MAP sur la Couverture et la Qualité de Couverture pour Sûr'Eau Premier Passage.* Social Marketing Research Series. Retrieved July 28, 2009, from http://www.psi.org/research/smr/539-madagascar_sureau_map_smrs.pdf

Quick, R., Venczel, L. V., Mintz, E. D., Soleto, L., Aparicio, J., Gironaz, M., et al. (1999). Diarrhea prevention in Bolivia through point-of-use disinfection and safe storage: A promising new strategy. *Epidemic Infections* 122, 83–90.

UN Development Program. (2006). *Beyond scarcity: Power, poverty and the global water crisis.* Summary Human Development Report. New York: Palgrave Macmillan.

UNICEF. (2005). *Madagascar revised country document,* p. 2. Retrieved July 28, 2009, from http://www.unicef.org/about/execboard/files/2004-PL3Rev1_Madagascar.pdf

UNICEF. (2007). *Global distribution of under-five deaths by cause.* Retrieved July 28, 2009, from www.unicef.org/media/files/Under_five_deaths_by_cause_2006_estimates3.oc

USAID. (2004). *Providing access to safe water in Madagascar.* Retrieved July 28, 2009, from http://africastories.usaid.gov/search_details.cfm?storyID=299&countryID=1§orID=0&yearID=4

USAID. (2005). *Demographic and health survey: Madagascar, 2003–2004* USAID. Retrieved July 28, 2009, from http://pdf.usaid.gov/pdf_docs/PNADC944.pdf

World Bank. (2008). *World Bank ICT at a glance: Madagascar.* Retrieved July 28, 2009, from http://devdata.worldbank.org/_ict/_mdg_ict.pdf

World Health Organization (WHO). (2003). *International network to promote household water treatment and safe storage.* Geneva, Switzerland: Author.

World Health Organization (WHO). (2005). *The world health report: 2005: Make every mother and child count.* Geneva, Switzerland: Author.

CHAPTER 11

Socialism Meets Social Marketing

Jump-Starting the Commercial Contraceptive Market in the Former Soviet Republic of Kazakhstan

Donald Ruschman, Randi Thompson, and Tatiana Stafford

Each success only buys an admission ticket to a more difficult problem.
—Henry Kissinger

This chapter examines how a comprehensive, multipronged, short-term effort to marshal, engage, and direct the considerable local talent and resources of the Republic of Kazakhstan was able to make contraceptives widely available commercially; convince women to adopt them as an alternative to abortion (helping to cut the rate in half); and then become largely self-sufficient by transferring principal responsibility for maintaining these newly found gains to the private, commercial sector.

The crash of the Soviet Union (USSR) in the early 1990s presented the West with once-in-a-lifetime challenges and opportunities. U.S. foreign policy toward the newly independent states was based on engagement and the provision of assistance to aid in the transition from communism and a command economy to democratic free markets (Tarnoff, 2002). Nowhere was the need more dramatic than in the Soviet public health system, where decades of massive entitlements, no longer affordable, were almost instantly abandoned. Layered beneath this problem was a Byzantine medical system and standards of practice that effectively encouraged the use of abortion as the principal method of fertility regulation, resulting in an abortion rate for the women of Kazakhstan that ranked among the highest in the world (Henshaw, Singh, & Haas, 1999). By the year 2000, that rate had been cut roughly in half (Westoff, 2000), and the social marketing effort that played an important role in that reduction was being sustained on a solely commercial basis by a network of private pharmacies.

KAZAKHSTAN: A COUNTRY OVERVIEW

Kazakhstan, largest of the Central Asian Republics and ninth largest country in the world, is situated between Russian Siberia to the north and the Indian sub-continent to the south. Populated by a mix of Mongol and Turkic nomadic tribes from the thirteenth century, Kazakhstan was conquered by Russia in the eighteenth century and became a Soviet Republic in 1936 (Central Intelligence Agency [CIA], 2009). With the country's annexation into the Soviet Union came the imposition of all the Soviet systems, both for the good and the not-so-good. Among the "good" was education. Literacy was near 100% in Kazakhstan (CIA, 2009), and education was a highly valued commodity. Among the "not-so-good" was the healthcare system. While offering virtually universal free access to health care, Soviet medicine evolved in a vacuum with little exposure to modern medical advances or standards-of-practice outside the USSR. The state healthcare system was responsible for all aspects of health services, including the determination of what drug regimens and drugs would be available, as well as their procurement, manufacture, and distribution through a central government pharmacy, Farmatsyia (Krakoff, 1997).

A Dependence on Abortion

The confluence of questionable Soviet medical practice, misconceptions about modern contraceptives, and a constricting supply of pharmaceuticals led to a dependence on abortion as a woman's top choice for fertility control (Popov, 1990). At the time of the collapse of the Soviet Union and the achievement of independence by Kazakhstan, Kazakhstani women could expect to average 1.8 abortions over their lifetime, and those living in the capital saw a rate of 3.1, close to double the national average (USAID/Macro International, 1995).

Another result of, or perhaps a reason for, the breakup of the Soviet Union was the state's inability to continue to deliver the massive entitlements that the socialist system had guaranteed. Consequently, provision of social services became the responsibility of each newly independent republic. In truth, the Soviet entitlement system had not been able to deliver its promised benefits for some time. At independence, the deficit became public and even more pronounced as the new republics' ability to meet the entitlement requirements were no better, and in most cases much worse, than the Soviet central government had been.

Kazakhstan's response was typical of the choices made by the newly independent republics. Farmatsyia, its central pharmacy, continued to be held responsible for providing most of its drugs free of charge to the majority of the population. At the same time, it was charged with becoming self-sufficient. From a Western perspective, this was clearly impossible, but without any real understanding of the fundamentals of business or markets, Farmatsyia forged ahead and attempted to resolve the two directives by increasing prices of those pharmaceuticals for which it was allowed to charge to cover the cost of those it was required to provide free. Prices skyrocketed, in some cases to more than 250% of world prices (Hausloner, 1995), and the market stalled, further cementing abortion as the principal means of fertility regulation available to the women of Kazakhstan.

U.S. Interest in Providing Assistance to the "Evil Empire"

U.S. foreign assistance, one of the primary funding tools for international social marketing programs in health, has traditionally been focused on the expressed needs of the governments of developing/third-world countries. However, the historic and unique nature of the dissolution of the Soviet Union (the "second world") and the challenges it presented, provided an unprecedented opportunity for the United States to influence what shape the broken "Evil Empire" would assume as it was reassembled. Consequently, the United States offered Russia and the newly independent republics a comprehensive assistance plan focused on aiding them in their transition from command economies to market-based ones (Tarnoff, 2002). While most of the assistance was concentrated on macro-economic concerns and the privatization of the vast assets of what had been the communist state government, it also came to be recognized that in order for these unprecedented fundamental changes to be accepted by the population, it was critical to address the well-being of individuals along with the massive failure of the public entitlement system. As a result, aid from the West included social sector components borrowed from traditional developing country approaches, warped to fit the truly unique nature of the failed Soviet Union and the time-limited window in which to apply them.

Social Marketing's Fit in the "Second World"

The U.S. Agency for International Development (USAID), the top U.S. foreign assistance supplier, has long been a proponent, funder, and believer in the efficacy of social marketing initiatives (USAID, 2007). Its worldwide Social Marketing for Change (SOMARC) project was, at the time of the work described in this case study, the agency's principal global social marketing effort in the field of reproductive health and the culmination of several decades of public health social marketing program design and funding evolution. Models were well established and typically calibrated to the needs and economies of USAID's traditional clients—less-developed countries (LDCs)—with a goal of reducing high population growth rates. Time horizons for the success of these models were often measured in decades, with a corresponding requirement for donor funding to support the project infrastructure and supply subsidized products for the expected lifetime of the effort.

However, for the second world of the former Soviet Union, few, if any, of these models were a good or direct fit. Nor were the traditional time lines appropriate. The United States, recognizing that the window of opportunity was small for the new republics to successfully implement the massive changes anticipated by the transition from a command economy to one based on demand, structured foreign policy and the aid that accompanied it as never before. Assistance efforts needed to be able to both show substantial results quickly and maintain those results when the short-term donor funding ended. These two parameters were largely new to the social marketing discipline as it had been applied to reproductive health. Meeting them necessitated both fresh approaches and implementers, with a standard "test" for the usefulness of a traditional tactic or program component being whether it could be expected to be maintained on a commercial basis once U.S. assistance ended.

The Kazakhstan SOMARC project, the "Red Apple Program" and the subject of this chapter, represents just such a revolutionary approach and implementation team.

THE REPRODUCTIVE HEALTH CRISIS IN KAZAKHSTAN

For most of the twentieth century, the principal method of birth control in the former Soviet Union was abortion (Popov, 1990). Although the Central Asian Republics did not have a population problem, the reliance on abortion for fertility regulation had created a reproductive health crisis (Darsky & Dworak, 1993). This continued through the early to mid-1990s, when Kazakhstani women nationwide were having an average of nearly two abortions (1.8) in their lifetimes. In the capital city of Almaty, the number of abortions was almost double the national rate, with women there having a lifetime average of three (USAID/Macro International, 1995; see Table 11-1).

The data also indicated a strong desire for family planning and need for contraceptives. More than half of all married Kazakhstani women reported they wanted no more children (59.4 percent said they had already reached the ideal family size), while an additional 20.2% said they wanted to space the births of their children (USAID/Macro International, 1995). It was this mismatch between desired behavior and a method to achieve it that the SOMARC Red Apple Program was charged with helping to resolve (see Figures 11-1 and 11-2).

TABLE 11-1   Abortions in Kazakhstan in the Mid-1990s

Abortions per lifetime per woman (nationwide)	1.8
Abortions per lifetime per woman (urban)	3.0 (Almaty)

Source: USAID/Macro International, *Demographic and Health Survey: Kazakhstan,* 1995.

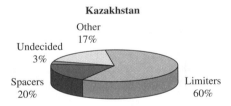

FIGURE 11-1   Need for Contraceptives (Married Women, Ages 15–49)
Courtesy of USAID/Macro International

CASE STUDY
The "Red Apple"

Krasnoye Yabloko ("Red Apple" in Russian) was the evocative name proposed by the local advertising firm, favored by focus groups, and chosen for the USAID-funded SOMARC Kazakhstan Social Marketing Project. The Red Apple program was focused on ending the near-critical reliance on abortion by women of Kazakhstan because of the virtual collapse of the Soviet pharmaceutical supply system along with a medical establishment that de facto discouraged nonclinical methods of birth control.

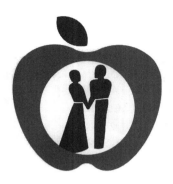

FIGURE 11-2 Red Apple Logo—Source: USAID

Courtesy of USAID/Akbar Public Relations

STRATEGIC APPROACH

The overarching strategy of the Red Apple program was to offer Kazakhstani women a contraceptive alternative to abortion that was readily available through commercial channels. While the program generally followed a traditional marketing model, because of the complex and evolving nature of the post-Soviet marketing environment, there were elements of the marketing mix that warranted special attention, especially the area of product procurement and distribution.

As a result, separate strategies were delineated for two principal program components: (1) consumers and (2) suppliers.

- *Consumer strategy:* Develop a comprehensive, branded, marketing/marketing communication campaign to encourage trial and continued use of contraceptives as the primary method of fertility regulation and a substitute for abortion.
- *Supplier strategy:* Make contraceptives available through the national network of newly privatized retail pharmacies by assuming market-entry risks on behalf of commercial pharmaceutical suppliers and distributors and by brokering commercial supply agreements between them and international pharmaceutical manufacturers.

Over time, specific program tactics varied significantly; however, they were consistently guided by the principle that the project had to be sustainable by the private sector in a short period of time. Often, that meant perhaps the easiest or most direct means to achieve a particular program objective was ruled out because it would not have been reasonable to expect the private sector to continue or maintain it at an appropriate level in the absence of donor support. This approach to the two main program components saw SOMARC contracting with local marketing service companies; providing technical assistance to design and execute a comprehensive consumer social marketing and marketing communications campaign; and filling the commercial marketplace with contraceptive products by absorbing market-entry costs and the associated risks of working in the newly independent states, on behalf of reluctant and skeptical pharmaceutical manufacturers, distributors, and retailers.

TARGET PROFILES

Consumer Targets

- *Primary targets:* Women aged 18 to 36 with long-term partners who wish to limit or postpone future pregnancies. This group comprises between 60% and 80% of the married women in the age group.
- *Secondary targets:* Reproductive health/medical professionals, primary targets' partners, and primary targets' key influentials. This group represents those individuals most likely to influence the primary targets' decision to use contraception instead of abortion as a method of fertility control.

Supplier Targets

- Newly privatized pharmaceutical distributors and retailers.
- Western pharmaceutical manufacturers and distributors.

MARKETING OBJECTIVES

Consumers

- *Behavior objectives:* Encourage trial and continued use of contraceptives as the primary means of fertility regulation by women of the target group.
- *Knowledge objectives:* Women of the primary target, as well as the individuals comprising the secondary target, should understand that contraceptives are a safe and reliable alternative to abortion.
- *Belief objectives:* Targeted women and the secondary targets should come to believe that hormones are not the dangerous substances old-style Soviet medicine depicted and modern, lower-dose contraceptives pose fewer health risks than the old formulas and much less risk than abortion.

Suppliers

- *Behavior objectives:* Conclude agreements for the purchase distribution and regular/consistent stocking in commercial/retail pharmacies of modern formulation contraceptives.

- *Knowledge objectives:* Targeted manufacturers, distributors, and retailers should understand that the usual risks of entering a new market will be borne by SOMARC.
- *Belief objectives:* Targeted manufacturers, distributors, and retailers should come to believe there is a commercially viable, unmet demand for modern formulation contraceptives that can be profitable and worth the investment of scarce resources.

BARRIERS, BENEFITS, AND COMPETITION

Consumers

The biggest barrier to be overcome by the Red Apple with regard to the targeted consumers was the long history of Soviet health care that effectively encouraged abortion through a professional/institutional misunderstanding of the fundamental method of action of hormonal contraceptives and a resultant fear of their use that was passed on to patients. This was coupled with a system that conferred healthcare entitlements almost solely through a hospital-based system of inpatient care/treatment, where abortion was often easier to access than contraceptives.

Choices outside of this entitlement system were limited and relatively difficult to access, even though abortion was understood to pose considerable reproductive health risks.

True to the paradoxical nature of most things Soviet, competitors to Red Apple products were also its collaborators. Structurally, the abortion-biased, hospital/inpatient care–based public health system, and its post-Soviet fragmented remnants, represented the largest obstacle to the substitution of contraceptives for abortion, because it was the largest abortion provider. However, it also was home to some of the Red Apple's biggest supporters: dedicated, enlightened, reproductive health physicians and public health policymakers, who recognized the many dangers from high abortion rates and were ready to embrace alternatives.

Suppliers

Kazakhstani commercial suppliers were, by definition, new to the workings of Western business and in almost all cases, new to commercial business itself. The most powerful and influential model was that of nearby developing Russian business, where fortunes were being made (and lost) at a breakneck pace. Relative to that "standard," the traditional return on money invested in the contraceptive market was very small—and not an especially attractive place to allocate scarce resources, even when market development costs were being borne by someone else.

The characterization of the breakup and transformation of the former Soviet Union as a once-in-a-lifetime occurrence fueled a strong bias toward high-risk/high-return short-term opportunities. These new entrepreneurs, fearful of missing out on the bonanza, made investment choices based primarily on how quickly they could turn a large profit and benefit in the shortest time possible from an unprecedented market that might well not be there tomorrow.

The Red Apple program's specific competition for suppliers' capital was every other drug category, almost all of which offered a greater profit margin than contraceptives. Coupled with the low return rate on contraceptives was a concern that in response to the abortion crisis, Western donors would provide free contraceptives for distribution through the public health system, thus effectively killing commercial market development, as well as investment in the industry.

POSITIONING

Consumers

Targeted consumers should see traditional Soviet reproductive health medical advice and practice as flawed and outdated. Modern formulation contraceptives are a safe and effective alternative to abortion, which poses substantial health risks and should be avoided.

Suppliers

Targeted suppliers should see a commercial opportunity to enter a new market with considerable growth potential, relatively free of risk or development costs. They should also see an opportunity to establish new commercial trade links with international pharmaceutical manufacturers and distributors.

STRATEGIES

The "Red Apple" brand was created to provide an overall identity to the SOMARC social marketing effort in Kazakhstan and to associate with that identity a level of standard of product quality and customer service not previously seen in the former Soviet Union. The brand also served as a focal point around which a variety of contraceptive products and services from a number of different manufacturers, suppliers, and commercial retail pharmacies could be supported.

Beneath the "umbrella" of the Red Apple was a comprehensive subset of campaigns targeted to the specific elements of each of the two major program components, consumers and suppliers. These campaigns included mass media (broadcast and print) advertising and public relations efforts, trade promotions, and training for key constituents that ranged from physician and pharmacist training in modern contraceptive technology to study tours to Western high-tech pharmaceutical plants for Kazakhstani drug manufacturers and distributors (see Figure 11-3).

Product

Physical Product

Initially, partnerships were brokered between four western and eastern European pharmaceutical manufacturers—Pharmacia/UpJohn, Schering, Organon, Gideon Richter—and local (Kazakhstani) distributors for the supply on a commercial basis at their best terms, of the following physical products:

- Oral contraceptive brands: Diane, Microgynon, and Triquilar from Schering; Marvelon from Organon; Rigevidon and Tri-Regol from Gideon Richter.
- Injectable contraceptive brand: DepoProvera from Pharmacia/UpJohn.

Each product included/imported under the Red Apple umbrella was labeled as such either by the manufacturer at the factory (as was the case with DepoProvera) or stickered with the Red Apple logo by the distributor.

Core and Actual Products

The core product was the benefit of dramatically improved reproductive health. The actual product was the choice of contraception over abortion—

SOMARC-*CAR's* The Futures Group International, SOMARC Project—Central Asian Republics

Framework for the strategic approach to the development of a sustainable private/commercial market for contraceptive.

STRATEGIC COMPONENT	TACTICS	ACTIVITIES (TYPICAL)	Kazakhstan

PROJECT ENVIRONMENT
- Creation/encouragement/maintenance of a receptive environment. (Policy level)

  Tactics: ● Identification of key individuals as advocates.

  Activities: ● Exposure to other models of government/private cooperation—**study tours**
  ● Creation/Training of **advisory boards**
  ● Direct **advocacy training** for both public and private sectors

  Tactics: ● Identification of information and service provision gatekeepers.

  Activities: ● **Training** of healthcare providers: doctors and pharmacists.

MARKET INFRASTRUCTURE
- Enlistment of western pharmaceutical manufactures and private distributors as project partners.

  Tactics: ● Survey/identification of national-level pharmaceutical distributors positioned to procure contraceptives from western manufacturers.

  Activities: ● Facilitation of commercial **distribution agreements**.

- Enlistment of private marketing service companies as project partners.

  Tactics: ● Survey/identification of marketing services resources.

  Activities: ● **Contracts** for marketing services: research, advertising, and PR.

- Creation/dissemination of communications materials.

  Tactics: ● Direct SOMARC creation of research-based, integrated communications campaign.

  Activities: ● **Technical assistance** targeted to the creation of materials.

  Tactics: ● Direct SOMARC purchase of media time/space.

  Activities: ● **Contracts** for media buying.

SUSTAINABILITY
- Facilitation of transition/assumption of marketing responsibilities to/by private, commercial organizations.

  Tactics: ● Build in-house marketing, research, and communications capacities of distribution companies.

  Activities: ● **Technical assistance** and training (including **media training**) for personnel.

  Tactics: ● Build and expand the capabilities of marketing service companies.
  ● Encourage/facilitate co-op advertising/ communications campaigns.

  Activities: ● **Leverage**/match SOMARC contract funds with distributor/manufacturer resources.

  Tactics: ● Develop franchise models.

  Activities: ● **Technical assistance** for distributor personnel.
  ● **Contracts** for design and construction.

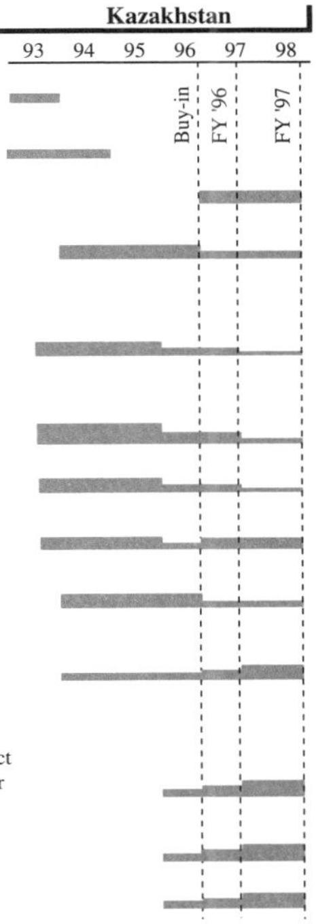

Timeline columns: 93 94 95 96 97 98 (Buy-in, FY 96, FY 97)

FIGURE 11-3 Red Apple Strategic/Tactical Framework

and all the information and access necessary to make that choice an informed and easy one.

Price

Monetary Costs

A key and integral part of the Red Apple strategy was the absolute requirement for the program to transition entirely to the private sector as a commercially viable effort. Prior to the deployment of SOMARC to Central Asia, exploratory research concluded that commercially profitable pricing of the contraceptive products SOMARC expected to offer would be reasonably affordable by the target market. Pricing for Red Apple–branded oral contraceptives ranged from

US$1.50 per cycle to US$3.00 per cycle. (As a comparison, a can of Coke cost between US$1.00 and US$2.00.)

Nonmonetary Costs

Although Red Apple contraceptive prices were well afforded by those the program targeted, these consumers were unaccustomed, under the Soviet entitlement system, to paying for reproductive health benefits. Additionally, in spite of Red Apple training to the contrary, one important nonmonetary cost was that the targeted women would have to potentially ignore their physician's or pharmacist's traditional/historic/likely advice against the use of hormones in order to buy Red Apple products.

To greatly reduce, if not eliminate, this last cost, SOMARC engaged in a large-scale effort to train both active pharmacists and physicians, as well as students of those disciplines, in modern reproductive health, contraceptive technology, and Western-style patient counseling and quality customer service.

Place

The place component of the marketing mix constituted a critically significant element of the Red Apple program. Procurement, distribution, and retail supply of contraceptives was the core of Red Apple strategy. SOMARC Kazakhstan worked throughout its tenure to ensure that, as promised by Red Apple communications/promotion efforts, a choice of Western standard contraceptive products would be consistently available on a national scale through an independent commercial pharmacy network.

The retail pharmacy was the intersection of Red Apple communication (promotion) and distribution/supply (place) efforts. As such, it was the focus of Red Apple attention and budget, and where Red Apple supplier strategy and tactics were largely executed.

Supplier

Place strategy/tactics included:

- Working with potential Red Apple distributors/retailers to broker supply agreements with Western pharmaceutical manufacturers at favorable terms.
- Providing training/technical assistance for Red Apple distributors/retailers in:

- Quality customer service (QCS).
- Inventory management and management information systems (MIS).
- Pharmacy management.
- Developing, with USAID privatization contractor Abt Associates, a franchising model (including funding to design and construct a model pharmacy) to assist in replicating successful businesses and leveraging business development investments.
- Designing, developing, and deploying a geographic information system (GIS) to provide near-real-time information about inventory levels of Red Apple products at individual pharmacies throughout the country.

Consumer

While most of SOMARC's place strategy was focused on suppliers, consumer place efforts were concentrated on building the pharmacy into an easily accessible, central repository of both accurate information about, and consistently available stocks of, Red Apple contraceptives. These strategy tactics included:

- Designing, developing, and producing a broad array of point-of-purchase materials to support Red Apple sales and counseling efforts in the pharmacies. Materials ranged from product displays to brochures with in-depth information about Red Apple products and their correct, appropriate use.
- Providing training/technical assistance to Red Apple pharmacies/pharmacists in modern contraceptive technology and customer counseling.

Promotion

When SOMARC began the project, there were no established marketing research, public relations, or advertising agencies. Prior to independence, the press was not open in Central Asia or anywhere else in the Soviet Union. Newspapers and reporters wrote about topics dictated by their employer, the state government. The concept of consumer marketing was not in the Soviet lexicon, because for decades the government had dictated the wants and needs of the country's consumers, based on multiyear "Central Plans" that forecast the necessary supplies of virtually every item produced or imported by the Soviet Union, thereby rendering Western-style professional marketing skills superfluous.

Consequently, before beginning to develop a campaign, SOMARC first identified resources in the region with some rough equivalent of expertise in critical marketing disciplines. Individuals and groups with experience in public opinion research, film/video production, and journalism were sought out and, if not formally incorporated as commercial businesses, were encouraged and assisted in doing so. SOMARC then began the job of working with them to transform their Soviet talent into Western marketing skills and to then use those new skills in the creation of a comprehensive consumer/target-directed communications campaign.

Because the SOMARC place strategy and tactics were focused almost exclusively on suppliers, promotion strategy and tactics were directed principally toward consumers, with suppliers benefiting from those efforts through sales of the Red Apple products they stocked.

Promotion

Messages

There were three initial goals, and messages were developed to:

- Launch the new brand and build awareness and acceptance of the program and its logo—and what they stand for.
- Begin to dispel Soviet medical practice myths about the safety and efficacy of modern hormonal contraceptives.
- Encourage purchase and trial of program contraceptives.

Message Development Protocol

1. *Research and analysis*
   a. Formative research: Focus groups were conducted among women in the target groups. The primary purpose of this research was to begin to understand the reasons women who said they did not want to become pregnant were not using reliable contraceptive methods. The groups were also used to add richness to some of the Soviet-era secondary data to test what arguments might be persuasive and to determine what specific language/ words/terms would be acceptable in convincing women in the target groups to try Red Apple products (BRIF, 1997a, 1997b; Futures Group International, 1994).

      Additionally, the focus groups were used to better understand the background and nature of both the perceived costs and personal benefits associated with modern contraceptive use for women in the target audiences (BRIF, 1997a, 1997b; Futures Group International, 1994).

b. Secondary research analysis: Reproductive health clinical data, amassed in great detail and stored as part of the former Soviet government planning system's statistical repository (Goskomstat), was analyzed to aid in the development of "typical" profiles of each of the Red Apple's target consumers.

2. *Creative development:* Early analysis showed that the Soviet mass media, although struggling for resources to remain solvent, continued to command attention and maintain much of the reach it had enjoyed during the Soviet era. That, coupled with an early decision to use program funds to purchase media time and space (in addition to the more traditional reproductive health social marketing practice of relying heavily on free/donated public service time), channeled Red Apple creative efforts primarily toward television and radio messages.

The formative and secondary research guided the development of creative material along two critical paths:

a. It was *not* necessary to devote Red Apple resources to educate target audiences about abortion's serious risk to a woman's health. In spite of its high rate of occurrence, abortion risks were well understood.

b. Correcting misinformation about hormones was imperative, as a poor understanding of essentially every aspect of hormonal contraception was the norm and a principal barrier to its trial and continued use.

A 50-minute introductory lifestyle feature was developed, centering on a series of peer recommendations from satisfied users as well as physician referrals. The "soap opera/feature" style was known to be popular among the target audience, and the added length allowed for in-depth treatment of the complex issues surrounding the misconceptions and benefits from using oral contraceptives, not possible in a 30- to 60-second ad.

Drawing on the materials developed for the introductory feature (and through careful production, directly using portions of the feature's scenes), SOMARC and the Red Apple agencies developed a series of television and radio ads featuring a main character (a woman from the primary target group) and her friends as they searched for, tried, and became satisfied users of Red Apple oral contraceptives. Behaviors/activities depicted in the ads included new users learning how to correctly take oral contraceptives; where, how, and from whom to obtain correct information; and how to behave when confronted with initial side effects.

Appearing on every piece of creative media was the Red Apple logo and the tag line: "*Safe, Effective Contraception for Today's Woman*" (see Figures 11-4 and 11-5).

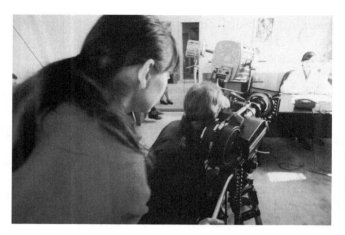

FIGURE 11-4 Producing Red Apple TV Advertising
Photo by chapter author

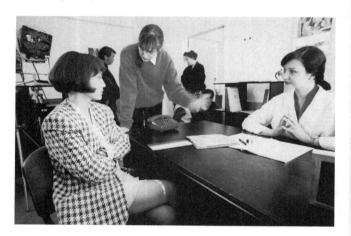

FIGURE 11-5 Producing Red Apple TV Advertising
Photo by chapter author

Messengers

SOMARC employed interpersonal communications (and messengers) to the greatest degree possible to address the difficult challenge of changing the target's long-standing, closely held beliefs and misconceptions about reproductive health. One-on-one conversations between target consumers and individuals representing trusted professionals, friends, and key family decision makers were modeled in Red Apple advertising in addition to the execution of a broad set of tactics designed to stimulate structured peer conversations/counseling.

SOMARC worked extensively with the newly formed and rapidly growing nongovernmental organization (NGO) community to determine which NGOs had access to target audiences and an institutional interest/ability to organize seminars and peer counseling efforts. The following represents a sample of the types of organizations and efforts SOMARC used to implement its interpersonal communications efforts.

Association of Business Women of Kazakhstan

The association worked with consumers, media, other NGOs, and government to improve the status and chances for successful business careers of Kazakhstani women.

It includes in its work:

- A local reproductive health project (door-to-door peer counselors, for whom they give monthly seminars).
- A monthly newspaper, *Women's World*.
- Twice-monthly open meetings, with speakers.

Medical and Pedagogical Association

The organization worked with physicians, teachers, and students in the area of reproductive health education. Its principal activity was the operation of reproductive health clinics in nine Kazakhstan cities. These and other NGOs partnered with the Red Apple in the following peer counseling efforts:

- *Training:* In key cities, NGO peer counselors were provided with introductory training in contraceptive technology and counseling. They were also offered, after appropriate screening, the opportunity to try Red Apple products free for six months. The counselors' activities were overseen by reproductive health physicians.
- *Seminars:* NGO representatives scheduled contraceptive seminars in locations frequented by the Red Apple's target audiences, such as health club facilities, and on campuses of colleges and universities. Speakers (from among the Red Apple's cadre of trained doctors and pharmacists; Red Apple distributors; and its NGO partner, the Medical and Pedagogical Association of Kazakhstan) addressed contraception and reproductive health issues.

Media Channels

In addition to the small but important number of seminars/special events conducted by SOMARC NGO partners was a full range of Red Apple communication efforts through both mass and interpersonal channels.

Mass Media

During the Soviet era, Kazakhstan's state-owned and state-controlled mass media (both broadcast and print) were well developed and provided virtually 100% national coverage through a handful of stations and newspapers. With independence and the transition to a market-based economy came a carving up of the state communications apparatus. At its height in late 1996, this "carving" produced as many as 50 TV and 30 radio stations (Katsiev, 2003). While still receiving feeds from the Russian network, programming options were greatly reduced, as were funds to purchase them.

The situation worked to the project's advantage, because it presented SOMARC with opportunities to structure favorable deals to provide original material in exchange for discounted air time. The local Red Apple advertising agency was especially skilled at negotiating Red Apple media buys and navigating through the plethora of stations and coverage/reach.

As a result of the combination of reach and cost and the agency's expertise in piecing together national coverage, television was the primary focus of the Red Apple mass media campaign, followed by radio and print. Comprehensive media plans were developed that incorporated a broad range of approaches to airing Red Apple material, from "traditional" buying of 30-, 45-, and 60-second commercial spots to producing and providing programming (such as the introductory feature and SOMARC-produced "call-in" TV and radio shows) for free in exchange for prime air time and a right to the surrounding commercials.

Public Relations

To extend and leverage the Red Apple communications effort, SOMARC worked with its public relations (PR) agency to develop a comprehensive public relations plan to complement the paid advertising effort. Included in it were a number of PR activities that were new to Kazakhstan's emerging commercial media market and directly led to the appearance of at least 300 broadcast and print stories about the Red Apple and Red Apple–related subjects.

Notable PR "firsts":

- Video and audio news releases, as well as programming (infomercials), written specifically to inform target audiences. TV and radio programs were produced by the Red Apple agencies using Red Apple spokespeople discussing issues surrounding contraception.
- Call-in radio programs (talk radio/TV) were developed as a forum for Red Apple issues and to provide cutting-edge information for adult audiences. Show topics covered included reproductive health, teenage sexuality, AIDS, and other relevant issues that were linked to the subject of contraception.

EVOLUTION OF STRATEGY AND TACTICS

Following the launch of the Red Apple, sales fluctuated at levels generally below the original program expectations, although government statistics showed that the abortion rate was declining. Monitoring and secondary research analysis revealed two problem areas where results were not at expected/needed levels. Trial and continued/sustained usage of Red Apple contraceptives were less than anticipated/ projected. Also, distribution was uneven, and consistent, broad availability of Red Apple products had not yet been achieved, contributing to the sustained usage problem. Consequently, following launch and 6 to 12 months of data collection, Red Apple strategy was refocused, and important adjustments made to two components of the marketing mix:

- *Communications:* Messages and dissemination activities were refined to more specifically address consumer fears of hormonal products in order to encourage product trial and sustained usage.
- *Distribution:* Support for core Red Apple participants (distributors, market service companies, and contraceptive manufacturers) was expanded to help provide for a reliable and consistent product supply and eventual project transition to viable, engaged partners.

This adjustment of strategy resulted in the introduction of SOMARC's most innovative efforts, and reproductive health social marketing firsts:

- The Red Apple hotline.
- Pharmacy detailing.

The hotline and detailing efforts were, by design, integrally linked. This linking allowed for considerable economy in the staffing and training plans for both activities and made their eventual commercial sustainability a more reasonably achievable goal. Additionally, although separate activities, each reinforced the other in their dual objectives of reaching both consumers and the medical profession to ultimately promote contraceptive sales. The program linkage between the two activities came in the dual role Red Apple personnel played. The operator-detailers split their time between staffing the hotline and calling on medical professionals.

The Hotline/Detailing Program was a collaborative effort among SOMARC, Medservice Plus (the largest of the Red Apple pharmaceutical distributors), Nursat (the telecommunication company that developed and provided the toll-free satellite phone network), and the Kazakhstan Medical and Pedagogical Association (the program technical adviser and trainer of the operator-detailers).

The hotline became operational in early 1998. It was linked to the Red Apple mass media communications campaign and promoted as a free and anonymous consumer information source. Designed to offer information and counseling about modern contraceptives and reproductive health topics and issues to both women and men, its operator-detailers could also direct callers to the closest pharmacies that stocked Red Apple products.

The hotline was an immediate "hit." Within the first 18 months of operation, hotline operator-detailers received more than 42,000 calls and answered more than 50,000 questions from callers throughout Kazakhstan. It was estimated that among Almaty residents alone, 1 in every 35 had used the service. SOMARC data suggested hotline calls were directly correlated to Red Apple sales (see Tables 11-2 and 11-3, as well as Figure 11-6).

The periodic reports of Red Apple operator-detailers also indicated a connection between hotline and detailing activities and sales growth/product interest. The operator-detailers noted that the pharmacies they contacted regularly ordered larger quantities of contraceptives when they were supported by the hotline.

TABLE 11-2   Calls to the Red Apple Consumer Information Hotline (January–May 1999)

	January	February	March	April	May	Total YTD
Hotline Cities:						
Almaty	868	879	958	1,164	1,178	**5,047**
Astana	9	6	2	5	79	**101**
Aktubinsk	3		22	19	19	**63**
Aktau	22	29	21	20	17	**109**
Atyrau		1	6	8	18	**33**
Karaganda	11	27	127	46	31	**242**
Pavlodar	36	43	96	47	53	**275**
Shymkent	17	9	22	23	29	**100**
Taraz	4	2	13	27	62	**108**
Uralsk	11	6	11	6	2	**36**
Total number of calls	*981*	*1,002*	*1,278*	*1,365*	*1,488*	*6,114*

Source: Author (hotline operator-detailer data collection record compilation).

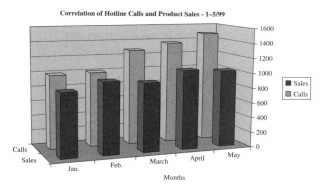

FIGURE 11-6   Hotline Calls vs. Sales

TABLE 11-3   Oral Contraceptive Sales (Almaty): From Hotline/Detailing Launch (March 1998–May 1999)

	March 1998	April 1998	May 1998	June 1998	July 1998	August 1998	September 1998	October 1998	November 1998	December 1998	January 1999	February 1999	March 1999	April 1999	May 1999	TOTALS
Marvelon	167	342	494	670	631	810	662	604	686	706	643	556	491	714	752	8,928
Microgynon	14	84	153	166	239	201	212	195	571	333	394	342	279	363	563	4,109
Tri-Regol	252	987	1,125	1,680	1,432	2,322	1,746	1,151	953	827	847	957	913	1,057	1,030	17,279
Regividon	591	1,371	1,704	2,412	1,797	2,869	2,197	1,850	1,530	1,628	1,525	1,560	1,282	1,432	1,769	25,517
Triquilar	576	1,419	1,995	2,988	1,845	3,584	2,991	1,458	1,081	917	807	912	638	862	1,041	23,114
Cilest								18	28	48	51	84	95	80	69	473
Diane-35		19	31	73	85	152	177	224	312	335	295	192	124	246	300	2,565
Excluton										39	32	39	28	40	92	270
Total OCs:	**1,600**	**4,222**	**5,502**	**7,989**	**6,029**	**9,938**	**7,985**	**5,500**	**5,161**	**4,833**	**4,594**	**4,642**	**3,850**	**4,794**	**5,616**	**82,255**

Source: Author (hotline operator-detailer data collection record compilation).

BUDGET

USAID funding of the Red Apple project was predicated on the assumption that it would be short term in nature and that any program costs remaining upon the expiration of U.S. assistance would be covered by Red Apple commercial partners. Because of the transitional/short-term nature of the planned assistance, none of the money was to be used to procure products (a typically large component of conventional reproductive health social marketing projects).

In the six years of USAID support of the Red Apple, it spent approximately US$3 million directly on contracted, in-country marketing services (including paid media buys). Project management and the provision of the large technical assistance component added as much as an additional US$10.5 million.

Even with those seemingly big numbers, the Red Apple budget was not large by U.S. commercial marketing standards, especially for a national program. However, it was commensurate with what was then being spent on similar private marketing efforts by the Red Apple commercial partners, in the expectation that it would ultimately be economically possible for them to continue the program on a solely commercial basis (see Table 11-4).

OUTCOMES

Going Out of Business (Mostly)

The Red Apple program was managed by USAID prime SOMARC contractor, The Futures Group International, until October 1998, when the program development contract ended. At that time, private sector manufacturers and distributors were commercially supplying Red Apple contraceptive products so that they were consistently available throughout the country in more than 80% of Kazakhstan's (then) 2,000 pharmacies (10 years later, the coverage was more than 90%; Kazakhstan Medical and Pedagogical Association, 2008). Moreover, basic marketing support activities for those products, piloted with USAID funding, were being undertaken and paid for by the manufacturers and commercial import and distribution companies.

There remained, however, two key communication and marketing components—the Red Apple Hotline and Red Apple Detailing efforts—that were not fully commercially sustainable at the end of the original contract. These

TABLE 11-4   Sample Budget: Final 8 Months (February–September 1998)

Sample Budget				
Market research	**Rate**	**Units**		**≥ Total**
Monitoring	$3,000	10		$ 30,000
Total				$ 30,000
Public Relations				
Events	$2,500.00			$0
Materials (printing, photocopies)	$ 0.10	1,000	copies	$ 100
Total				$ 100
Training				
QCS Training	$1,000	8	sess.	$ 8,000
Materials (reprints)	5	50	items	250
Other direct costs (ODCs) (communications)	62.5	6	months	375
Seminars	7,000	1		7,000
Detailing teams				5,000
Total				$ 20,625
Advertising				
Production (60-second spots, TV)	$5,000	1.0	spots	$ 5,000
Media time: TV	1,200	100	spots	120,000
Media time: radio	500	58	spots	29,000
Hotline	25,000	1		25,000
Production (point-of-sale material)	125	2	items	250
Printing promotional material (brochures)	2.5	2,000	copies	5,000
Total				$184,250

Source: Author (draft/sample budget prepared for USAID funding extension, 1998).

two activities were introduced as a tactical adjustment in direct response to research indicating a need for more detailed information by both consumers and health professionals if they were to become and remain Red Apple customers (both users and advocates). It was clear at the time of their development that these two linked activities would likely not be fully adopted and maintained by the Red Apple commercial partners. However, the value demonstrated by the Hotline/Detailing Program to both the Red Apple and potentially other reproductive health education efforts was sufficient enough, even after only a few months of operation, for USAID to allow an exception to its requirement that all activities be commercially viable, and funding was extended an additional two years through USAID's Commercial Market Strategies (CMS) project.

The money was well spent. During that extension of support, the Red Apple Hotline/Detailing Program continued to expand its activities and achieved the following:

- Detailed an increasing number of service delivery points so that more than 1,600 pharmacies were selling Red Apple products around the country.
- Added three new products to the Red Apple family of contraceptives.
- Expanded the Red Apple hotline to another city and trained hotline operator-detailers on additional reproductive health issues.
- Responded to increasing numbers of hotline calls: from January to September 2000, Red Apple operator-detailers talked to more than 23,000 callers, answering 28,800 questions on reproductive health issues.
- Made more than 1,000 referrals per month, directing hotline callers to Red Apple pharmacies and clinics.
- Tracked a dramatic threefold increase in sales of Red Apple products in a little more than a year from the launch of the hotline.

A HARD-EARNED SUCCESS

USAID funding of the full Red Apple program in Kazakhstan lasted for approximately six years, with an additional two years of support for the hotline and detailing efforts. When the Red Apple finally transitioned entirely into nongovernment hands, the two major goals of the project had been largely met.

- *Goal 1—Consumers:* Encourage trial and continued use of contraceptives as the primary method of fertility regulation and a substitute for abortion.

  By the time USAID support ended, the Red Apple was responsible for a significant portion of a public health effort that saw Kazakhstan's total abortion rate drop by approximately 50%, while there was a parallel increase of a similar magnitude in the use of modern contraceptive practice. (Westoff, 2000)

- *Goal 2—Suppliers:* Make contraceptives available through the national network of newly privatized retail pharmacies.

    From a starting point that saw sporadic availability of old formulation, high-dose oral contraceptives and Russian-produced, failure-prone, condoms, through a network of approximately 400 state pharmacies (many existing on paper only), to a consistently available supply of Western standard, modern formulation hormonal contraceptives through a commercial network of more than 1,600 privately owned and operated/licensed pharmacies.

    The ultimate success of the Red Apple program was determined largely by the close relationships established and built among pharmaceutical manufacturers, distributors, and retailers.
- The manufacturers cooperated by accepting market-entry risks, extending their best terms to previously unknown/untested new distributors, printing the Red Apple logo on their products, providing information updates about products to hotline operator-detailers, and collaborating on promotional activities.
- Distributors supplied the contraceptives at a reasonable price and serviced/supported the market by using a percentage of their profits to continue Red Apple marketing efforts.
- Pharmacies/pharmacists maintained stocks of Red Apple products, counseled users/purchasers in their safe correct use, and provided the critical link between consumers and suppliers of quality reproductive health products.

SUMMARY

By all important measures, the Kazakhstan Red Apple program was a success. The principal program objectives were met: Kazakhstani women were having fewer abortions, contraceptives were widely available through commercial channels, the private sector had adopted and continued much of the market support effort, and the client was pleased. Why and how had this happened, and more importantly, what can be learned from it?

Universal Lessons from a Once-in-a-Lifetime Setting

Many of the challenges faced by the newly independent states of the former Soviet Union were unique to the time and place. Kazakhstan and the other republics were not developing countries. They had talented resources—with many capabilities—but lacked the necessary means to take advantage of them in the radically new, market-based environment. However, even with the marked differences of Kazakhstan from the more typical development/social marketing setting and the program adaptations required to address them, important lessons emerge from the work of the Red Apple that are directly applicable to other environments where social marketing efforts may be considered.

Build Capacity

Perhaps the most important of the lessons to come from the SOMARC Red Apple Program was its approach to the issue of sustainability. Whether by design or by default, the constraints imposed by the intended short-term/transitional nature of U.S. assistance were fundamental in shaping program design and execution decisions that led directly to the successful transfer of key program components to the private sector.

Central to this approach was the idea of building capacity, not infrastructure, as the path to sustainability. The Red Apple's sustainable successes were a direct result of using program resources to identify, support, and develop the already considerable capabilities of the local professionals who, following the collapse of the Soviet Union, would become marketing service providers in the fields of market research, advertising, public relations, and pharmaceutical sales and distribution.

The challenges to this approach were considerable. A more traditional strategy of establishing (and funding) a dedicated organization to develop and manage the social marketing effort might have yielded quicker and more quantifiable initial results. While an especially tempting prospect given the relatively short-term nature of the assistance, the likelihood of such an organization continuing to exist and serve its intended function in the absence of donor funding was low, particularly in the freewheeling, capitalism-on-steroids environment of post-Soviet Central Asia, where the return from investing scarce resources in relatively low-margin, single-product pharmaceutical ventures was not especially attractive. Instead, considerable time was devoted (risked) to select and assemble a commercial team that would integrate the new social marketing functions with commercially motivated ones.

This process was not easy, smooth, or quick. In the program development stage, more than 50 companies were approached as potential participants in the Red Apple program before stable partnerships were established. Adherence to the strategy was rewarded when the result proved the effort worthwhile by delivering a life to the program that has now extended more than a decade beyond the initial donor funding period.

Choose Appropriate Measures

While, as previously noted, the Red Apple was a success on virtually every level, it was not always viewed that way. Because of its nonstandard hybrid design and the extended time period needed to identify, recruit, and train the various program partners, the Red Apple initially lacked not only the more traditional reproductive health program measures of success, but marketing information of all sorts. The extended period between the start of program activities and the actual launch of product sales created a "dataless" window during which concern over the wisdom of the approach grew. Ultimately, as the case study showed, the concern was unfounded. However, with any new social marketing effort comes an opportunity to introduce measures that not only return timely, actionable information to the program, but also serve to provide funders with evidence their money is being well spent. Because of a tendency to rely on established or accepted measures, this opportunity is often overlooked initially—and in all too many instances, not considered at all. This can be especially true if it appears the assistance effort will be a long-term one, where success tends to be gauged more by traditional development measures that may not correlate well with standard marketing tactics and the specific feedback needed to tune the marketing mix.

In the case of the Red Apple, because of the reliance on newly established businesses for virtually all the marketing components of the program, the generation of marketing information was necessarily a function of these young businesses' ability and interest to deliver. As these organizations gained experience in both the marketplace and Western business practice, the breadth and depth of useful information that could be contracted for and/or found from open/public sources increased markedly. Until that occurrence though, program managers and donor evaluators had only anecdotal and/or inferential methods of determining whether funding was being used effectively. With that lack of traditional measures of success came a hesitancy to endorse the new approach.

Some, if not all, of this early conflict over program direction and effectiveness could have been lessened by introducing new measures more appropriate to both the early capabilities of the program partners and the new approach being undertaken.

Conclusion

It has long been the authors' contention that social marketing has the best chance for success when it most resembles commercial marketing in its adherence to the fundamental details of the marketing discipline, from its initial strategic design to daily tactical decisions. The success of the Red Apple program offers strong support for that premise. The key programmatic choices that it guided should serve as a model for social marketing efforts elsewhere—especially where managers of emerging economies are seeking ways to stimulate the private sector and in places where long-term commercial sustainability may be a possibility.

QUESTIONS FOR DISCUSSION

1. Is program self-sufficiency something to strive for? Funding for social marketing efforts, as with most if not all public social programs, continues a historic decline. For programs where revenues are present, self-sufficiency (or at least the possibility of covering some of the program's costs) may be a real possibility. Is this a reasonable goal? Should self-sufficiency and/or cost recovery be a delineated objective where it might be possible? If it is, how can/might/will this parameter affect the strategy and tactics of the program both positively and negatively?

2. What are the benefits and drawbacks (if any) to having a physical "product"? Public health social marketing programs, by their nature, often include some sort of physical product. Having a tangible "product" can make strategic and tactical development and planning more closely match commercial marketing practice. Is this necessarily a good thing? Conventional wisdom suggests that the closer social marketing can come to its commercial roots, the greater the chances are for success; however, there may be drawbacks as well. The presence of a "product" facilitates the adoption of commercial success measures, like sales revenues, that can overpower social objectives. How can (and should) programs balance these two measures?

REFERENCES

BRIF. (1997a). *Kazakhstan provider study—Preliminary summary of findings.* Washington, DC: The Futures Group International.

BRIF. (1997b). *Kazakhstan tracking study—Summary of findings.* Washington, DC: The Futures Group International.

Central Intelligence Agency (CIA). (2009). *The World Factbook.* Retrieved July 28, 2009, from https://www.cia.gov/library/publications/the-world-factbook/geos/kz.html

Darsky, L., & Dworak, N. (1993). *Kazakhstan: Fertility indicators and characteristics of the potential market for contraception.* Washington, DC: The Futures Group International.

The Futures Group International. (1994). *Kazakhstan baseline survey.* Washington, DC: Author.

Hausloner, P. (1995). *Privatizing the pharmaceutical sector in the former Soviet Union.* Bethesda, MD: Abt Associates.

Henshaw, S., Singh, S., & Haas, T. (1999). The incidence of abortion worldwide. *International Family Perspectives* 25(Suppl.).

Katsiev, O. (2003). *Television and radio companies, operating in the Republic of Kazakhstan.* Retrieved July 28, 2009, from http://old.internews.kz/eng/stations/index.htm.

Kazakhstan Medical and Pedagogical Association. (2008). *Pharmacy survey.* Almaty, Kazakhstan: Author.

Krakoff, C. (1997). *Pharmacy sector privatization and restructuring in Kazakhstan.* Bethesda, MD: Abt Associates.

Popov, A. (1990). Sky-high abortion rates reflect dire lack of choice. *Entre Nous* 16, 5–7.

Tarnoff, C. (2002). *U.S. assistance to the former Soviet Union 1991–2001: A History of Administration and Congressional Action.* (CRC-Report for Congress. CRS-Web Order Code: 30148.) Washington, DC: Congressional Research Service, the Library of Congress.

USAID. (2007). *Our work: Health: Family planning: Technical areas: Contraceptive social marketing.* Retrieved July 28, 2009 from http://www.usaid.gov/our_work/global_health/pop/techareas/contrasocial/index.html#

USAID/Macro International. (1995). *Kazakhstan demographic and health survey—DHS.* Calverton, MD: Author.

Westoff, C. (2000). *The substitution of contraception for abortion in Kazakhstan in the 1990s* (DHS Analytical Studies, No. 1). Calverton, MD: ORC Macro.

CHAPTER 12

"Love Your Liver, Improve Your Health"

A Hepatitis B Prevention and Educational Campaign in China

Hong Cheng, Jun Qiao, and Huixin Zhang

In this chapter, major public health issues in China and its government strategies and policies on those issues are first reviewed. After that, a nationwide campaign on hepatitis B prevention and education is explored in the case study.

CHINA: A COUNTRY OVERVIEW

General Information

China, formally called the People's Republic of China since 1949 when the Communist Party of China came to power, is one of the oldest civilizations in the world, with a recorded history of more than 4,000 years (*Encyclopedia Britannica*, 2009). Situated in East Asia, China has a total area of 9.6 million square kilometers (about 3.7 million square miles), second only to Russia in land area, and is the fourth largest in the world—after Russia, Canada, and the United States—in total size (including water area). Home to 1.34 billion people, China is the most populous nation in the world today (Central Intelligence Agency [CIA], 2009; China quick facts, 2009).

Of the 56 ethnic groups in China, Han Chinese comprise 91.6% of the nation's population. By far the most common Chinese tongue is Putonghua (Mandarin), which literally means "ordinary or common language." Many of the Han speak some mutually unintelligible dialects, but they are unified by their traditions and cultural traits, as well as the written characters of their language. The other 55 ethnic groups account for 8.4% of China's total population (China quick facts, 2009; CIA, 2009).

China also is a country with multiple religions, mainly including Buddhism, Daoism, Islamism, Catholicism, and Christianity. In accordance with the Constitution of the People's Republic of China (2004), Chinese citizens are entitled the right to "enjoy freedom of religious belief" (p. 10).

Administratively, China is divided into 23 provinces, five autonomous regions, four centrally administered municipalities, and two special administrative regions (SARs; *Chinese cities and provinces*, 2009). Directly under the administration of the central government, Beijing, Shanghai, Tianjin, and Chongqing have "the same political, economical, and jurisdictional rights as a province" (*Chinese cities and provinces*, 2009, p. 1). The sovereignty of Hong Kong and Macao, the two SARs, was handed over to the PRC from the United Kingdom and Portugal in 1997 and 1999, respectively. China regards Taiwan as one of its provinces (China quick facts, 2009). Conventionally, China is also divided by regions—North, Northeast, South, Southwest, West, Northwest, Central, and East—based on their geographical locations in the country (Regions, 2008).

A new era in contemporary Chinese history began in late 1978 when a national policy of economic reform and opening up to the outside was adopted, which ushered in an economic boom that has lasted for three decades so far. Leading the world in terms of the growth rate in gross domestic product (GDP), China had an average annual growth of 9.7% from 1978 through 2008 (Chinability, 2008; China's GDP grows, 2009). This increase rate made China's 2008 GDP more than 70 times the 1978 figure (You, 2008). Despite a global economic recession, China's GDP in 2009 was still expected to grow about 8% (China's 2009 GDP, 2009). Measured on the basis of purchasing power parity (PPP), estimated at US$7.8 trillion in 2008, China is the second largest economy in the world today, trailing only the United States. In per capita terms, however, China is still a lower-middle-income country (CIA, 2009).

The economic development in China is quite unbalanced, with the coastal areas in the east far more developed than the regions in the west. To help western regions to catch up, the Chinese government currently is implementing a large-scale Western China Development program, seen as "a Chinese version of Germany's 'rebuilding the east'" by some in Western countries (Schüller, 2005, p. 89).

Major Public Health Achievements and Issues

As a developing nation, China has made enormous efforts to improve public health and proclaimed "momentous achievements" (Wen, 2008, p. 5). Between 2003 and 2007, for example, total government expenditures on medical and health care in the country reached 629.4 billion yuan (about US$78.6 billion), a 127% increase from the prior five-year period. While infant and maternal mortality rates dropped significantly, average life expectancy reached 73.5 years in 2009 (CIA, 2009), a nearly 3-year increase from 2001 and a 38-year shoot-up from 1949 (Chinese people's, 2001). Females (75.5 years), on average, live about four years longer than males (71.6 years) (CIA, 2009).

Over the years, the government has set up an extensive medical network for public health—at national, provincial, municipal, and townish levels, and from urban to rural areas. By the end of 2008, there were about 300,000 medical setups in China, including more than 60,000 hospitals; 28,000 community medical centers/stations; 3,560 disease prevention and control centers/stations; and 2,591 medical supervision centers, among others (Development, 2009).

With its large population and uneven regional economic development, however, China is faced with many pressing issues in public health. Take, for example, HIV/AIDS, tuberculosis, and malaria—the three contagious diseases worrying the World Health Organization (WHO) most (WHO, 2009) or addressed in the UN Millennium Declaration (2000). Since 1985 when China discovered the first case of HIV/AIDS, the disease has spread quickly in the country (Med8th, 2009). In 2006, the Ministry of Health (MOH; the government body overseeing public health in China), UNAIDS, and WHO jointly estimated that the country had 650,000 HIV carriers and 75,000 AIDS patients. By 2007, the figure increased to 700,000 and 85,000. According to a more recent MOH report, the number of HIV carriers and AIDS patients reduced, fortunately, to 264,302 and 77,753, respectively, in 2008. Although "the spread of AIDS has generally slowed down in China," it is still "highly prevalent among specific groups such as migrant workers, and in some regions, particularly remote areas and the countryside" (China reports, 2008, p. 1).

With help from the World Bank and WHO, China launched a series of pilot projects involving the use of the directly observed treatment short course, commonly known as DOTS, in 1991 (DOTS prevents, 2009; DOTS program helps, 2004). The DOTS program in China has become the largest in the world today, preventing about 30,000 deaths a year from tuberculosis (China halves, 2009). Despite the great success of the program, tuberculosis has become a severe epidemic killer in China, with more than 130,000 people dying from the disease yearly. The country has about 5 million TB patients; 80% of them live in rural areas (China steps up, 2007).

Malaria is a major parasitic disease with a wide distribution in China. The prevalence gradually decreases from south to north. The provinces of Hainan and Yunnan, in South China and Southwest China, respectively, are the areas where malaria has been the most endemic with high transmission of *Plasmodium falciparum*, a protozoan parasite that causes malaria in humans. Since 2000, a malaria resurgence has occurred in some other parts of the country. Anhui Province in East China is the most seriously affected area, with the highest number of malaria cases in 2006 (Zhang, Wang, Fang, Ma, Xu, Tian, et al., 2008).

In addition to these three major diseases, another public health issue—hepatitis B—severely threatens people's health in China. Of the 350 million chronic hepatitis B virus (HBV) carriers worldwide (WHO, 2009), about 120 million are in China, including 20 million patients[1] (Fusu, 2006). Every year 280,000 Chinese die of hepatitis B–related diseases (Ge, 2006). China has the heaviest burden of hepatitis B in the world (So, 2004).

Public Health Strategies and Reform

Since the founding of the People's Republic, the central government's overall strategy for public health has been an emphasis of preventive rather curative medicine on the premise that the former is "active" whereas the latter "passive." Before 1978, when the economic reform in China started, all expenditures for public health system development were provided by the government. After 1978, the central finance system gradually decentralized; after 1994, the financial system was further devolved to local governments (Claeson, Wang, & Hu, 2004). From the late 1990s to 2008, government expenditure hovered between 15% and 18% of total health spending, the equivalent of 1% of China's GDP, way down from prior decades (Zhang, 2008).

As a result, "the public health system and its core functions were crucially weakened, with less attention given to routine immunization, surveillance, and health promotion activities" (Claeson et al., 2004, p. 11). "Soaring medical costs in recent years have plunged many rural and urban Chinese back into poverty" (Zhang, 2008, p. 1). Inadequate government financial support has led to a change in the nature of hospitals, from institutions that "heal the wounded and rescue the dying," which Mao Zedong, late chairman of the Communist Party of China, called for, to businesses that "seek profits above all and provide medicine and medical services as expensively as possible" (Zhang, 2008, p. 1). According to a 2007 survey by China's National Bureau of Statistics (NBS) on "unsafe" factors upsetting the

---

[1]While a *hepatitis B virus carrier* only "carries" HBV in the body, a *hepatitis B patient* has developed chronic liver disease that reduces the functioning of the liver. "Not all carriers of the virus develop chronic liver disease; in fact, a majority have no symptoms" (Hepatitis B, 2009, p. 1).

public, "rising medical costs have become the top concern among Chinese people" (Zhang, 2008, p. 1).

Amid mounting concerns from the public, the Chinese government started a medical reform in 2006, with a focus on the improvement of public health service. The main purposes of the reform are:

- To ensure the nonprofit nature of the nation's public medical service.
- To speed up building a health insurance network in both urban and rural areas.
- To set up a state catalog, production, and distribution of basic medicines.
- To improve disease prevention and control, public health monitoring, and the management of public health emergencies. (Wang, 2006; Zhang, 2008)

In 2008, the central government allocated 83.2 billion yuan (about US$11.7 billion) to support the reform and healthcare development, an increase of 16.7 billion yuan (about US$2.4 billion) over the year before. The money was spent mainly on facilities at the urban community and village level (Zhang, 2008). Some experts still suggest the government increase its spending on public health from the current 1% of GDP to 3% (Zhang, Y., 2008).

Over recent years, the central government has also promoted public health through advancing laws and regulations: Infectious Disease Prevention Law, Public Health Emergence Ordinance, SARS Prevention and Control Management Protocols, Guidance on the Strengthening of SARS Prevention and Treatment in Rural Areas, and Protocols for the Management of Public Health Emergencies and Infectious Disease Monitoring Reports.

As far as the control of hepatitis B is concerned, the disease has been listed in the Chinese government's 11th five-year plan (2006–2010). The mention of hepatitis B in the Chinese government's current economic development guidelines indicates that the control of this disease has become a national priority. In response to the central government's guidelines, the Ministry of Health also issued a five-year plan (2006–2010) particularly for hepatitis B control. In the plan, the MOH promises:

- To set up sound systems to monitor hepatitis B prevalence, the vaccination rate of newborns, and infections in high-risk groups.
- To have all medical institutions work to eliminate spread of the virus by blood transmission, one of the three major channels for virus diffusion (the other two being sexual intercourse and mother-to-child transmission).
- To reduce the positive rate of all Chinese from the current 9% to 7% and of children under 5 years old to 1% by 2010.
- To have the vaccination rate of newborns reach beyond 90% by 2010. (Chinese Health Ministry, 2006)

The MOH also highly stresses the roles of the media and other social sectors in the development of public health. Over the years, the ministry has run public service advertisements through China Central Television (CCTV), the national TV network in the country, to promote the prevention of AIDS, viral hepatitis, tuberculosis, and malaria. It has cooperated with several most influential Chinese Web sites (such as Sina, Sohu, Xinhua, and the Chinese Medicine Net) to publicize public health events and initiatives.

At the same time, many professional organizations and social groups have volunteered their service to public health. The China Advertising Association, for example, has, since 1996, hosted public service advertising (PSA) contests during its annual advertising festivals, which have played a positive role in the prevention of diseases (Cheng & Chan, 2009). Other media outlets (like *Beijing Youth Daily*, *Nanfang Metropolitan News*, and *Yangcheng Evening News*) have also organized or participated in various public health–related PSA contests (e.g., Exhibition, 2008; Second, 2006). In recent years, some enterprises have actively sponsored public health programs in the country (e.g., Healthy China, 2007). In short, public health in China involves support from the government, the media, nonprofit organizations, and the commercial sector.

CASE STUDY
The "Love Your Liver, Improve Your Health" Campaign

BACKGROUND, PURPOSE, AND FOCUS

Background

One might think HIV/AIDS, SARS, and the avian flu are the major health problems in China nowadays, due to the focus of international reports and media coverage. It is true that they are serious public health problems in the country, but "the greatest health threat and the 'silent killer' in the Chinese community" is actually hepatitis B (So, 2004, p. 1). As mentioned earlier in the chapter, there are 120 million HBV carriers in China (accounting for about 9% of the nation's total population), of which 20 million are hepatitis B patients (Fusu, 2006). Hepatitis B kills 808 people in China daily (Pettypiece, 2007). The killer of hepatitis B is "silent"—mainly because the government, the media, and the society paid little attention to it in the past (So, 2004).

"Hepatitis B is transmitted the same way as HIV/AIDS and not by food or casual contact" (So, 2004, p. 1). Many Chinese became infected at childbirth when the mother is a hepatitis B carrier. Others became infected by injections or cuts with needles, syringes, medical, or dental instruments; blood contaminated with HBV; or from unprotected sex. Most chronically infected individuals do not know they have been infected because they often feel perfectly healthy. By the time symptoms have developed, it is often too late. The reason chronic hepatitis B is so dangerous is because "without treatment or regular screening for liver cancer, one in four chronically infected persons will eventually die of liver cancer or liver failure" (So, 2004, p. 1).

Hepatitis B is preventable. The hepatitis B vaccine is a safe and effective vaccine that can protect the uninfected from HBV infection and the development of liver cancer. For this reason, the HBV vaccine is often called "the first anti-cancer vaccine" (So, 2004, p. 1). Even for those who have chronic HBV infection (often referred to as HBV carriers), most could lead normal, working lives. Many will not die if they receive treatment for hepatitis B to prevent further damage to the liver and regular monitoring to detect the cancer at an early stage when it could be successfully treated (So, 2004).

Despite the prevalence of hepatitis B, doctors interviewed in China said most people were more aware of AIDS than hepatitis B (Pettypiece, 2007). Many are not aware of the risk, the association of hepatitis B and liver cancer, the importance of HBV vaccination to prevent liver cancer, and the need for HBV carriers to have regular liver cancer screening (So, 2004).

Due to the fear caused by the lack of adequate knowledge about hepatitis B, discrimination against hepatitis B patients, and even HBV carriers, has become a widely spread social problem. According to a 2005 survey by Synovate Healthcare, a London-based research firm, 52% of Chinese hepatitis B patients lost a job or education opportunity due to their infection. The Chinese government later revised its policy to allow hiring of people who carry the virus but do not show symptoms (Pettypiece, 2007).

Suffering the disease of hepatitis B is also a major reason for poverty in many families. According to Chinese economists, patients inflicted with HBV-related liver diseases in China suffer direct economic losses of more than 26 billion yuan (nearly US$4 billion) in their personal or family lives (Sociological reading, 2007). Hepatitis B's impact on economic development and social stability cannot be underestimated.

Campaign Purposes and Rationale

As reviewed earlier, many hepatitis B–related problems (such as the public's broad unawareness of the importance of vaccination and regular screening for liver cancer, the widely spread discrimination against HBV carriers, and the lack of confidence on the part of the hepatitis B patients in overcoming the disease) warrant an anti–hepatitis B campaign in the nation. The purpose of the campaign was to decrease incidence of hepatitis B in the country with a focus on vaccines, screening, and safe sex, as well as to eliminate discrimination against HBV carriers in society.

SWOT ANALYSIS

Strengths

The campaign has a "tripartite strategic alliance" among the government (represented by China's MOH), nonprofit organizations (such as the China Foundation for Hepatitis Prevention and Control [CFHPC]), and marketing professionals (in this case, McCann Healthcare China). Given China's unique social system, the direct and strong government involvement in this campaign would help with the promotion of hepatitis B prevention and education. (Government involvement in China indicates the attention the government gives to hepatitis B problems and adds to the credibility of the campaign due to constant misleading and even deceptive information about hepatitis B treatment on the market. The Chinese government also has the power to mobilize various sectors in society for the campaign.) As part of McCann Worldwide, a New York–headquartered global advertising network, McCann Healthcare China has strong health marketing expertise and extensive experience in designing and managing health-related campaigns in China.

Weaknesses

Although this anti–hepatitis B campaign was jointly run by the MOH and the CFHPC, partially sponsored by the Bristol-Myers Squibb company (a two-year grant of US$378,000 in total to the CFHPC; Bristol-Myers Squibb, 2006), total funding (estimated at 7 million yuan, or less than US$1 million) for the campaign was still lacking, which could affect the depth of campaign activities.

Opportunities

The grim reality caused by hepatitis B rampancy in China has received great attention from the Chinese government. As mentioned earlier, in the 11th five-year plan (2006–2010) for national economic development, the government has made the strict control of hepatitis B spread a national priority. To implement this priority, the MOH has formulated a plan of hepatitis B prevention and control

(2006–2010), as well as the implementation of the "Healthy China 2020" strategy. To eliminate discrimination against HBV carriers and patients, the Ministry of Labor and Personnel issued the "General Standards on Physical Examinations for the Employment of Civil Servants (Trial Implementation)" in 2004, in which it was made clear that an applicant for a civil servant position would be disqualified only if infected with HBV, but those who are carriers of the virus should pass the physical examination so long as a contagious infection could be ruled out through further tests. Many in China welcomed the new regulations, "hailing them as a solution offered by policymakers towards resolving the issue of discriminatory hiring practices against HBV carriers" (Liu, 2006, p. 1). All these government plans, strategies, and policies regarding hepatitis B have created a favorable regulatory environment for the anti–hepatitis B campaign.

Before this campaign, the China Medical Association had appealed several times to the public through the media to perceive and prevent hepatitis B in a correct and scientific manner. These appeals were certainly helpful for this campaign.

Threats

Not only are there a large number of HBV carriers in China, but there are also people who have little knowledge about the disease. Surveys conducted by the China Medical Association in early 2006 indicted that the majority of HBV carriers did not know the basics of hepatitis B and its treatment. Besides, the society as a whole holds severe discrimination against hepatitis B patients and even virus carriers. With the fear of being discriminated, most hepatitis B patients and virus carriers do not want people around them to know about their health situation, adding to the difficulty in hepatitis B prevention and control. Furthermore, deceptive information on hepatitis B treatment is rampant, which not only misled the public but also created resistance to correct and accurate information about the disease and its treatment from more reliable resources.

SIMILAR PROGRAMS IN THE PAST

National Children's Vaccination Day

Since 1978, the national day for promoting vaccinations for children and disseminating related information has been April 25. In 2005, the General Office of the Ministry of Health issued a "Circular on National Children's Vaccination Information Day." Themed "Implement Immunization Program, Protect Children's Health," this circular further stressed the importance of vaccination for children (Lingling, 2006).

Bristol-Myers Squibb Foundation Donations

In 2002, this U.S.-based foundation donated US$510,000 to the CFHPC for "the China Rural Area Hepatitis B Prevention and Educational Project" (Press releases, 2004). In 2005, the Bristol-Myers Squibb Foundation (BMSF) donated US$50,000 to fund CFHPC's report on the prevalence of hepatitis in China and related issues. In 2006, the BMSF contributed US$200,000 to the CFHPC to carry out a two-year project on hepatitis B education and advisory activities for women of reproductive age in rural areas of Gansu and Shaanxi, two provinces in the underdeveloped West China. In 2007, BMSF spent another US$371,000 in its collaboration with the Shanghai Charity Foundation and the Shanghai Center for Disease Control for awareness programs for 200,000 people, including migrant workers, high-risk groups, schoolchildren and teachers, and hepatitis patients and their families (Hepatitis in Asia, 2009).

These prior programs and activities paved the way for this nationwide anti–hepatitis B campaign. They made many people aware of the importance of vaccination and had many, especially children, vaccinated. They also provided valuable experience to the upcoming anti–hepatitis B campaign, in terms of campaign planning and partnering with the BMSF. Nevertheless, these prior programs were either short term (one day a year only) or regional in scope. Thus, a large-scale national campaign was still called for.

TARGETED AUDIENCE

Primary Target

According to a "Study on the Cognitive Status of Chinese Hepatitis B Patients" released by the Chinese Medical Association in 2006, those aged 20 to 50 were 89% of the sample; those who had been married and/or had children accounted for 62% of the sample; and men and women were almost equally represented in the sample. Thus, the primary target of this anti–hepatitis B campaign was determined as men and women aged 20 to 50.

- *University students.* China has about 2,300 colleges and universities, with a total enrollment of more than 23 million undergraduates (typically aged 18 to 24) and graduates (typically up to 30 years old; Higher education, 2007). This segment in the population is not only at high risk of hepatitis B (due to increasing sexual liberation among the youth), but also directly faces discrimination against HBV carriers on campus and in society. It is critical to provide these young people with essential knowledge on hepatitis B prevention and orient them with the correct attitude toward HBV carriers among them.

- *Hepatitis B virus carriers and patients in the general public.* As mentioned earlier, there are 120 million HBV carriers (including 20 million chronic hepatitis B patients) in China. According to formative research, these people need basic information and knowledge about hepatitis B as well as appropriate and timely screening. This segment of the population also suffers widespread discrimination in society.

Secondary Target

- *The 20- to 50-year-olds in the general public.* According to formative research, fundamental information and knowledge about hepatitis B was essential for the prevention and control of the disease in China. Prevalent discrimination against hepatitis B patients and virus carriers in society was also found to be related to the lack of basic knowledge and information about the disease.

CAMPAIGN OBJECTIVES

The overall objectives of the campaign were to promote hepatitis B prevention and treatment across the nation. Specifically, the campaign was designed to achieve the following:

Behavior Objectives

- To pay due attention to hepatitis B by getting vaccinated and/or tested for hepatitis B prevention and treatment.
- To prevent oneself from hepatitis B virus infection by using condoms during sex.
- To avoid discriminating HBV carriers and patients.
- To resort to appropriate approaches (like legal means, if necessary) and avoid inappropriate ones (such as violence) when facing hepatitis B–caused discrimination.

Knowledge Objectives

- To realize the importance of liver health.
- To appreciate appropriate and timely vaccinations, especially for children.

- To know the necessity of regular screening for hepatitis B virus carriers and patients.
- To understand how the disease is transmitted.
- To become familiar with hepatitis B–related government regulation.

Belief Objectives

- To believe that hepatitis B is preventable.
- To believe that discrimination is not a solution for the hepatitis B problem.

CAMPAIGN BARRIERS, BENEFITS, AND COMPETITION

Barriers

- Deep-rooted unhealthy lifestyles among some people, especially high-risk groups.
- Lack of adequate knowledge about hepatitis B—its transmission and treatment—which gives rise to many people's lack of attention to the disease and/or their ungrounded fear for it.
- Costs for hepatitis B vaccination, screening, and treatment, especially for low-income individuals and families.
- Lack of convenient access to hepatitis B vaccination, screening, and treatment.

Benefits

- A healthy lifestyle contributes to good health.
- Availability of the information and knowledge needed to prevent oneself properly from hepatitis B and help others, especially family members and children.
- Free hepatitis B vaccines for many, especially children under age 5 in underdeveloped areas.
- A healthier and happier society for everyone to live in, when this infectious disease and the discrimination it has caused are both under control.

Competition

- Misleading and deceptive information on hepatitis B treatments.

- Competing needs for government and public attention and resources from other diseases (such as HIV/AIDS and avian influenza, commonly known as "bird flu") and other national priorities (such as economic development and poverty alleviation for the low-income population).

CAMPAIGN POSITIONING

This nationwide anti–hepatitis B campaign is one filled with care and love—care about one's own liver health and one's loved ones'. With "Love Your Liver, Improve Your Health" as its slogan—and through its caring and loving tone—the campaign provides the target audiences with the fundamental information and knowledge they need to care for their own liver health and free them from unnecessary fears of hepatitis B virus carriers and patients.

CAMPAIGN STRATEGIES AND IMPLEMENTATIONS

Product Strategies and Implementations

Core Product

- A healthy liver makes you and your loved ones healthy and happy.

Actual Product

- Protected sex helps reduce the danger of being infected by hepatitis B.
- Appropriate and timely hepatitis B vaccinations are the most effective way to prevent hepatitis B, especially for newborns.
- Hepatitis B patients and virus carriers should go to hospitals for appropriate and timely screening.
- Family members and/or friends of hepatitis B patients or virus carriers should urge them to get appropriate and timely medical assistance.
- Discrimination is no protection for hepatitis B.
- Hepatitis B vaccines.

Price Strategies and Implementations

- The major "costs" for hepatitis B prevention and control are good personal lifestyles.

- Hepatitis B vaccinations are free for children in many parts of the country, especially those underdeveloped ones. In the underdeveloped western region, for example, the government started an immunization project for children. More than US$30 million in project funding came from abroad, while the central government allocated 100 million yuan, or some US$12.5 million, for this project (Ge, 2006).
- Hepatitis B vaccinations are not costly (about 20 yuan, or less than US$3, per shot); one only needs three shots for lifelong immunization (Fusu, 2006).

Place Strategies and Implementations

The People's Great Hall in Beijing was selected to launch the campaign. (The Hall to China is like what the Capitol Hill is to the United States: where many important national affairs are discussed and many important national and international conferences and events are held.) This high-profile venue should give the campaign a strong start, attracting large media coverage and public attention.

- In cities and well-developed rural areas, hepatitis B prevention and control information and knowledge were made easily available and accessible to the primary target audience.
- In underdeveloped regions, special efforts were made to deliver such information and treatments, including free hepatitis B vaccinations. For example, the CFHPC delivered free vaccinations to children in 331 primary schools and kindergartens in Qinghai Province and offered information sessions on hepatitis B prevention to rural women of childbearing age in Gansu and Shaanxi provinces during the campaign (Hepatitis in Asia, 2009; Zhang Weijian appointed, 2007). (The free hepatitis B vaccination delivery was an integration of the 4Ps.)

Promotion Strategies and Implementations

The promotion strategies for the campaign were mainly twofold: (1) it took an integrated marketing communications approach, involving advertising, public relations, and special events, among other communications means, and (2) it resorted to celebrities who are popular among the target audience, especially the young. These celebrities are also HBV carriers, who would function as role models for those suffering from the disease both physically and psychologically on how to fight the battle against it.

Celebrity Endorsement

- McCann Healthcare China, the designated marketing company for the campaign, invited Andy Lau—LIU Dehua, as he is known in the Chinese mainland—to be a voluntary "Ambassador of Hepatitis B Prevention and Control." A Hong Kong pop singer and film actor/producer, Lau is called a "superstar" by the Chinese media. He "came out" himself, confessing that he has been an HBV carrier since his childhood. Lau's confession was perceived as a risky act, because in the showbiz world, "any unfavorable rumor can destroy a star's career." But Lau did not waver in his commitment. Many see his confession and commitment "a true milestone in the battle against the daily discrimination suffered by HBV carriers across the country" (Stars show, 2007, p. 2; see Figure 12-1).

- Lau composed "Darling," the campaign theme song, and wrote its lyrics, which sound like his whispers to his liver—his "Darling." A few lines of the lyrics are translated from Chinese into English here to give you an idea of the song:

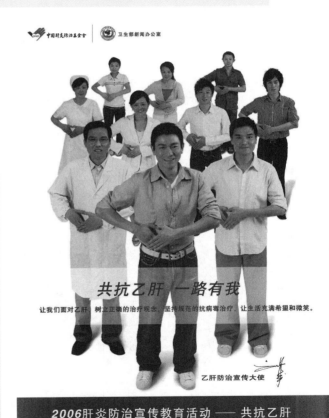

FIGURE 12-1 Hong Kong Superstar Andy Lau, Front Center, Featured in a Campaign Advertisement
Photo courtesy of *China Advertising*

Darling
I, I give you everything I could
My care, my sweetness, and my breath
. . .
Because of you, I understand how valuable life is
Did you know, your carelessness will make me sad for the rest of my life
. . .
You, you are the one and only in my life
Your voice, your encouragement, the meanings [of life] to me
. . .
If we don't have a good health
How can we be together
. . .
(Darling, 2006)

- As the campaign's publicity ambassador, Lau visited HBV sufferers in hospitals and publicly criticized schools that refused to enroll HBV students (see Figure 12-2).
- From June through August 2006, a hepatitis B prevention and educational TV spot starring Andy Lau was completed by TIAN Zhuangzhuang, a renowned film director in China. Lau invited Tian and LIN Jiadong (a well-known artist in China) to take part in the anti–hepatitis B campaign. It was the first time that Tian directed a PSA. The celebrities' participations captured enormous media and public attention.

Press Conference

- After several months' preparations, on August 30, 2006, this nationwide anti–hepatitis B campaign was kicked off in Beijing. A press conference titled "the Launch of China Hepatitis B Prevention and Educational Activities" was held in the People's Great Hall. It was at the press conference that Andy Lau was officially appointed the publicity ambassador of this campaign (see Figure 12-3).

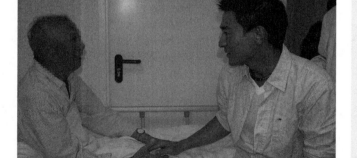

FIGURE 12-2   Andy Lau, right, Hong Kong Superstar and Campaign Ambassador during a Hospital Visit with Hepatitis B Patients

Photo courtesy of *China Advertising*

Public Service Advertisements

- The aforementioned PSA had two versions—a 30-second clip and a 15-second spot. The story told in the PSA went that when Andy Lau had learned his friend and co-worker got hepatitis B, he comforted him, encouraged him, and helped him rebuild his confidence and courage for life, and was even willing to accompany him to fight against the disease. This storyline had strong emotional appeal, reinforced by strong visuals, the campaign song composed and written by Lau, and his encouraging voice-over. This PSA narrowed the distance between TV viewers and the campaign and brought the theme of the campaign to life: "Mobilize all people, care for our health, and combat hepatitis B together."

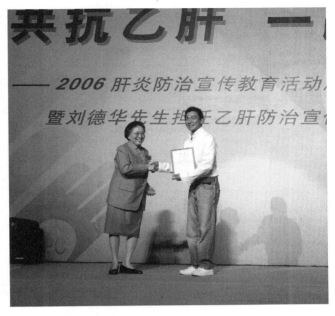

FIGURE 12-3   Hong Kong Superstar Andy Lau, right, Appointed the "Ambassador of Hepatitis B Prevention and Control"

Photo courtesy of *China Advertising*

Media Synergy

- Various media outlets, national or local, participated in the campaign promotion. Coordinated by Universal McCann China, McCann Healthcare China's media partner, publicized the campaign song through the TV and radio stations across the country, including those economically underdeveloped areas. Those TV stations that broadcast the campaign song in their MTV programs also aired the PSA spot that Andy Lau starred.
- Universal McCann China also won free or discounted space from newspapers, magazines, the Internet, and out-of-home advertising media (such as billboards) for the campaign.

- McCann Healthcare China designed a flyer on hepatitis B prevention and control, having it inserted into Lau's CD, *Andy Lau Voice 2006*, in which the campaign song "Darling" was included. The CD was distributed nationwide, and in many Asian countries, by Lau's publishing company. (Making the campaign visible overseas not only created broader visibility for the campaign, but also attracted donations from other countries.) The campaign song was the only Mandarin song on this album. Although Lau's fans in the Chinese mainland like his songs in Cantonese, his "mother tongue," a song sung by Lau in Mandarin, "the common language" in the Chinese mainland, added cultural proximity to the song that emotionally appeals to the target audience (see Figure 12-4).

Campaign Poster Contest

- The CFHPC hosted a "Love Your Liver, Improve Your Health" poster design contest among campuses. Students from more than 100 colleges and universities across the country participated in the competition.

Corporation Sponsorships

- BMSF donated nearly 600,000 yuan (more than US$80,000) to the CFHPC-hosted student contest.
- As mentioned earlier in the chapter, BMSF has been a major donor to various anti–hepatitis B programs in China. In 2006, when this campaign was ongoing, BMSF donated another US$200,000 to the CFHPC to carry out a two-year project on hepatitis B education and advisory activities for women of reproductive age in the underdeveloped rural areas in West China.

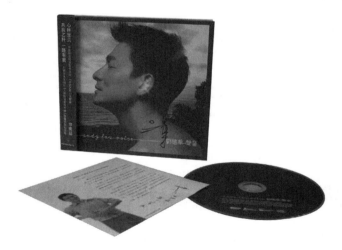

FIGURE 12-4 Flyer and CD for Andy Lau's Newly Released Album

Photo courtesy of *China Advertising*

CAMPAIGN OUTCOME AND EVALUATION

Media Impressions

- When the press conference was held in the People's Great Hall on August 30, 2006, to launch the campaign, more than 200 media outlets (television, radio, newspapers, magazines, and online media) across the country (including those from Hong Kong and Taiwan) covered the event and created enormous publicity for the campaign.
- Within the first week of the campaign, 51 TV stations, 95 radio stations, 79 newspapers, eight magazines, and seven major news Web sites reported the campaign. Newspapers alone carried 93 stories; some of them made more than two reports. CCTV coverage was even more extensive. Its eight news channels all reported the campaign multiple times within that week. The term "Ambassador of Hepatitis B Prevention and Control" alone received 659,000 hits on Baidu, the largest Chinese search engine, and 106,000 hits on Google China, just within the first week of the campaign.

Campaign Effects

To identify the effect of the campaign, the authors had a survey conducted in five cities (Beijing, Shanghai, Nanjing, Xi'an, and Xining) across the country, coordinated by *China Advertising*, a Shanghai-based trade magazine of the Chinese advertising industry. The survey was conducted in January 2008 when this 28-month (September 2006–December 2008) campaign was halfway through.

Survey Conducted

The five cities selected for the survey are the same ones where the China Medical Association conducted its formative campaign research in early 2006. The five cities represent different regions and different levels of economic development in China. Beijing, the national capital, is in North China. Both Shanghai (China's commercial center) and Nanjing (the capital city of Jiangsu Province) are in East China. Xi'an, the capital city of Shaanxi Province, is in Central China. Xining, the capital city of Qinghai Province, is in West China. While Beijing and Shanghai are among the most developed areas in China, Xining is within the most underdeveloped region in the country.

Convenient samples were collected through intercepts on 17 university campuses, in four hospitals, and on the streets of these five cities by volunteer university students. A total of 927 questionnaires were distributed; 862 were completed.

The survey had three focuses: (1) people's awareness of the campaign, (2) their knowledge of hepatitis B and related topics, and (3) their behavior changes or intentions to change.

Survey Findings

Campaign Awareness and Recalls

- Half of the respondents were aware of the hepatitis B prevention and educational campaign co-organized by the CFHPC and China's MOH. This awareness is quite high considering the media clutter the target audience is exposed to nowadays in this age of information overflow.
- At least 57% of the respondents recalled correctly that Andy Lau was the campaign ambassador.
- More than two-thirds of the respondents recalled correctly that "Darling" was the campaign song.
- Only about 15% of the respondents recalled correctly the campaign slogan, "Love Your Liver, Improve Your Health."

Campaign Impact on Knowledge

Our questions for identifying the target audience's basic knowledge about hepatitis B responded to those raised in the survey released by the Chinese Medical Association in early 2006 (hereafter, "pre-campaign survey"). We found through our survey (hereafter, "mid-campaign survey") that for those correct statements, there was a clear increase in the percentage of correct answers; for those wrong statements, there was an obvious decrease in the percentage of those who regarded them as correct. These differences (see Table 12-1) indicate the strong impact of the campaign on the target audience's basic knowledge about hepatitis B.

As indicted by our respondents, doctors, television, and newspapers were the top three sources for their information and knowledge on hepatitis B. Among all media types, the Internet was the third most frequently used medium for such information and knowledge, after television and newspapers. These findings indicate the important role doctors play in hepatitis B prevention and education due to the credibility they have among the public. These findings also indicate the need to further improve medical professionals' quality and service to ensure that they provide accurate information, timely diagnoses, and appropriate treatments for hepatitis B patients.

TABLE 12-1   Respondents' Knowledge on Hepatitis B: A Pre-Campaign and Mid-Campaign Comparison

Knowledge on Hepatitis B	Pre-Campaign (%)	Mid-Campaign (%)	Change (%)
Hepatitis B virus carriers are not chronic hepatitis B patients.	62	78	+16
Hepatitis B vaccines play a decisive role in hepatitis B prevention.	20	34	+14
To eat or work together or shake hands with hepatitis B patients will cause infection by the hepatitis B virus.	50	37	−13
Hepatitis B mothers will transmit the disease to their newborns.	61	82	+21
Blood transfusion from hepatitis B virus carriers or patients will cause hepatitis B transmission.	70	89	+19
Having unprotected sex with chronic hepatitis B virus carriers or patients will facilitate transmission of the disease.	54	69	+15
Kissing hepatitis B virus carriers or patients will facilitate transmission of the disease.	50	31	−19
One should have concerns about one's own health when working with a hepatitis B virus carrier.	69	65	−4
It is a violation of the law to fail a candidate for a civil service position simply because he or she is a hepatitis B virus carrier.	51	71	+20
It is a violation of the law if a company refuses to hire a candidate simply because he or she is a hepatitis B virus carrier.	56	75	+19

Campaign Impact on Behavior

From our survey questions on major hepatitis B–related behaviors, we obtained the following results:

- 80% of our respondents indicated that they would take a hepatitis B vaccine if they had not done so yet.
- 88% of them indicated that they would use condoms in sexual intercourse with hepatitis B virus carriers, if they had not used them before.

- 65% of them said they do not mind studying with or working with HBV carriers.
- 92% of hepatitis B patients or virus carriers among our respondents answered that they would resort to legal procedure, if necessary (rather than violence), when facing discrimination from others.

Although we do not have comparable data from the pre-campaign survey to compare with, it is evident that most of our respondents are very much aware of how to prevent hepatitis B in their daily life and the appropriate way to deal with the disease-caused discrimination. Given the significant increase in people's familiarity with the effectiveness of hepatitis B vaccination and the major ways for the disease to transmit, we could infer that this anti–hepatitis B campaign exerted some positive influences on our target audience's behavior. Because the campaign was still ongoing when our survey was conducted, we have every reason to believe that this large-scale national campaign will exert an even stronger impact on target audience behavior by its completion.

SUMMARY

In this chapter, we reviewed the major public health issues in China and the Chinese government's recent policies for dealing with these issues, especially those caused by hepatitis B. The national anti–hepatitis B campaign examined in this chapter is a success story of social marketing in this socialist country, where the concept of social marketing is well received and actively practiced. The campaign was successful because, based on our mid-campaign survey, it largely achieved its objectives (in terms of knowledge, belief, and behavior). In our view, several worthy lessons can be learned through this campaign:

- *Strong multisector partnership.* The partnership for the anti–hepatitis B campaign was multifaceted involving the government (i.e., the MOH), nonprofit organizations (like the CFHPC), private companies (such as Bristol-Myers Squibb), the media (at both national and local levels), and citizens (like Andy Lau). Due to China's unique social environment, the government has played a strong leadership role in providing policies and long-term planning for hepatitis B prevention and control, as well as handling related social issues (such as discrimination against HBV carriers and hepatitis B patients). Another critical role the government played in the anti–hepatitis B campaign was to provide part of the funds for free vaccines to children in underdeveloped regions and ensure vaccination is affordable to other average citizens.

Meanwhile, the CFHPC played a pivotal role in the campaign, coordinating all parties involved. For example, donations from various sources, both domestic and overseas, all went through the CFHPC. It also worked closely with the Chinese Medical Association and McCann Healthcare China to ensure the campaign success. Obviously, the multisector partnership had direct impact on the integration of all the 4Ps in the marketing mix strategies for this campaign.

- *Synergy of the campaign promotion.* Another major lesson that can be learned from this campaign is the integration of various communication efforts. These efforts included press conferences, PSAs, and special events in terms of communication formats and involved television, radio, newspapers, magazines, the Internet, and billboards as far as communication media were concerned. The impact of Integrated Marketing Communications (IMC) in this campaign was clearly documented by the broad awareness of the campaign and the high percentage of recalls of campaign messages. Our mid-campaign survey indicates that both television and newspapers are still highly effective for public health information dissemination in China, while the Internet is showing great potential.

- *Celebrity endorsement.* It is obvious that this anti–hepatitis B campaign was celebrity-driven and celebrity-intensive, from having Andy Lau as the campaign publicity ambassador to featuring him in the campaign PSAs (including the campaign song he created and performed) and from inviting him to the campaign press conference to covering his visits to hepatitis B patients in hospitals. Our survey respondents' much higher recalls of Lau and his song than the recall of campaign slogan indicate that celebrity endorsement and edutainment can be two more effective ways to reach out to the target audience than some traditional advertising executions.

It goes without saying that our conclusions in this case study are subject to further tests via more social marketing campaigns as well as more empirical studies. One thing for sure is that social marketing is actively used in China as a more audience-oriented and multipronged tool for public health, with great impact on behavior.

QUESTIONS FOR DISCUSSION

1. Based on the anti–hepatitis B campaign reviewed in this chapter, what similarities and differences have you noticed between the practice of social marketing for public health in China and that in your home country? In your opinion,

what has given rise to those similarities and differences? What implications could those similarities and differences have for social marketing for public health in a global scope?

2. How did the multisector partnership among the government, nonprofit organizations, private companies, the media, and citizens affect the 4Ps in the marketing mix strategies in this anti–hepatitis B campaign in China? On which of the 4Ps do you think this multisector partnership had the greatest impact?

3. Why did celebrity endorsement appear more effective than some conventional promotional executions (such as the campaign slogan in this campaign)? Do you have similar experience from your media consumption and/or social marketing practice?

ACKNOWLEDGMENTS

The authors wish to thank Xiaolu Ma of Northwestern University (China), Minli Gong and Xiong Chen of the Qinghai University of Finance and Economics, Jue Lü of the Nanjing University of Finance and Economics, and Xiang Zhang of the Beijing University of Industry and Commerce for their assistance in the mid-campaign survey in China.

REFERENCES

Bristol-Myers Squibb. (2006). *Foundation and corporation philanthropy*. Retrieved July 28, 2009, from http://www.bristol-myers.com/sr/foundation/health_disparities/hepatitis/content/data/hepatitis_current_grants.html#prevent

Central Intelligence Agency (CIA). (2009). *World Factbook*. Retrieved July 28, 2009, from https://www.cia.gov/cia/publications/factbook/geos/ch.html

Cheng, H., & Chan, K. (2009). Public service advertising in China: A semiotic analysis. In H. Cheng & K. Chan (Eds.), *Advertising and Chinese Society: Impacts and Issues* (pp. 203–221). Copenhagen, Denmark: Copenhagen Business School Press.

China halves TB deaths through DOTS. (2009). Retrieved July 28, 2009, from http://www.who.int/inf-new/tuber2.htm

China quick facts. (2009). Retrieved July 28, 2009, from http://www.chinagate.cn/english/e-changshi/index.htm

China reports 264,000 people living with HIV/AIDS. (2008, November 30). Retrieved July 28, 2009, from http://news.xinhuanet.com/english/2008-11/30/content_10433172.htm

China steps up efforts to fight tuberculosis. (2007, March 21). Retrieved July 28, 2009, from http://french.china.org.cn/english/health/203649.htm

Chinability. (2008). *GDP growth 1952–2008*. Retrieved July 28, 2009, from http://www.chinability.com/GDP.htm

China's 2009 GDP growth seen at 8%: Think-tank. (2009, August 5). Retrieved August 18, 2009, from http://www.cnbc.com/id/32307109

China's GDP grows 9% in 2008. (2009, January 22). Retrieved July 28, 2009, from http://www.china.org.cn/business/news/2009-01/22/content_17169174.htm

Chinese cities and provinces information and links. (2009). Retrieved July 28, 2009, from http://www.chinatoday.com/city/a.htm

Chinese Health Ministry. (2006, February 13). *Chinese Health Ministry issues new plan to control hepatitis B.* Retrieved July 28, 2009, from http://www.redorbit.com/news/health/388214/chinese_health_ministry_issues_new_plan_to_control_hepatitis_b/#

Chinese people's average lifespan. (2001, January 5). Retrieved July 28, 2009, from http://www.primasia.com/News/hk/2001/01/05d.htm

Claeson, M., H. Wang, & S. Hu. (2004). *A critical review of public health in China.* Retrieved July 28, 2009, from http://ceh.resourcehub.ssrc.org/a-critical-review-of-public-health-in-china/resource_view

Constitution of the People's Republic of China. (2004). Retrieved July 28, 2009, from http://english.gov.cn/2005-08/05/content_20813.htm

Darling. (2006). Retrieved July 28, 2009, from http://asianfanatics.net/forum/index.php?showtopic=286761

Development of public health in China. (2009). Retrieved from July 28, 2009, from http://www.gov.cn/test/2005-09/21/content_65516.htm

DOTS prevents TB deaths in China. (2009). Retrieved July 28, 2009, from http://www.who.int/inf-new/tuber2.htm

DOTS program helps reduce tuberculosis rates in China. (2004, August 8). Retrieved July 28, 2009, from http://www.voanews.com/specialenglish/archive/2004-08/a-2004-08-08-2-1.cfm?renderforprint=1&pageid=76027

Encyclopaedia Britannica Online. (2009). China. Retrieved July 28, 2009, from http://search.eb.com/eb/article-9117321

Exhibition for the award-winning works in the Third Shenzhen Public Service Advertising Contest open to the public. (2008, December 18). Retrieved July 28, 2009, from http://jingsai.chda.net/show.aspx?id=2521&cid=15

Fusu. (2006, October 20). *Facing 120 million hepatitis B virus carriers.* Retrieved July 28, 2009, from http://news.cctv.com/china/20061020/106866.shtml

Ge, T. (2006, October 31). *China launches hepatitis B campaign.* Retrieved July 28, 2009, from http://www.cctv.com/english/20060831/102132.shtml

Healthy China Long March Program. (2007). Retrieved July 28, 2009, from http://www.sm114.com.cn/s/addzlg/143937817.htm

Hepatitis B. (2009). Retrieved from July 28, 2009, from http://medical-dictionary.thefreedictionary.com/hepatitis+B

Hepatitis in Asia. (2009). Retrieved July 28, 2009, from http://www.bms.com/foundation/reducing_health_disparities/hepatitis/Pages/default.aspx

Higher education in China: A review of its rapid growth. (2007, March 7). *China Education News*, p. 9.

Lingling. (2006, April 24). *April 25: The National Children's Vaccination Day.* Retrieved July 28, 2009, from http://www.cph.com.cn/Gtgov/200604/20060424103551.htm

Liu, H. (2006). *Voices against discrimination: An update of recent cases and developments.* Retrieved July 28, 2009, from http://www.chinareview.info/pages/case.htm

Med8th. (2009). *Data on HIV/AIDS.* Retrieved July 28, 2009, from http://www.med8th.com/medinfo/category/hivaid.htm

Pettypiece, S. (2007, December 25). *Deaths in China from hepatitis B prompt Bristol, Glaxo urgency.* Retrieved July 28, 2009, from http://www.bloomberg.com/apps/news?pid=20601109&sid=aGFNm0ebdzZk&refer=home#

Press releases. (2004, November 1). *Bristol-Myers Squibb Foundation and China Foundation for Hepatitis Prevention and Control collaborate to fight one of China's most pressing health problems.* Retrieved July 28, 2009, from http://www.businesswire.com/portal/site/bms/?ndmViewId=news_view&newsId=20081211006022&newsLang=en

Regions. (2008). Retrieved July 28, 2009, from http://chinasite.com/Regions/regions.html

Schüller, M. (2005). China's Western Development Program: A Chinese version of Germany's "Rebuilding the East"? *Provincial China* 8(2), 89–117.

Second "Responsible China, Save Health" Public Service Advertising Contest. (2006, February 13). Retrieved July 28, 2009, from http://www.4a98.com/news/zjzb/2006-02-13/article_5754.html

So, S. (2004). *Why eradicating hepatitis B and liver cancer should be a national priority in China.* Paper presented at the China National Conference on Hepatitis Prevention and Control, Hangzhou, China, April 26–29.

Sociological reading of hepatitis B. (2007, June 15). Retrieved July 28, 2009, from http://hbv.jiankang163.com/news/xinwenzhiji/840.html

Stars show their hearts in 2006. (2007, February 25). Retrieved July 28, 2009, from http://www.cctv.com/program/cultureexpress/20070225/105416_1.shtml

UN Millennium Declaration. (2000). Retrieved July 28, 2009, from http://www.un.org/millennium/declaration/ares552e.htm

Wang, P. (2006, October 25). *President Hu promises bigger government role in public health.* Retrieved July 28, 2009, from http://www.cctv.com/english/20061025/100280.shtml

Wen, J. (2008, March 19). *Full text: Report on the work of the government.* Retrieved July 28, 2009, from http://www.cctv.com/english/20080319/105209_4.shtml

World Health Organization (WHO). (2009). *Data and statistics.* Retrieved July 28, 2009, from http://www.who.int/research/en/

You, N. (2008, December 18). *Time to rejoice—and reflect.* Retrieved July 28, 2009, from http://www.chinadaily.com.cn/bizchina/2008-12/18/content_7318338.htm

Zhang. (2008, April 16). *Wen: China's health care reform focuses on public service.* Retrieved July 28, 2009, from http://www.cctv.com/english/20080416/100727.shtml

Zhang Weijian appointed "Hepatitis Ambassador," calling for public attention to hepatitis prevention and control. (2007, October 9). Retrieved from July 28, 2009, from http://health.cnhubei.com/jbdq/2007-10/09/cms468411article.shtml

Zhang, W., Wang, L., Fang, F., Ma, J., Xu, J., Jiang, J., et al. (2008). Spatial analysis of malaria in Anhui province, China. *Malaria Journal* 7: 206.

Zhang, Y. (2008, December 8). Expert demands government boost health spending. Retrieved July 28, 2009, from http://www.china.org.cn/china/national/2008-12/08/content_16916972.htm

CHAPTER 13

Integrated Corporate Social Initiatives in Japan

From Product Development to Healthcare Information

Morikazu Hirose

In the early 1940s, the major causes of death in Japan were tuberculosis, pneumonia, and cerebrovascular disease. The leading causes of death in 2007 were cancer, heart disease, and cerebrovascular disease (Ministry of Health, Labour, and Welfare [MHLW], 2007). Improvements in medicine and lifestyles have contributed significantly to these changes. However, over the past 60 years, Japanese dietary habits have switched from traditional Japanese dishes that mainly include rice, fish, and vegetables to Western dishes that contain more meats, oils, and fats. This change has caused a rise in lifestyle diseases. This chapter reviews how the government has tackled lifestyle diseases and presents a case study of Terumo, which is a major medical company, Shibuya-ku, Tokyo, Japan. It has developed a painless needle for diabetic patients and provided more healthcare information to the people of Japan. The case offers a promising direction and good example of exploring effective corporate social marketing initiatives.

JAPAN: A COUNTRY OVERVIEW

Japan is situated in eastern Asia and is made up of an island chain that lies between the North Pacific Ocean and the Sea of Japan, east of the Korean Peninsula. Japan comprises 47 prefectures and a total area of 377,923 square kilometers (about 234,000 square miles, or slightly less than the size of California). Japan is home to a population of more than 127 million (Central Intelligence Agency [CIA], 2009). Japan is the second most technologically powerful economy in the world after the United States and the third largest economy in the world after the United States and China, based on purchasing power parity, or PPP (CIA, 2009).

The problems that Japan faces, as pointed out in the "2008 State of the State" address from its prime minister, include a sluggish economy experiencing the pressures of fast-changing globalization, a social security system under severe financial stress, a declining birthrate, a harsh employment situation, global competition in technology, global environmental changes, and global resources/energy issues (Fukuda, 2008).

The life expectancy in Japan is 78.73 years for males and 85.59 years for females (Japanese life span, 2008); the life expectancy of Japanese women is the highest in the world, and that of men is the third highest after Iceland and Hong Kong (Japanese life span, 2008). According to Japan's Ministry of Health, Labour, and Welfare (MHLW), improved treatments for cancer, heart disease, and stroke have increased the life expectancy in the country (MHLW, 2007).

Public Health in Japan

Japan's MHLW has identified nine public health–related priority areas in Japan: (1) nutrition and eating habits, (2) physical activity and exercise, (3) rest and mental health, (4) smoking, (5) alcohol, (6) dental health, (7) diabetes, (8) cardiovascular disease, and (9) cancer (MHLW, 2002). In addition, Japanese society currently faces problems associated with a declining birthrate, an aging population, escalating demands for nursing care, an increase in lifestyle diseases, and an increase in medical spending.

Lifestyle diseases are largely caused by unhealthy lifestyle behaviors, including inappropriate dietary habits, smoking, drinking, lack of exercise, and excessive stress. These poor lifestyle habits can lead to such diseases as visceral adiposity, which includes diabetes, high blood pressure, and hyperlipemia. Unhealthy lifestyle behaviors are also likely to cause more severe diseases, such as heart attack and stroke. Such serious diseases result in declining life functions and an increased demand for nursing care in the country.

A universal healthcare system, where medical expenses were paid for, was introduced in Japan in 1961, thus limiting the personal medical expenses of individuals. As a result, public health has improved. For example, the average life span of men and women, respectively, improved from 50.16 and 53.96 years in 1947 to 65.32 and 70.19 years in 1960 and 73.35 and 78.76 years in 1980 (Japanese life span, 2008).

In the past, the percentage of senior citizens in Japan has remained at a stable level; however, today the number of people over age 65 has reached a record high of 26 million, accounting for 20.8% of the Japanese population (MHLW, 2007).

Emerging Health Problems

As noted earlier, the current major causes of death in Japan are cancer, heart disease, and cerebrovascular disease. Since the late 1940s, the major causes of death have changed, largely as a result of changes in dietary habits. The Japanese people today eat more high-calorie foods that contain meat, oil, and fat compared to six decades ago. In addition, many individuals do not exercise as frequently. Thus, lifestyle diseases are now widespread. Although some of these diseases, such as diabetes, are not immediate causes of death, they can trigger fatal diseases.

The country's aging society has produced increased medical expenditures. These expenditures increase drastically with age in Japan. Medical expenditures per elderly person are five times those of other age groups in the country. Lifestyle diseases account for about 60% of the illnesses that cause death and about 30% of medical expenditures (MHLW, 2007).

It is very important for individuals suffering from lifestyle diseases to improve their lifestyle substantially if they are to improve their health. If lifestyle is improved, pathogenesis for such diseases can be reduced, and good quality of life can be maintained. Such lifestyle improvement will also reduce overall medical expenditures for the elderly (MHLW, 2007).

Healthcare Policy in Japan

The healthcare policy of the Japanese government—especially the policy implemented by the Ministry of Health, Labour, and Welfare—is meant to enhance the management of citizen health and place more emphasis on prevention rather than treatment of illness. If successful, such a policy can help maintain and operate the health insurance system efficiently and at a lower cost.

Over the years since 1978, the Ministry has undertaken a variety of campaigns to help the country cope with lifestyle diseases. For example, the First Measure for

Enhancing Citizens' Health, launched in 1978, had three objectives: (1) lifelong health management, (2) development of a foundation for health enhancement, and (3) education and diffusion of health enhancement. All three objectives were designed to detect and treat diseases at their early stages through regular health checkups. In addition, by applying the assumption that appropriate nutrition, exercise, and rest are three major factors for good health, physical checkup systems for all age groups—from infants to the elderly—were implemented, municipal healthcare centers were developed, and nurses and nutritionists were employed at each municipality across the country (MHLW, 2006).

The Second Measure for Enhancing Citizens' Health, launched in 1988, focused on physical exercise, one of the three major factors leading to good health. Numerous instructors were trained in healthy exercise through this campaign, named the "Active 80 Health Plan." These personnel were effective in helping citizens prevent the onset of lifestyle diseases by treating them at early stages, as well as in developing healthcare facilities in various municipalities (MHLW, 2006).

In 1996, Japan's public health policy changed. The term *seijin-byo* (adult disease), which was closely related to aging, was renamed *seikatsu-shuukan-byo* (lifestyle disease) in order to refine the government's focus on the significant role that lifestyle plays in one's health (MHLW, 1996).

Based on these measures, the Ministry of Welfare (now the Ministry of Health, Labour, and Welfare) launched the "Japanese National Health Promotion in the 21st Century" (or Healthy Japan 21), an 11-year campaign that lasted from 2000 to 2010. With this campaign, it is hoped that individuals will define specific personal goals for improving their lifestyles in terms of eating, exercise, and rest to prevent lifestyle diseases, such as cancer, heart disease, stroke, and diabetes. To promote Healthy Japan 21 comprehensively and effectively, the Japanese government supports proactive efforts of local governments and related staff (Japan Health Promotion & Fitness Foundation [JHPFF], 2008).

Healthy Japan 21 includes numerical goals that differ from those in previous public health measures. The goals address 70 items in nine fields, including eating habits, exercise, smoking, alcohol intake, cardiovascular diseases, and cancer.

The Health Promotion Law was enacted in 2003 to complement Healthy Japan 21. The Health Promotion Law stipulates that:

1. In order to promote health enhancement comprehensively, the Japanese government shall produce a basic policy for setting national goals and basic objectives.
2. In order to promote health enhancement, local governments shall produce plans for health enhancement based on the situation of each region.
3. In order to provide health checkups in workplaces, communities, and schools for health enhancement, common guidelines for those checkups shall be produced.

4. The managers of frequently used facilities shall be obliged to make an effort to prevent secondhand smoke. (MHLW, 2007)

The Health Promotion Law requires not only the Japanese government, but also insured persons, healthcare institutions, educational organs, firms, and volunteer groups, to engage in the development of an environment that addresses improved health. Especially with respect to smoking, its theme is set forth in law, so that the related audience is aware of the smoking issue. Health evaluation is carried out with reference to these goals, and the results are based on scientific data. This law also addresses the importance of providing information to assist citizens in voluntary activities and defines the effective utilization of the mass media in that effort (MHLW, 2007).

Health Information Shows

Around 2006, the mass media began using the words "metabolic syndrome" (Thirteen million people, 2006). With or without use of these words, the Japanese people were becoming increasingly conscious about their health. The desire to maintain good health, prevent sickness, and treat existing illnesses, as well as the need to relieve fatigue and reduce weight, have remained high today.

In the mid-1990s, a big change occurred in the way health information was disseminated in Japan. Mass communication, especially television, had a substantial effect on information propagation and delivery in Japan in the mid-1990s.

For example, Mino Monta, a famous Japanese emcee, first introduced health food products and diet food in an information show called *Gogo Wa Marumaru Omoikkiri Television* (meaning "Let's enjoy watching TV throughout afternoon" in Japanese). The show was aired on weekday afternoons and targeted middle-age and older housewives.

In 1995, cocoa, introduced on the show, became incredibly popular. Cocoa has a large amount of polyphenol in it, which helps metabolize cholesterol and prevent gastric ulcers. The same day that Mino Monta introduced cocoa as an antidote for such conditions, some Japanese grocery stores sold out of cocoa (Omoikkiri effect, 1996).

One can interpret the reason for one product to become popular so quickly. In fact, the makers of the product had not given enough information on the product previously, and these kinds of information shows were giving consumers appropriate information that they wanted. Even though the boom only occurred for a short period of time, cocoa makers were able to boost sales, and the show that introduced the product became popular, producing an increased number of similar TV shows. Consumers began to buy into any health information heard on TV—but without paying attention to its accuracy (The price of health, 1997).

Food Faddism and the Media

If it becomes clear that a single ingredient in a food has a particular dietary effect or causes blood elements to normalize, television shows often make it seem as though one can live a healthy life just by eating such a food. This tendency, also seen in the West, is called "food faddism" (Takahashi, 2007). Defining the concept as "exaggerating and believing in the effect that foods and nutrition have for health and sickness" (p. 20), Takahashi pointed out that Japanese consumers were becoming confused by the wealth of health foods that were continuing to pop up, one after the other.

In January 2007, fictitious statements of health information on Fuji TV's *Hakkutu!! Aru-Aru Dictionary* surfaced, creating a problem for the show. They stated a false dietary effect of natto, reporting the effect as truth. Due to the story, local grocery stores soon had a shortage of natto, beginning the next day. However, to report on the positive health effects of natto, producers of the television show had misused an American scholar's opinion and recorded fake comments concerning that opinion in Japanese. It was discovered upon investigation that there were many exaggerations, fictitious statements, and falsifications provided on the show. The show was canceled because many viewers sent complaints to the TV station (Aruaru problem, 2007).

CASE STUDY
Terumo

With regard to smoking, global awareness of anti-smoking has produced concrete measures to be put in place to prohibit smoking, which has led to good results. However, in the case of other lifestyle diseases, such factors as aging, lifestyle, and inheritance (which are intricately related to each another) are difficult aspects for a government to affect directly. It is impractical to restrict lifestyles to cope with lifestyle diseases, and such choices are thus left to individuals. It is especially important, therefore, to explain to citizens the details about health at various stages of life; infuse the society with sufficient knowledge of health; and promote reasonable, ongoing personal actions that will help prevent lifestyle diseases.

To compensate for public health measures communicated by the government, well-designed corporate social initiatives can play an important role in providing healthcare information. According to Kotler and Lee (2005), corporate social responsibility (CSR) is "a commitment to improving community well-being through discretionary business practices and contributions of corporate resources" (p. 3). They also define corporate social marketing as how "a corporation supports the development and/or implementation of a behavior change campaign intended to improve public health, safety, the environment, or community well-being. The distinguishing feature is the behavior change focus, which differentiates it from cause promotions that focus on supporting awareness, fundraising, and volunteer recruitment for a cause" (Kotler & Lee, 2005, p. 23).

A corporation may conduct this campaign in partnership with a governmental agency or a nonprofit organization, or—as is the case for the discussion in this chapter—the corporation may be the primary or sole sponsor of the campaign.

The rest of this chapter addresses the corporate social marketing initiatives of Terumo, one of the largest manufacturers of healthcare products and equipment in Japan. This review covers Terumo's development of painless syringe needles for diabetic patients and its efforts to enhance the public's understanding of diabetes and other lifestyle diseases, by using communication strategies, an advertising campaign, and educational TV programs.

CAMPAIGN BACKGROUND, FOCUS, AND PURPOSE

The number of diabetes patients in Japan has rapidly increased. The Ministry of Health, Labour, and Welfare estimates that 18.7 million people are potential diabetes patients in Japan (MHLW, 2008). In 2005, about 2.47 million people took continuous treatments (MHLW, 2005). It is difficult for potential patients to realize they have diabetes. It is also painful for patients to inject themselves with traditional needles, so some stop their treatment. To motivate and encourage patients and the general population, there should be more healthcare information out there for them.

Unlike in the United States, the advertising of prescription drugs and medical devices, so called DTC (direct-to-consumer) advertising, is heavily restricted in Japan. Advertisers are not allowed to show or mention the names of their products or the brands in their advertisements. Therefore, advertisers for medical devices typically do not use mass media advertising campaigns to promote their products. Most advertising campaigns developed by medical device advertisers are aimed at raising public awareness and enhancing company images—not selling brand names.

Over the years, Terumo has "done well by doing good," infusing its business expertise into the development of corporate social initiatives that contribute to Japan's public health. For example, Dr. Shibasaburo Kitazato (1853–1931), the

physician who founded Terumo in 1921, designed and produced superior ther-
mometers for medical use. Dr. Kitazato had a larger goal in life, however. He
wanted to bring healthier living to the common people through greater utilization of superior medical technology. His desire was to contribute to society by
providing better health care, and this goal still drives Terumo today.

Terumo introduced cutting-edge healthcare products, including disposable
medical instruments, blood bags, infusions, artificial organs, and catheters. The
company's innovative achievements have improved medical practices in Japan.
The will of its founder remains the basis of its corporate philosophy:
"Contributing to Society through Healthcare." Terumo provides value-added
products and services in the healthcare industry and has earned the trust of
both health workers and patients (Terumo, 2002).

In the 1990s, Terumo, like other Japanese companies, faced financial difficulties. At the time, the Japanese economy was experiencing the collapse of an
economic bubble. This era is now called "the lost decade" in Japan. Terumo
struggled to respond. In an effort to turn the situation around, Tetsuo Akutsu
became the president and Takashi Wachi (currently the chairman and CEO) became its executive director in 1993.

These two executives reformed the company corporate culture and focused on employee satisfaction. In Terumo's corporate statement, they stressed
corporate citizenship (Terumo, 2007b, p. 5). Terumo believes in being a
provider of total healthcare solutions in terms of both products and information and in creating products that are gentle to people. Terumo's CSR (corporate social responsibility) as well as its marketing initiatives are based on this
corporate philosophy.

Terumo's focus is on how people can live a healthy life even they have diseases. It is trying to provide not only less painful needles to encourage patient
diabetic care, but also useful information for prevention and treatment of disease in their daily lives.

CAMPAIGN TARGET

There are two major types of diabetes: insulin-dependent diabetes mellitus
(IDDM) and non-insulin-dependent diabetes mellitus (NIDDM). IDDM is
characterized by an absolute insulin deficiency and occurs in children aged 3 or
4 to 18 and is also called "juvenile diabetes." Its etiology is uncertain, and the incidence is 1 to 2 per 100,000. NIDDM, on the other hand, can be caused by unhealthy eating habits, lack of exercise, mental stress, and obesity. While insulin

therapy is also used for NIDDM patients when neither diet nor exercise therapy is effective to control the blood-sugar levels, all patients with IDDM diabetes are required to have insulin injections.

The main targets of this campaign are the estimated 18.7 million potential diabetes patients who have some risk factors in their blood tests and the 2.47 million patients who take continuous treatments (MHLW, 2005, 2007). In particular, painless needles focus on patients who need to inject every day, and who experience pain every time they inject themselves. According to the Ministry of Health, Labour, and Welfare, the number of potential diabetes patients increases among individuals in their 50s (MHLW, 2004). To prevent diabetes, the general public, mainly those who are over 40, were included as a target.

The other targets are families and friends of patients. Those patients who need to inject every day suffer from pain and inconvenience from having to treat themselves. Especially in the case of children, daily treatments are painful. Support from families and friends is highly important for continuous treatment. If families and friends have enough knowledge about the disease, they can support the patients more easily.

CAMPAIGN OBJECTIVES

Marketing strategies were developed to enhance commitment to campaign targets as follows.

- *Behavior objectives.* Encourage diabetes patients who need continuous treatment to inject as prescribed; raise awareness among friends and families to support patients mentally; and encourage the general public to take preventive action, including healthy diet or sufficient exercise to prevent lifestyle diseases.
- *Knowledge objectives.* Educate patients about new needles that can reduce the pain from daily injections; provide friends and families with information about what lifestyle diseases are and how patients can best treat themselves; and provide the general public with reliable and useful healthcare knowledge for better public health.
- *Belief objectives.* Help patients understand that daily injections are not painful with the use of the new needles; help potential patients understand that proper knowledge is important to prevent lifestyle diseases; and inform friends and families of patients that understanding the disease will help them offer greater support to patients.

CAMPAIGN, BARRIERS, BENEFITS, AND COMPETITION

It is not easy for patients to switch to new needles. There are many factors to consider when patients decide which needles to use. They may hesitate to switch from the needles they have been using to new ones. They may prefer conventional needles because these are less expensive. Furthermore, it is difficult to provide the target audience with proper information that gets noticed in the cluttered environment of television shows, infomercials, and commercials that deliver healthcare information. As a result, people without proper knowledge may become confused.

The benefits of the new needle—Nanopass 33—are numerous. Nanopass 33 is painless and very gentle to the skin. Especially for IDDM patients, the painless needle lets patients eliminate fear and pain about daily treatment and allows them to continue their self-treatment as prescribed, thus adding to their health and longevity. Families and friends of patients can share their knowledge about diabetes to support the patients. Further, commercials, television shows, and healthcare information offered by Terumo in its corporate social initiatives are beneficial because the general public will gain proper knowledge about the different diseases in their daily lives.

While Nanopass 33 is a very unique product at this moment, 31G and 32G needles still exist in the market and are competitive. Information without empirical evidence may mislead or not inform the target audience properly.

CAMPAIGN STRATEGIES (4Ps) AND IMPLEMENTATION

Product Strategy and Implementation

As Wachi (2004) explained, "a company cannot survive without securing good sales and yet does not deserve to exist without making contributions to society" (p. 149). Terumo is committed to both securing sales and contributing to society. This idea is fully embodied in Nanopass 33, an insulin syringe needle for diabetes patients.

People who have diabetes and need insulin must inject that insulin three or four times per day. Thus, many want each injection to be as painless as possible. Terumo had wanted to introduce very fine needles as a gentle alternative to enter a new market. Terumo decided to manufacture new needles for diabetes patients. In an effort to secure its position in the market, Terumo needed to create more innovative needles.

To have a less painful needle, the needle tip should be as fine as possible. The finer it is, however, the higher the injection pressure, which means that more force is required to push the needle through the skin. If so, the elderly and children have difficulty using the syringe. Tetsuya Ohyauchi, chief engineer for this product, came up with the possibility of using the Hagen-Poiseuille law, a physical law concerning incompressible flow: When the needle tip is conical, not cylindrical as typical needle tips are, the upper part of the needle is made broader, and the injection pressure then is lower (Higurashi, 2006).

However, in manufacturing such needles, Terumo hit a wall. There was a problem. Terumo searched all across Japan, looking for companies that utilize a high-precision, deep-drawing process. Eventually, the company found Okano Industrial (Higurashi, 2006).

In 2000, Terumo approached Okano Industrial with a proposal to manufacture the syringe needle. The internal diameter of the world's finest needle, Nanopass 33, had to be 0.08 mm, as fine as a mosquito's proboscis.

At the time, Okano Industrial was just a back-street factory, but its technological excellence was known worldwide, especially for its development of a lithium-ion battery housing that had facilitated the miniaturization of cellular phones. Terumo explained to Okano Industrial, "Patients with diabetes and other diseases have to inject a drug with great frequency. We want to lessen their burden, so we want the thickness of the needle to be reduced to two-thirds" (Masayuki Okano, 2004). The process was technically very difficult, and Terumo did not know where to begin—even after a one-year effort in development. Without any realistic ideas about the process, Okano accepted the proposal with "mechanics wits" (Masayuki Okano, 2004, p. 11).

Masayuki Okano, president of Okano Industrial, had another idea. He once hated hospitals because he hated injections. In his late teens, he developed peritonitis because he had refused to undergo an appendectomy. He had been close to death. Although the eventual surgery was successful and he escaped death, he required many nutrient injections in his thigh during his hospitalization, and those injections required the use of a thick needle. He frowns even now, remembering the severe pain. Due to this personal experience, he decided, "I'll carry out this challenging project" (Masayuki Okano, 2004, p. 11).

Okano Industrial spent five years developing the needle. Its conventional line was capable of producing similar needles, but the cost per needle exceeded 100 yen (approximately US$1.00). This cost was too expensive to commercialize the product. After a number of unsuccessful efforts, Okano Industrial finally hit upon the idea of rolling up a very thin sheet of stainless steel to make a cylinder. The manufacturing cost per needle then was estimated at less than 10 yen (approximately 10 cents in U.S. currency).

The company's "painless syringe needle" won the 2005 Good Design Award sponsored by the Japan Industrial Design Promotion Organization.

An advertisement for the product also won the Minister of Economy, Trade, and Industry Award in the TV Commercial Division of the "Advertisement Beneficial to Consumers" contest organized by Japan's Advertisers Association.

For diabetes patients who must inject insulin every day, the "painless syringe needle" enhances the quality of life. What was once thought to be natural and expected and unavoidable—that this treatment should be painful—is now an outdated idea. The healthcare industry is expected to help provide a better life for people, and Nanopass 33 has undoubtedly helped meet this goal.

Terumo was unable to keep up with the overwhelming demand for its painless syringe needles from patients with diabetes and those with other diseases who must inject a drug several times a day. The tip of Nanopass 33 is extremely fine, 0.02 mm in diameter, and less painful than typical needles. Terumo has invested approximately 1 billion yen (US$10 million) into the expansion of its production line and doubled its monthly production of Nanopass 33 to 7 million needles. The sales of Nanopass 33 are now estimated to be more than 1 billion yen for the fiscal year ending March 2008, up 40% from the previous year (Terumo decides, 2007).

In addition to this tangible product, Terumo provides healthcare information as part of its ongoing corporate social initiatives. They inform the general public about lifestyle diseases as well as valuable daily healthcare information through television programs, advertising, and its homepage. Terumo has also organized a series of prevention of lifestyle-related diseases seminars with medical experts as presenters. These other initiatives are explained in more detail in the following section.

Price Strategy and Implementation

The price of needles is completely controlled by the Japanese government. The MHLW determines the price according to its performance as well as the price for any other prescription medical equipment in Japan. The Japanese government has introduced a universal healthcare system so all prescription drugs and medical devices are covered by medical insurance. Therefore, any price discount strategy is not applicable in this industry. That is why patients can take the latest medical treatments in Japan.

Terumo developed not only innovative needles, but also an innovative process to reduce production costs. However, it still costs patients 18 yen (approximately 18 cents) per needle even with medical insurance. It is still 5% to 6% more expensive compared to the old type of needle. Diabetic patients usually have to inject four times a day. The difference in the price amounts to 1,460 yen (approximately US$15) a year.

Place Strategy and Implementation

The general public does not have an opportunity to see the Nanopass 33 because the needles are distributed only through medical institutions. Because it is prescribed by doctors and sold behind-the-counter, doctors and pharmacists are the strongest influencers on the distribution channel.

In Japan, the distribution channel of prescription drugs and medical devices is also strictly controlled by the government. The reason is that highly specialized goods and services are dealt with only by specialists such as doctors and pharmacists. These goods are sold at the hospital or an ethical pharmacy. Therefore, patients cannot buy any needles by mail or online.

Promotion Strategy and Implementation

Targeting both patients and the general public with different information encourages continuous treatment and improves the lifestyle of the general public. The MHLW has studied the information resources available to patients. Male information resources are television and radio (63.7%), newspapers (33.0%), and hospitals (25.8%); for females, information comes from television and radio (74.1%), newspapers (35.9%), and magazines (33.1%; MHLW, 2004). It seems that communication through the mass media still has a great impact on the Japanese people.

Mass Media Advertising

Some people will develop a disease, whereas others will not. Patients generally suffer when treatment is painful or when others do not see how painful it is. Whether friends and family understand the disease or not may affect the patient's will to fight that disease considerably.

The following script is an award-winning TV commercial for the Painless Syringe Needle, Nanopass 33 (see Figure 13-1):

> *There are so many diabetes patients around the world. And they must inject insulin by themselves every day.*
> *Terumo developed the world's finest needle for an insulin syringe for diabetes patients to free them when battling diabetes from this painful experience.*
> *Mother: How was it?*
> *Son: It didn't hurt at all!*
> *There are so many patients in need of our needles.*
> *Gentle Health Care Terumo*

The boy in this TV commercial is fighting IDDM (juvenile diabetes). Despite his young age, he has to inject himself every day to protect his own life.

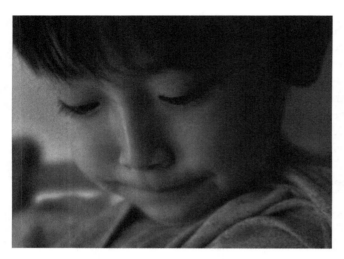

FIGURE 13-1   Television Commercial of Terumo
Courtesy of Terumo

After the injection, he smiles and says, "It didn't hurt at all!" This remark communicates what the Nanopass 33 is all about as well as Terumo's pledge to help enhance every patient's quality of life.

While patients with diseases other than IDDM also have to inject insulin, this young boy's appearance in the TV commercial was very effective in increasing public understanding of diabetes. Some people believe that those who develop diabetes do so as a result of unhealthy lifestyle habits, but such a prejudice or misunderstanding is removed once people see how patients cope with the disease. You can also imagine how painful treatment is for patients with diseases other than IDDM.

Begun in 1961, the Japan Advertisers Association's Advertisement Beneficial to Consumers contest is a prestigious competition. While most Japanese advertising contests feature judges from advertising agencies and advertisers, the judges in the Advertisement Beneficial to Consumers contest are customers and academic experts. Thus, the advertisements are evaluated from a consumer viewpoint. An advertisement for Nanopass 33 won the Minister of Economy, Trade, and Industry Award in the TV Commercial Division of the 2006 Advertisement Beneficial to Consumers contest.

Kazue Shimamura (2006), chairperson of the awards committee, explained, "the Nanopass 33 advertisement won because it informed patients about newly

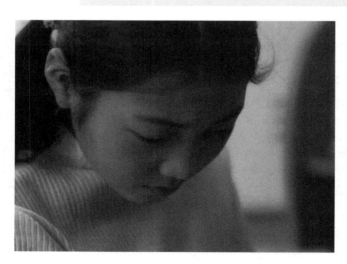

FIGURE 13-1   *(Continued)*

developed syringes for frequent injections and also about the painless Nanopass 33 while it raised general public awareness about the difficulties associated with diseases requiring daily injections."

The TV Program "Karada no Kimochi" (Body Feels)

In recent years, many Japanese TV programs have provided information on health, but not all provide reliable, accurate information. Some shows feature folk remedies whose efficacy is dubious, and others exaggerate the ef-

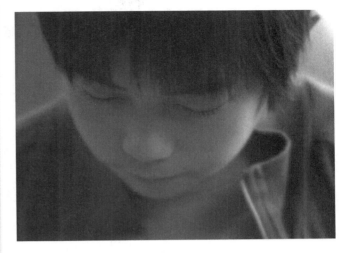

FIGURE 13-1   *(Continued)*

ficacy of a specific food. Recent TV programs have had a tendency to provide information in a somewhat sensational and jocular manner. Information on health and health care should be taken seriously.

In April 2006, Terumo exclusively launched a TV program called *Weekly! Healthcare Calendar Karada no Kimochi (Body Feels)* that has provided information on health and health care. The program is broadcast on Sundays from 7:00 to 7:30 a.m. on the CBC/TBS channel (Terumo, 2006).

With its catch phrase, "Lead a healthy life doing what you can on a daily basis," the program offers viewers tips for a healthy lifestyle. Some of the tips are:

- "Walking changes your body: Live a healthy life by walking."
- "More moisture for your eyes! Clear eyes for you! Ophthalmologist advises how to treat and prevent dry eyes."
- "Reduce visceral fat in 120 million people! The latest

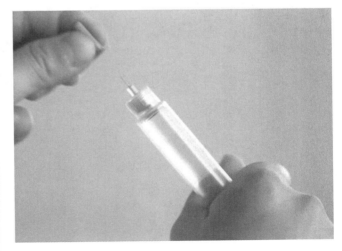

FIGURE 13-1   *(Continued)*

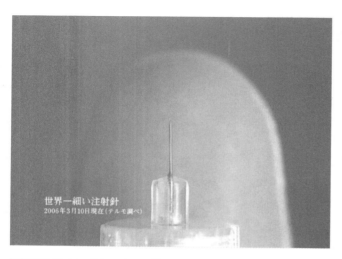

FIGURE 13-1   *(Continued)*

news on prevention and treatment of the metabolic syndrome!"
- "Early detection saves lives! The must-know basics of breast cancer."

Back in 2004, Terumo launched *Kenko Tenki Yoho (Health Weather Forecast)* as a TV and radio program. It is still available on Terumo's Web site. Warnings about changes in physical conditions, such as arthralgia, heat stroke, influenza, asthma, blood pressure, pollen (which causes hay fever), and ultraviolet (UV) rays are provided, along with the weather forecast (Terumo, 2004).

At the same time, Terumo hosts a column called "That's Interesting! A Doctors' Column" in newspapers and magazines to provide expert medical advice on the relationships between seasonal changes and physical conditions. The experts advise individuals about how to take care of themselves during seasonal changes. In the winter and spring, for example, they talk about how to prevent hay fever or to take drugs during the pollination period, how blood pressure and temperature are related, and why arthralgia and the cold are connected. In summer and autumn, they explain how to prevent heat stroke, food poisoning, and UV damage.

The information that the medical device manufacturer Terumo provides regarding health care is both accurate and seriously valuable. Although the TV program that airs on

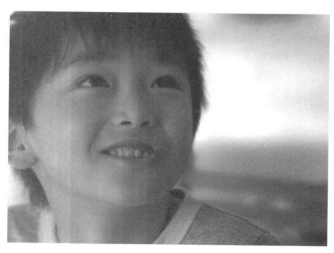

FIGURE 13-1   *(Continued)*

Sundays at 7:00 a.m. does not draw a large audience, Terumo is steadfast in its efforts to practice its corporate philosophy: Contributing to Society through Healthcare.

Other Promotions by Terumo

In addition to its medical devices, Terumo provides healthcare information on the Internet and in brochures (including those at shops) because the company believes self-care in health is important to preventing lifestyle-related diseases. Since

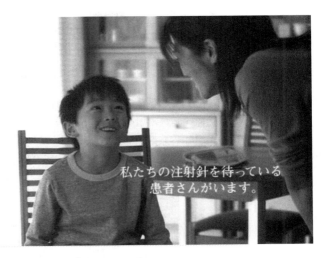

FIGURE 13-1   *(Continued)*

2005, Terumo has also organized a series of seminars on preventing lifestyle-related diseases, at which medical experts deliver lectures on lifestyle diseases, such as hypertension and diabetes. The seminars give the public more accurate knowledge about these diseases and encourage individuals to improve their lifestyle habits. These seminars are held in collaboration with professional associations in medicine and other medical groups along with the media and distributors, including drug stores. While other healthcare companies host similar events, Terumo has taken the initiative in providing both cutting-edge medical products and information to the Japanese public (Terumo, 2007b).

人にやさしい医療へ

⊕TERUMO®

FIGURE 13-1   *(Continued)*

OUTCOME

Usually, diabetes patients do not decide which needles they want to use. That choice is decided mainly by doctors. In the case of Nanopass 33, most users now decide by themselves (Painless needle, 2006). Nanopass 33 has been changing the belief that injection is painful.

Research by Terumo shows the effectiveness of its initiatives. In the research, respondents were found not only to hold favorable attitudes toward Terumo, but also to pay attention to health care in general as seen in the following comments:

"I had not had any idea about Terumo before I saw the commercial. However, it made me think that Terumo really cares about health care."

"I like 'Weekly Healthcare Calendar.' It's very unique. Now I pay great attention to my physical conditions in various seasons."

"I like the commercial for painless needles by Terumo. This commercial made me realize there are children who have to give a shot by themselves every day." (Terumo, 2007a)

Nikkei Corporate Image Research, one of the largest and the most-referenced corporate image and reputation research in Japan (Watabe, 2007), provides still more evidence of the success of Terumo's initiatives. According to Nikkei, advertising awareness, corporate awareness, and the corporate reputation of Terumo have increased in the last decade (Nikkei, 2007) (see Figure 13-2). These findings indicate that Terumo's corporate social initiatives not only increased corporate awareness for Terumo but also enhanced the general public's awareness of healthcare issues related to diabetes patients.

LESSONS LEARNED

In this chapter, healthcare problems in Japan are reviewed, including issues that range from political measures taken to consumer confusion. Japanese public healthcare measures have resulted in failure when those measures do not take into account the consumer point of view. It is clear that social marketing is useful when developing effective public health campaigns.

The Terumo case provides direction, in particular, for corporate social marketing in the constrained environment that exists in Japan. Terumo developed Nanopass 33, a cutting-edge product that reduced the pain of injections. That development was based on the company's basic philosophy and communicated through their corporate advertising. Further, Terumo provided the general public with healthcare information on how to monitor one's health in daily life. This

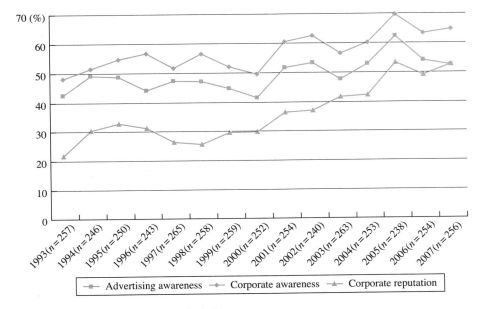

70 (%)
60
50
40
30
20
10
0

1993(*n* = 257)
1994(*n* = 246)
1995(*n* = 250)
1996(*n* = 243)
1997(*n* = 265)
1998(*n* = 258)
1999(*n* = 259)
2000(*n* = 252)
2001(*n* = 254)
2002(*n* = 240)
2003(*n* = 263)
2004(*n* = 253)
2005(*n* = 238)
2006(*n* = 254)
2007(*n* = 256)

—■— Advertising awareness   —◆— Corporate awareness   —▲— Corporate reputation

FIGURE 13-2   Impact of Terumo's initiatives
Courtesy of Nikkei

integration of product development with providing healthcare information thus made Terumo's corporate social initiatives even more effective.

In Japan, advertisements for prescribed devices have strict restrictions. Advertisers cannot appeal directly to the general public with product names and prices. Therefore, communications by the medical industry are focused on raising the awareness of public health and providing knowledge about diseases or the latest treatments rather than directly promoting specific products and services. While the industry operates with huge budgets and develops many drugs and devices for public health, most of these products are delivered only to doctors and certain patients.

Once medical companies successfully develop excellent products to help patients reduce their pain from treatments, they should communicate that advance clearly to the general public. Medical companies could raise awareness of public health while still providing information on their products by applying corporate social initiatives.

QUESTIONS FOR DISCUSSION

1. What information is needed to raise the awareness of a lifestyle disease in your country?

2. Based on this chapter, how did the government, industry, and media in Japan collaborate in their pursuit of improved public health? What do you think of this collaboration?

3. In the Terumo case, how were corporate advertising and corporate social initiatives integrated? What do you think of this integration? Was it successful?

ACKNOWLEDGMENT

The author thanks Terumo and Nikkei for providing information and images needed for this chapter.

REFERENCES

Aruaru problem—Continuing improper shows, strict viewers, check programs strictly. (2007, April 4). *The Nikkei*, p. 16.

Central Intelligence Agency (CIA). (2009). *The world factbook.* Retrieved July 28, 2009, from https://www.cia.gov/library/publications/the-world-factbook/geos/ja.html

Fukuda, Y. (2008, January, 18). *Policy speech by Prime Minister Yasuo Fukuda to the 169th Session of the Diet.* Retrieved July 28, 2009, from http://www.kantei.go.jp/foreign/hukuda speech/2008/01/18housin_e.html

Higurashi, R. (2006). Terumo: The combination of epoch-making approach and technology into a painless needle. *Weekly Toyo Keizai, 6007,* 70.

Japanese life span reached a record high last year. (2008, August 1). *The Nikkei*, p. 38.

Japan Health Promotion & Fitness Foundation (JHPFF). (2008). *About Healthy Japan 21.* Retrieved July 28, 2009, from http://www.kenkounippon21.gr.jp/kenkounippon21/about/index.html

Kotler, P., & Lee, N. (2005). *Corporate social responsibility: Doing the most good for your company and your cause.* Hoboken, NJ: John Wiley & Sons.

Masayuki Okano, president of Okano Industrial: Painless needle. (2004, August 29). *The Nikkei*, p. 11.

Ministry of Health, Labour, and Welfare (MHLW). (1996). *Basic directions toward disease control and prevention based on lifestyle diseases.* Retrieved July 28, 2009, from http://www1.mhlw.go.jp/shingi/1217-1.html

Ministry of Health, Labour, and Welfare (MHLW). (2002). *White paper on the labour economy.* Tokyo: Gyousei, Author.

Ministry of Health, Labour, and Welfare (MHLW). (2004). *Diabetes fact research.* Retrieved July 28, 2009, from http://www.mhlw.go.jp/shingi/2004/03/s0318-15.htm

Ministry of Health, Labour, and Welfare (MHLW). (2005). *Patients research.* Retrieved July 28, 2009, from http://www.mhlw.go.jp/toukei/saikin/hw/kanja/05/index.html

Ministry of Health, Labour, and Welfare (MHLW). (2006). *White paper on the labour economy.* Tokyo: Gyousei, Author.

Ministry of Health, Labour, and Welfare (MHLW). (2007). *White paper on the labour economy.* Tokyo: Gyousei, Author.

Ministry of Health, Labour, and Welfare (MHLW). (2008). *White paper on the labour economy.* Tokyo: Gyousei, Author.

Nikkei. (2007). Nikkei corporate image research. Unpublished raw data.

Omoikkiri effect. (1996, April 9). *The Nikkei Daily*, p. 16.

Painless needle gets off to a flying start. (2006, July 25). *Nikkei Kinyu Shimbun*, p. 5.

The price of health and safety the boom that TV makes the overheating sales of uncertain effects. (1997, May 29). *The Nikkei*, p. 29.

Shimamura, K. (2006). *Advertisement beneficial to consumers 2006.* Unpublished manuscript, Tokyo.

Takahashi, K. (2007). *Food faddism—A diet not affected by the media.* Tokyo: Chuohoki.

Terumo. (2002). *For gentle medical care: From 1991 to 2001.* Tokyo: Terumo.

Terumo. (2004). *Terumo sponsors "Kenko Tenki Yoho."* Retrieved July 28, 2009, from http://www.terumo.co.jp/press/2004/005.html

Terumo. (2006). *Terumo sponsors new style healthcare program "Karada No Kimochi."* Retrieved July 28, 2009, from http://www.terumo.co.jp/press/2006/006.html

Terumo. (2007a). *The research on Karada no Kimochi.* Unpublished manuscript. Tokyo: Author.

Terumo. (2007b). *Social and environmental report 2007.* Tokyo: Author.

Terumo decides to produce more painless needles. (2007, April 18). *The Nikkei*, p. 13.

Thirteen million people have metabolic syndrome. (2006, May 9). *The Nikkei*, p. 38.

Wachi, T. (2004). Growth is achieved from cutting edge and basic business fields. *Weekly Toyo Keizai, 5878*, 146–149.

Watabe, K. (2007). Corporate image research. *Nikkei Advertising Note*, pp. 12–15.

CHAPTER 14

Successful Contraceptive Social Marketing Attempts in India

Sameer Deshpande, Jaidev Balakrishnan, Anurudra Bhanot, and Sanjeev Dham

INDIA: A COUNTRY OVERVIEW

India is the second most populous country in the world, with a population of more than 1.1 billion living in an area of 1.27 million square miles, an area slightly more than one-third the size of the United States. India is a federal republic comprised of 28 states and seven union territories. With a bicameral parliament, it is the largest democracy in the world, having held elections regularly since 1951. The president is the head of the country, although the prime minister manages the day-to-day administration (Central Intelligence Agency [CIA], 2009). "India is pluralistic, multi-ethnic, and multi-lingual" (World Health Organization [WHO], 2007, p. 81). The major ethnic groups are Indo-Aryan (72% of the population) and Dravidian (25%); religions include Hinduism (80.5%), Islam (13.4%), Christianity (2.3%), and Sikhism (1.9%), while representing a host of other religions such as Jainism, Buddhism, and Zoroastrianism. There are 23 official languages, of which English and Hindi are the most common (CIA, 2009).

For five decades after achieving independence, India followed a mixed-economy model, utilizing both capitalist and socialist economic thoughts. However, due to financial pressures, the country liberalized its economy in 1991. Since then, it has increasingly embraced the capitalist model. Since 1997, after years of sluggish growth, the country has experienced rapid annual growth at an average rate of 7% (CIA, 2009). India has become one of the world's fastest-growing economies and is slated to become the third largest in the world by 2050 (Goldman Sachs, 2003), dominant in the areas of information technology, business processes outsourcing, pharmaceuticals, and telecommunications (CIA, 2009). The country is experiencing a boom in ownership of consumer durable and nondurable goods, and this growth is expected to continue in the future (National Council of Applied Economic Research [NCAER], 2005).

Though impressive, India's economic development has been uneven: an estimated 25% of the population continues to live below the poverty line. Gains in development are threatened by the significant social, economic, and environmental challenges posed by India's large and growing population and by ethnic and regional strife (CIA, 2009).

Major Public Health Issues

India suffers from public health challenges normally associated with both developed and developing worlds. The key public health issues identified by the government of India include overpopulation; high maternal mortality and child mortality; and communicable and noncommunicable diseases such as malaria, filariasis, kala-azar (visceral leishmaniasis), dengue, tuberculosis, leprosy, HIV/AIDS, cancer, cardiovascular diseases, diabetes, and blindness. Other common public health challenges include acute respiratory infection, water supply, and sanitation, diarrhea and malnutrition, substantial regional inequalities in health status and quality of health care, and lack of health insurance for 90% of the population (Ministry of Health and Family Welfare [MOHFW], 2005; WHO, 2007). Relevant to a contraceptive social marketing context, India bears the double burden of overpopulation and a high incidence of HIV/AIDS.

These issues are echoed in the World Health Organization's Country Cooperation Strategy 2006–2011 for India (WHO, 2006), which outlines three main health challenges: (1) dealing effectively with unfinished agendas of communicable diseases, maternal and child health, and health systems strengthening; (2) dealing with emerging challenges such as the premature burden of noncommunicable diseases; and (3) dealing with globalization-related issues while contributing to the management and shaping of the global policy environment.

Trends in the Use of Social Marketing and Health Communication

There have been several social marketing attempts by central and state governmental bodies, as well as international and domestic nonprofit organizations, to address the myriad public health problems. In recent years, social marketing principles have been employed to promote immunization, oral rehydration therapy, treated bed nets, micronutrients, public toilets, and water conservation.

However, the most prominent efforts in India have centered on contraceptive social marketing—historically to promote family planning and, more recently, to prevent HIV/AIDS. In the 1960s, India was the first country to introduce the concept of contraceptive social marketing to its family planning program, thanks to the efforts of Peter King and his colleagues at the Indian Institute of Management, Calcutta (Harvey, 1999). Over the years, the government program has undergone several changes, with an increased reliance on voluntary organizations in recent years.

Currently, the government of India's national contraceptive social marketing program supplies condoms and oral contraceptive pills to consumers who cannot afford to buy them at full market price and who, at the same time, are not reached by the free public distribution program. The government of India sources condoms and oral contraceptive pills from local manufacturers and supplies them at a subsidized price to nonprofit social marketing agencies. The government also provides a marketing subsidy to these agencies, which distribute the products through existing commercial networks and use the mass media and other retail marketing techniques to advertise and promote the products. At present, India's contraceptive social marketing program is the largest in the world, with condom sales having increased from less than 10 million per year in the late 1960s to more than 1 billion (Thapa, Prasad, Rao, Severy, & Rao, 1994).

The Indian contraceptive social marketing addresses a variety of public health issues related to the twin burden of overpopulation and the high prevalence of HIV/AIDS. This chapter highlights two such social marketing efforts.

CASE STUDY 1
Population Services International's
Emergency Contraception Campaign[1]

CAMPAIGN BACKGROUND AND ENVIRONMENT

Population Services International (PSI) has been a partner in India's national contraceptive social marketing program since 1988. In addition, with the permission of the government of India and support from bilateral donors and U.S.-based foundations, PSI has implemented social marketing programs to

[1]This case is based on project reports presented by Population Services International to its donors.

encourage the use of emergency contraception (EC) for birth spacing and re-productive health, as well as other social marketing products. PSI also applies social franchising concepts and techniques to improve utilization of quality services for maternal and child health, voluntary counseling and testing for HIV, and the diagnosis and treatment of sexually transmitted infections (STIs).

With approximately 115,000 women dying each year from complications related to pregnancy and childbirth, India accounts for more than 23% of ma-ternal deaths in the developing world. The global maternal mortality ratio in 2005 is estimated at 400 per 100,000 live births. The adjusted UN estimate for India in 2005 was 450, which classified India in the *high* category (UNICEF, 2007). The high maternal mortality in India is fueled by high rates of unin-tended pregnancy, complications of pregnancy and childbirth, and unsafe abor-tions, which in turn are driven by the following factors:

- Social and cultural constraints on women, such as opposition to contraceptive use by husbands and mothers-in-law.
- Early-age marriage, which exposes young girls to the risk of early and repeated pregnancies.
- Sexual violence and coercion, including rape within marriage.
- Lack of access to safe abortion procedures. (Mallik, 2003)

According to a recent study, complications of unsafe abortion alone account for 13% of all maternal deaths in India (Ganatra & Johnston, 2002). EC plays an important role in the reduction of maternal mortality by providing women a safe, effective, and affordable method to prevent pregnancy after unprotected sex. The pills must be taken within 72 hours after intercourse. As its name im-plies, EC is intended for emergency use when the primary means of contracep-tion fails (i.e., if the condom slips or tears or if the woman forgets to consume the pill), or in the case of forced, unprotected sex (International Consortium for Emergency Contraception [ICEC], 2004).

Social Marketing Emergency Contraception in Rajasthan

The state of Rajasthan, located in the northwestern part of India with a popula-tion of 56 million, has relatively poor health indicators, with a total fertility rate of 3.2 children born per woman (International Institute of Population Sciences [IIPS] & Macro International, 2007) and maternal deaths of 607 per 100,000 live births (MOHFW, n.d.).

As an implementing partner in the government of India's contraceptive social marketing program, PSI has marketed condoms and oral contraceptive pills in the state of Rajasthan since 1989. In partnership with the William and Flora Hewlett Foundation, PSI created, managed, and promoted a branded network of qualified medical doctors to provide affordable, high-quality family planning choices to low-income women and men in Rajasthan, under the brand name *Saadhan* (translated as "a medium," although it is also referred to as a "contraceptive").

In 2004, with the continued support of the Hewlett Foundation, PSI launched a pilot program to increase trial and use of EC in eight districts in Rajasthan. Because emergency contraceptive pills (EC pills) were categorized as a prescription drug in India at that time, the original strategy was to add EC to the family planning and birth spacing services provided by Saadhan clinics. In 2005, when EC pills became an over-the-counter drug, the program strategy was accordingly modified.

SWOT Analysis

Strengths

- Levonorgestrel (the EC regimen available in India) has a high efficacy rate and limited side effects.
- The commodity cost was sufficiently low that price subsidization was unnecessary to render the product affordable. This increased the sustainability of the program.

Weaknesses

- Repeated use of EC pills lowers their efficacy and raises the risk of hormonal imbalances, disrupted menstrual cycles, and increased risks of complications in pregnancy. For these reasons, EC pills are to be used in emergency situations only.

Opportunities

- EC pills were introduced as part of the national Reproductive and Child Health Program in 2002. This demonstrates government of India support for EC.
- EC pills acquired over-the-counter status in India in 2005, enabling wider access through pharmacies.
- During the project period, the government's national contraceptive social marketing program had not expanded to include EC pills. Such inclusion would significantly increase access to and demand for EC pills.
- A 2004 population-based survey commissioned by PSI in the project area revealed that 78% of the 2,700 respondents mentioned frequent instances of unprotected sex. The mean number of such instances in one month prior to the survey was 10. A high risk of unwanted pregnancy and the potential need for EC lay with this group.

- By increasing access to EC, health services provide a point of contact for women facing unintended pregnancy due to nonuse of other spacing methods. With increased information, products, and appropriate counseling, these women may become regular users of birth spacing methods.

Threats

- The use of EC pills was subject to the same constraints as regular birth spacing methods—for example, a lack of available choices and little support from family.
- The concept of a postcoital contraceptive was very new, even among qualified medical practitioners. Therefore, dissociating EC pills from abortifacients (drugs used specifically to abort) was an uphill task.
- For additional target-audience-oriented challenges, refer to the "Barriers" section.

Past and Similar Efforts

PSI's EC social marketing program in Rajasthan, which promoted EC as part of a broader spectrum of choices in reproductive technologies, was the first of its kind in India. In similar efforts, social marketing organizations Parivar Seva Sanstha and Janani distributed and promoted their own brands of EC pills. The Family Planning Association of India also introduced EC pills on a pilot basis as part of its choices in select districts in the state of Madhya Pradesh.

TARGET AUDIENCES

The program's primary target audience consisted of married unsterilized women and men intentionally or unintentionally indulging in unprotected sex, aged 15 to 34, living in urban slums in eight districts in Rajasthan: Jaipur, Tonk, Alwar, Sawai Madhopur, Udaipur, Bhilwara, Chittor, and Sirohi. This age demographic contributes to more than 70% of total fertility in Rajasthan, and women undergo sterilization after completing their families at the median age of 27 years (IIPS & ORC Macro, 2001). The program focused on urban slums for two reasons. First, qualified doctors were more readily found in urban and peri-urban areas than rural areas; the program succeeded in building a network of 178 Saadhan clinics to serve the target beneficiaries. More importantly, recent studies have shown that the lifetime risk of maternal death in India is substantially higher (up to three times) in urban areas than in rural areas (Ranjan, 2006), with urban slums reporting significantly poorer reproductive health indicators than the urban average.

The program's secondary target audience consisted of pharmacists and doctors in the public and private sectors. In view of the low awareness of EC, pharmacists and doctors play an important role as trusted, authoritative sources of information and effective behavior change agents. For this reason, it was essential to build their knowledge and endorsement of EC.

CAMPAIGN OBJECTIVES AND GOALS

Behavior Objectives

For the target beneficiaries, the program's overarching behavior goal was to increase use of modern contraceptive methods from 25.6% to 32.8% in order to space births and plan their families; the specific behavior objective was to increase trial and correct use of EC pills through the sale of 50,000 EC doses to prevent unintended pregnancy after unprotected sex, and subsequent graduation to regular birth spacing methods. The time frame provided by the donor for achieving these was 28 months. For doctors and pharmacists, the behavior objective was to increase accurate communication and appropriate counseling for EC and regular birth spacing methods. An additional behavior objective for doctors was to increase the appropriate screening and prescription of EC pills.

Knowledge Objectives

The program sought to increase knowledge of the following key facts among target beneficiaries as well as doctors and pharmacists:
- Pregnancy is established 72 hours after having unprotected sex.
- EC pills must be taken within three days of the unprotected sex act.
- EC pills are the solution when a contraceptive method fails or no method was used.
- EC pills are postcoital contraceptives that prevent pregnancy after sex. EC is not abortion; EC helps avoid abortion. The campaign countered the prevalent perception that contraceptives were methods used only before or during sexual intercourse and that any method used after intercourse was an abortifacient, a much prevalent technology.
- EC pills are effective and low on side effects.

For the target beneficiaries, objectives also included communicating that even one act of unprotected sex can result in pregnancy and that EC pills are available at Saadhan clinics (when EC pills were prescription only) and at pharmacists (when EC pills became available over the counter).

For doctors, further knowledge objectives included the government's endorsement of EC pills and their favorable impact on women's health, as well as guidelines for the screening and counseling of EC clients.

Belief Objectives

The belief objective for the target beneficiaries was to promote the idea that the use of contraceptives, including EC, to space births and plan your family will contribute to the physical, mental, and financial well-being of the family. This objective was important for building the husbands' support for the use of EC pills and regular contraceptive methods, which is crucial in view of the low decision-making power of women in Indian households, and specifically in Rajasthan.

TARGET AUDIENCE BARRIERS, MOTIVATORS (BENEFITS), AND COMPETITION

Barriers

Through segmentation analysis based on survey, the program identified two key barriers to the use of EC pills among the target beneficiaries: (1) opposition or little support from the spouse for the adoption of any modern contraceptive method and (2) ignorance or skepticism of the fact that a single act of unprotected sex can result in pregnancy.

Additional barriers to the timely and correct use of EC pills include (1) a lack of awareness of EC pills and where to get them, (2) low product availability at clinics and pharmacies within a manageable distance, (3) reliance on missing periods rather than the occurrence of unprotected sex as the indicator of risk of pregnancy, and (4) a lack of experience in using other modern contraceptive methods.

Motivators and Perceived Benefits

Perceived benefits for the use of EC pills were the physical, mental, and financial well-being of the family resulting from well-spaced births.

Competing Behaviors

Behavior that competes with the desired behavior of using EC pills is to do nothing and leave the pregnancy to fate. If the woman becomes pregnant there are two choices: terminate the pregnancy or accept it.

Both options can result in several negative financial, mental, and health-related consequences. However, the woman considers the benefits of these options to be better than the costs. A pregnant woman weighs aborting the fetus or accepting the pregnancy with the benefit of retaining the company of her spouse. In the Indian context, especially in low socioeconomic classes, women are prominently dependent on their spouses both financially and for social identity. As a result, they have no choice but to leave the decisions to their husbands.

POSITIONING STATEMENT

We want our target audience to perceive that the use of EC (and other modern contraceptives) will result in marital bliss and is a better option than undertaking potentially unsafe abortions or living with unwanted pregnancies.

CAMPAIGN STRATEGIES, IMPLEMENTATION, AND EVALUATION

Product Strategies

For the purposes of the program, PSI obtained the distribution rights of Preventol in Rajasthan. Preventol, manufactured by Hindustan Latex Limited, consists of two 0.75-mg levonorgestrel pills in a blister strip, packaged in a box featuring an abstract male and female silhouette. Due to the low awareness of EC and EC pills, the program's priority was to promote this little-known technology—that is, to increase the use of the method rather than the brand. The product was promoted using the phrase "Emergency Goli-Teen Din Wali" ("the three-day emergency pill"). A logo bearing this phrase (see Figure 14-1) featured prominently on the product's outer packaging.

Training of Doctors and Orientation of Pharmacists

To increase accurate knowledge and enthusiastic support of EC among this important group, the program provided training in the technical aspects of EC,

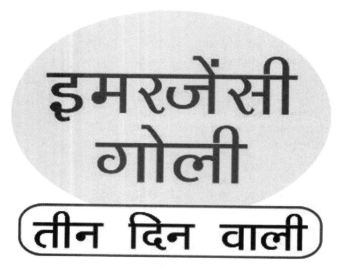

FIGURE 14-1　The "Emergency Goli-Teen Din Wali" phrase

Courtesy of Population Services International, India

client screening, history taking, and counseling regarding the family planning options to 562 doctors and organized 28 group meetings to orient pharmacists in EC knowledge and issues.

Pricing Strategies

The program negotiated a favorable purchase price with the manufacturer. After covering the production cost, distribution costs, and the margins required by wholesalers and retailers, the program was able to offer Preventol to consumers at the affordable maximum retail price of 20 rupees (US$0.50) per dose. This compared to the maximum retail price ranging from 50 to 75 rupees (US$1.25–$1.88) per dose for commercial brands.

Place Strategies

In the initial stage of the program, when EC pills were a prescription-only drug, the program added EC pills to the family planning and birth spacing services provided by the 178-clinic Saadhan network. The program focused on offering quality EC screening, counseling, and prescription services to the target beneficiaries and distributed the product mainly through Saadhan clinics and nearby pharmacists. One year into the program, it became clear that this strategy was not cost-effective in attaining the level of product availability and visibility required for popularizing such a new technology. Accordingly, the distribution strategy was amended to expand coverage of pharmacists and doctors outside the Saadhan network.

Even with the newly gained over-the-counter status, EC pills could only be sold in pharmacies and not at nonpharmaceutical outlets (where oral contraceptive pills and condoms could be sold). To make EC pills widely available to the target beneficiaries, the program built a distribution network of 1,200 pharmacists and 562 doctors in the private and public sectors in the eight program districts.

Promotion Strategies

The promotion strategy differed with the over-the-counter status of EC pills. During the prescription-only phase, the objective was to raise awareness of EC and its availability at Saadhan clinics primarily through outdoor and print media as well as interpersonal communication. After the drug achieved over-the-counter status, the program stepped up radio and TV promotion of EC pills and their availability at pharmacies, while maintaining interpersonal outreach activities in the slum communities.

Prescription-Only Strategy

During this phase, a mix of print ads, billboards, and interpersonal outreach in the target slum areas was used to promote EC as part of a broader spectrum of modern contraceptive methods. The campaign focused on directing target beneficiaries to Saadhan clinics for EC information, counseling, and prescription. Print ads were placed in mainstream dailies with high circulation, and billboards advertised in prominent locations in the target slums to promote the benefits of EC pills (see Figure 14-2) and the Saadhan doctor network (see Figure 14-3).

Saadhan doctors, who were trained in EC screening, counseling, and prescription, displayed illuminated sign boards bearing the Saadhan logo (see Figure 14-4) outside their clinics to indicate the availability of modern birth spacing options, including EC.

The outreach campaign was also employed to achieve EC pill–related campaign objectives as well as to popularize Saadhan doctors nearest to the slums and to convince the target group to visit them for products, services, and information related to modern contraceptive methods.

Over-the-Counter Strategy

Media Selection

EC attaining over-the-counter status paved the way to greater accessibility for this new technology. To create a greater and more focused reach of its communication campaign among the targeted population, PSI based the selection of its media channels on the National Readership Survey 2002 findings. Because a husband's support for adoption of any form of modern contraception was critical, the media plan was formulated to reach males. TV ads were placed on a private channel, E-TV, that runs state-specific programs and has a reach restricted to the state. To ensure high viewership, the campaign's TV spots were placed around state news and movie song–based programs that aired during prime

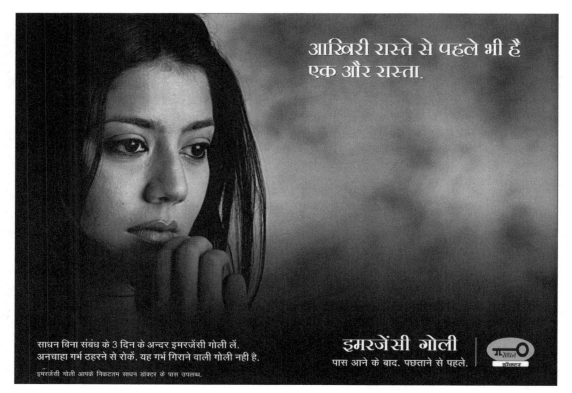

FIGURE 14-2   Print and billboard campaign—EC focus
(Translation: There is still one option left before you resort to the last course. After unprotected sex, use EC within three days. It prevents unwanted pregnancies. It is not an abortifacient. EC is available at your nearest Saadhan doctor. Emergency pill. After you get close, before you regret. Saadhan Network logo.)
Courtesy of Population Services International, India

time. Radio spots were broadcast on the government-run FM radio station; the All India Radio; and leading mainstream state dailies, namely, *Dainik Bhaskar*, *Rajasthan Patrika*, and *Navjyoti*.

Point of purchase communication was utilized by placing "Emergency Goli-Teen Din Wali available here" banners and posters at pharmacies, and EC information brochures for distribution to consumers. The banners and posters formed part of the integrated communication campaign; they featured the same character and tagline as the TV spot described next.

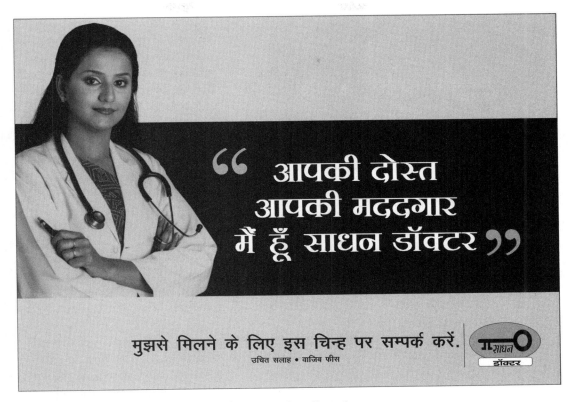

FIGURE 14-3   Print and billboard campaign—Saadhan focus
(Translation: Your friend, whom you can count on for help. I am a Saadhan doctor. To meet me, contact at this sign. Right advice, affordable fees. Saadhan Network logo.)
Courtesy of Population Services International, India

Message Design

The TV spot was based on a popular Hindi movie song "Kahi Der Na ho jaye" (Hope it doesn't get too late). The story begins with a couple and infant, preparing to board a train, encountering a variety of people—a porter, a tea vendor, and a folk singer singing this song to them. Finally, the husband quizzically asks the folk singer what he means by this, at which point the folk singer sings to him that even a single instance of "coming close" without protection could lead to the risk of his wife getting unintentionally pregnant. After hearing this, the husband and wife look at each other in dismay. The folk

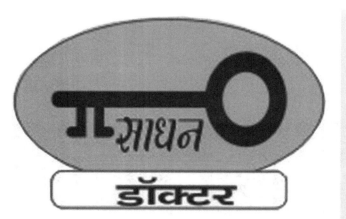

FIGURE 14-4 Saadhan network logo
Courtesy of Population Services International, India

singer continues that in such a situation if within three days of such a situation he gives his wife "emergency goli," they can avoid such an outcome. The husband and wife heave a sigh of relief. The TV spot ends with a voice-over recommending the use of this pill only in an emergency and advocating the use of condoms or oral contraceptive pills for regular contraception. The viewer is directed to the nearest pharmacist for the EC pill. The radio spots adopted a similar theme. Print advertisements used the same female model as in the television spot, portraying her in a pensive mood after an act of unprotected sex and then in a relieved mood on knowing that a solution (EC) exists.

The female outreach campaign used specially designed interpersonal communication tools and made 425,124 contacts with the female target beneficiaries through household visits or women's group meetings.

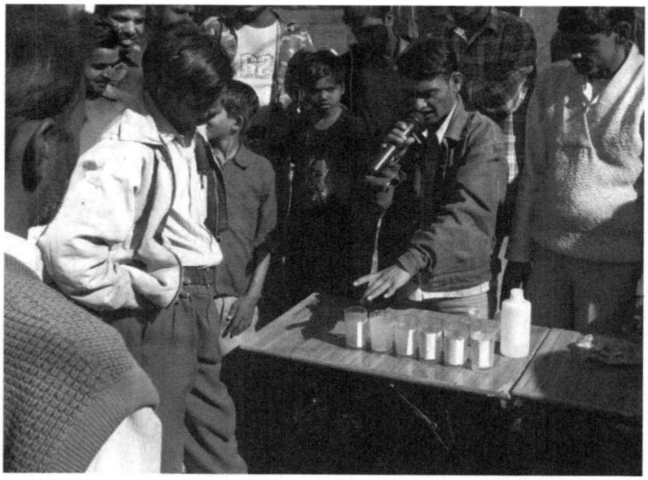

Lack of support from the husband was identified as a significant barrier to the trial and use of modern contraceptive methods, including EC. To address this barrier, the project launched an interpersonal outreach campaign targeting men in 38 towns in the eight program districts. Outreach activities took the form of interactive games (see Figure 14-5) and quizzes in places where men congregate. A total of 47,347 men were reached in this campaign.

FIGURE 14-5 Interactive games with men
Courtesy of Population Services International, India

Other Important Strategies

Advocacy at the State Level

The program organized a state-level workshop on EC in the state capital of Jaipur in close coordination with the Jaipur Obstetrics and Gynaecological Society, the Indian Medical Association, and other medical associations across Rajasthan. The state government of Rajasthan played an active role by instructing chief medical officers and health officers from all 32 districts to nominate participants for the workshop. The workshop was attended by more than 600 physicians from the public and private sector and received generous coverage in the media. This high-profile event gave much-needed momentum to the popularization of EC in Rajasthan by demonstrating the state government's endorsement of EC and by providing participants and the media with accurate information.

The state government has requested to use the project's information, education, and communication material to popularize EC in the public health system. The project's banner and leaflet have been included in the government's quarterly magazine for public health providers.

Advocacy at the National Level

PSI is an active member of Advocating Reproductive Choices (ARC), an alliance of nongovernmental organizations (NGOs) working in the field of reproductive health in the country. When EC pills were a prescription-only drug, ARC's advocacy efforts focused on obtaining over-the-counter status for EC pills. With the granting of over-the-counter status in August 2005, and the Ministry of Health and Family Welfare's ensuing announcement that EC pills would be included in the national contraceptive social marketing program, the focus of ARC's advocacy with the government of India has switched to the design of the national social marketing program for EC (lifting the current restriction against EC pill sales by nonpharmacists) and government investment in the mass media promotion of EC. Specifically, ARC has advocated for a multistate EC social marketing program with an extensive promotional campaign that is co-sponsored by the government and international donors to raise awareness and acceptance of EC. PSI has contributed to the discussion by sharing the research results, communication strategy, lessons learned, and other information from the project.

CAMPAIGN BUDGET AND TIME FRAME

The program budget was US$1.2 million. The program took place over 28 months, from January 2004 to April 2006.

TABLE 14-1   Impact of the EC Campaign

Indicators	Baseline	Endline
Ever heard of EC	5.9%	44.7%*
Ever used EC	0.3	2.9*
Current use of modern birth spacing method	25.6	32.8*
Belief that even a single act of unprotected intercourse can cause pregnancy	56.2	74.6*
Support from husband for contraceptive use and/or EC	62.7	77.2*

*Significant at $p < 0.05$

EVALUATION

For measurement of project performance, a baseline survey was conducted by the research agency Synovate India among the female target group in the project area in December 2004 ($n = 2,700$); an endline survey was conducted by the research agency Mode Modellers in May 2006 ($n = 1,988$). A comparison of the survey results shows a significant increase in EC awareness and use, and substantial improvement in the key factors influencing the target group's ability and motivation to use EC (see Table 14-1).

Separately, surveys conducted by PSI among pharmacists in the project indicated significant popularization of the concept of "emergency goli." Consumers asking for emergency goli when seeking a method to avoid pregnancy after unprotected sex increased from 55% in March 2005 to 95% by March 2006. In the 28-month period, the program sold 73,420 doses of Preventol. The increased awareness and demand for emergency goli has prompted the entry of five other brands of EC pills into the Rajasthan market, while Hindustan Latex Limited has increased its marketing effort for Preventol—all of which will contribute to improved availability and visibility of EC pills. More importantly, the program has improved long-term demand for modern contraceptive methods by building spousal support and by significantly strengthening knowledge and belief that pregnancy can result from even a single act of unprotected sex.

LESSONS LEARNED FROM THE PSI CAMPAIGN

By increasing access to one kind of contraceptive (EC), the program established contact with women and men facing unintended pregnancy due to nonuse of other spacing methods and motivated them to use modern contraceptive methods through follow-up counseling.

Interpersonal outreach to women, in the form of recurring household visits and women's group meetings, provided the depth of communication and follow-up necessary for debunking myths regarding fertility; building women's confidence about modern contraceptive methods, including EC; and generally supporting them through the different stages of the behavior change process, from pre-contemplation to maintenance.

Similarly, interpersonal outreach to men, in the form of interactive games and quizzes in places where men congregate, created an opportunity for men to think and talk about the benefits of birth spacing, an issue that they rarely discuss openly but in which they are the prime decision maker.

Mass media played a crucial role in providing credibility to ground-level activities. This was evident at the initial stage of implementation, when the campaign was restricted to interpersonal communication activities. Outreach workers faced considerable difficulties in convincing the target beneficiaries to try EC pills because the target beneficiaries had not seen or heard about this new technology.

In the initial stage of the program, when EC pills were a prescription-only drug, the strategy was to provide access to EC pills and quality EC counseling through the Saadhan network and pharmacists in the program area. After a year of implementation, it became clear that this was not a cost-effective way to attain the high level of product presence required to achieve a "tipping point" in EC use. The strategy was amended to focus on advocacy for over-the-counter status for EC pills, wide orientation of pharmacists in EC, and extensive detailing of EC pills to healthcare providers within and outside the Saadhan network. After EC pills became an over-the-counter drug, the strategy was further amended to increase the focus on mass media promotion and coverage of pharmacists to maximize product visibility and availability.

CASE STUDY 2
BBC World Service Trust HIV/AIDS Campaigns[2]

This case examines how the concept of entertainment-education—that is, *edutainment* (Singhal & Rogers, 2002)—was applied to create behavioral change communication when dealing with the HIV/AIDS challenge in India.

[2]This case is based on information available at the BBC World Service Trust Web site: www.bbc worldservicetrust.org

CAMPAIGN BACKGROUND AND ENVIRONMENT

According to recent estimates by the National Family Health Survey (IIPS & Macro International, 2007), 0.36% of the general adult population in India has HIV, or between 2 million and 3.1 million people. The survey found HIV to be heavily concentrated in the 15-to-49 age group (88.7% of all infections), among the high-risk groups (injecting drug users, men who have sex with men, and commercial sex workers), and among men more than women. The first AIDS case in India was detected in 1986; since then HIV infection has been reported in all states and union territories. However, the epidemic is the most extreme in the southern half of the country and in the far northeast.

The government of India, states, and prominent cities (State AIDS Prevention and Control Societies) are actively addressing this epidemic through a network of units set up at the National AIDS Control Organization (NACO). Private-sector social marketing organizations are similarly helping the government in these efforts. The BBC World Service Trust (BBC WST), the international charity of BBC, has actively supported the government of India's HIV/AIDS prevention and control efforts using the creative power of the media. Between 2002 and 2007, the BBC WST produced and broadcast three HIV/AIDS–related health campaign programs aired on the national TV channel Doordarshan (DD-1) in India: (1) a detective drama serial titled *Jasoos Vijay* ("Detective Vijay"), (2) a youth reality show titled *Haath Se Haath Mila* ("Let's Join Hands"), and (3) a series of public service announcements aired during commercial breaks on the two programs.

Funded by the British government's Department for International Development (DFID), the campaigns were implemented in partnership with India's national broadcaster Doordarshan and NACO. As Nielsen's Television Audience Monitoring (TAM) data show, even in a highly competitive TV audience market, DD-1 still enjoys high viewership with a nationally representative sample. It had a 17% share of viewers in 2006, nearly three times that of its closest competitor. The profile of DD-1 audiences matched with that of the project's target audience: middle- and lower-middle-class households from semi-urban towns and villages.

CAMPAIGN OBJECTIVES AND GOALS

The purpose of the campaigns was to reduce the growth rate of HIV infection in India. The campaign objectives were as follows:

Behavior Objectives

The behavioral objectives included promoting open discussion of sexual health issues, influencing behavior regarding the means of preventing HIV (including the use of condoms), and promoting behavioral change with regard to reducing stigma and discrimination against people living with HIV/AIDS.

Knowledge Objectives

The knowledge objectives included educating people about the routes of HIV transmission and ways of preventing the disease. The objectives also included education about the availability and application of methods of HIV/AIDS treatment (including anti-retroviral drugs).

Belief Objectives

The belief objectives of the campaign were to promote an attitudinal shift toward discussion of sexual health issues and to reduce stigma and discrimination against people living with HIV/AIDS.

TARGET AUDIENCE BARRIERS AND MOTIVATORS

Barriers

Formative research identified the following barriers to the practice of safe sex:

- Myths and misconceptions—particularly among women, the less educated, and rural populations—about the routes of HIV transmission, methods of prevention, testing for HIV, treatment, care, and support for people living with HIV/AIDS.
- Lack of accurate knowledge, leading to the low perception of risk to self, increased risk of infection, and enhanced stigma and discrimination toward those living with HIV/AIDS.
- Negative perceptions associated with condoms—beliefs that condoms are "dirty" things, reduce pleasure, are not very effective (slip, tear, leak), are meant for contraception, and imply mistrust if suggested by a partner.
- High dependence, particularly among the rural populations, on traditional cures, quacks, and myths about cures for HIV.
- Shame and embarrassment associated with discussions around sexual health, HIV/AIDS, STIs, and the purchase and usage of condoms.

Motivators

- The reliability of the information provided through the government channel—the perception that it is without commercial motives.
- The influence of role models in creating aspirational values and lifestyles—particularly among the youth and those from rural areas.

CAMPAIGN STRATEGIES, IMPLEMENTATION, AND EVALUATION

Product Strategies

The core benefit promoted to the primary audience (sexually active males and females) was the reduced risk of HIV/AIDS transmission from or to their partners through unprotected sex. The tangible product promoted was a condom as a method of preventing HIV/AIDS transmission.

Price and Place Strategies

The BBC WST efforts were part of a larger condom promotion campaign. The TV programs informed audiences about places they could obtain subsidized condoms distributed under NACO's social marketing program. The TV shows also attempted to communicate reduction in HIV/AIDS–related stigma and discrimination by creating awareness among the general population and changing their attitudes toward people living with HIV/AIDS (PLHAs). The public service announcements (PSAs) also gave information to the audiences on how and where to get people tested for HIV/AIDS. The PSAs informed the audiences that the tests are conducted free of charge at government hospitals/dispensaries and that pre- and post-counseling are available at voluntary counseling and testing centers.

Promotion Strategies

The product, price, and place strategies were promoted through three TV vehicles. Each one of them, along with their objectives, is now described.

Jasoos Vijay ("Detective Vijay"): Drama Serial

The *Jasoos Vijay* serial TV drama was designed for semi-urban small towns and rural audiences. The weekly drama was telecast on Sunday nights during prime time (8:30 p.m.) and re-telecast on Monday mornings. Although created specifically to communicate information and awareness of HIV/AIDS, *Jasoos Vijay* addressed a broad range of issues of concern to rural audiences within an "entertaining and interactive drama format" (see Figure 14-6).

Detective Vijay, the lead character in the program, solved a crime story over four episodes, assisted by his fiancée and two friends. The central character himself was portrayed as HIV-positive, allowing the program to address issues of the care and treatment of those living with the virus and tackling stigma and discrimination. In addition to HIV/AIDS issues, which remained central to the messaging across the series, the program addressed other themes like superstition, "quack" doctors, gender inequality, and crimes against women (e.g., domestic violence, rape, practice of dowry) during different episodes. Messaging on various themes was woven into the plot, and each story line was pretested to gauge audience reaction.

Om Puri, a renowned theater and cinema personality, anchored the interactive part of the program. Toward the end of each episode, he would challenge the audience to solve the crime before Detective Vijay did. He would invite their comments and feedback on each episode along with their questions, clarifications, and experiences related to HIV/AIDS. The viewers were also invited to write for a booklet about HIV/AIDS. At the peak of its run, the program received

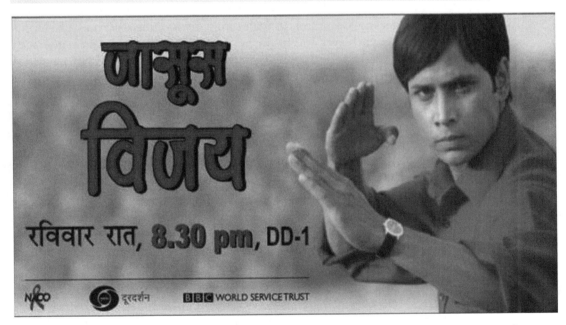

FIGURE 14-6   (Translation: Detective Vijay, Sunday night, 8:30 pm, [channel] DD-1)

more than 1,500 audience letters per month. In its last year alone, the program received more than 15,000 letters from engaged audiences.

The program also created a website (www.jasoosvijay.com) to provide additional information about HIV/AIDS and to encourage people to write in with their questions and experiences. The Web site received 50 to 100 e-mails per month from audiences all over India.

Haath Se Haath Mila ("Let's Join Hands"): Youth Reality Show

Haath Se Haath Mila was conceived as a mainstream family entertainment show with a focus on Indian youth. The program format was primarily a reality show, including movie clips and songs, documentary drama, discussions, challenges, vox populi, travelogues, and interviews with Indian movie stars.

Central to the show were young achievers who had made a difference in their communities for people with HIV/AIDS. These "real" people came from different walks of life: doctors and healthcare workers, people who ran NGOs and support groups, lawyers, activists, educators, counselors and communicators, and people living with HIV/AIDS. Also common to all these people was their love for Indian movies and movie stars.

Over three episodes, the show told the story of one young achiever, journeying through his or her life—family and friends, work and colleagues, fears and struggles, dreams and aspirations. A major ingredient of the story was a face-off between the young achiever and his or her favorite Hindi movie star—interaction between the real-life and "reel"-life heroes—regarding each other's worlds and work, youth concerns, and issues relating to HIV/AIDS. For young achievers, it was a dream come true to be able to join hands with their favorite movie stars and to draw them into their work and campaigning. The show leveraged the appeal of movie stars by weaving their movie clips and songs seamlessly into the narrative.

HIV/AIDS messaging was naturally embedded in the story of young achievers in each episode. However, specific themes (such as stigma and discrimination, voluntary blood testing, care and counseling, anti-retroviral therapy) were discussed in different episodes in context with each young achiever's story. *Haath Se Haath Mila* was telecast every Thursday during prime time (see Figure 14-7).

The project team augmented the reach of the programs through two innovative strategies:

1. A road show featuring *Haath Se Haath Mila* "branded buses" created a buzz around the campaign theme by reaching out to young people in small towns, in the first two phases.

2. A music album and a video featuring the title track of the show and other popular songs were created. The video brought together a large number of Indian movie actors, lyricists, singers, and music directors on a single platform.

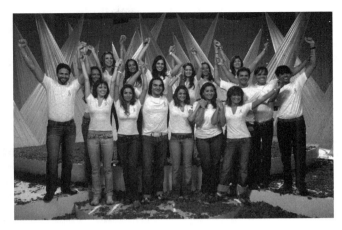

FIGURE 14-7 *Haath Se Haath Mila* star cast

Public Service Announcements

PSAs were a key part of BBC WST's campaign against HIV/AIDS: "Understand AIDS, Choose Life." BBC WST produced more than 30 PSAs covering a range of HIV/AIDS prevention, treatment, and support issues (see Figure 14-8).

The PSAs were aimed at viewers across India and were dubbed into a range of widely spoken languages. Each PSA was inserted strategically to reinforce the themes of the main shows, *Jasoos Vijay* and *Haath Se Haath Mila*.

The PSAs carried a mix of creative strategies while using cricketing personalities, Indian movie stars, and clay animation to communicate messages to relevant target groups. The advertisements used a mix of humor, empathy, and sheer conviction for raising awareness, dispelling myths, and creating an enabling environment for discussing taboo topics.

CAMPAIGN BUDGET AND TIME FRAME

The BBC WST project ran from 2002 to 2007. One hundred and eighteen episodes of each program, *Jasoos Vijay* and *Haath Se Haath Mila*, were telecast on a

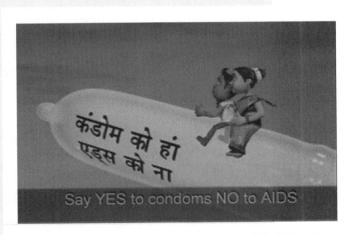

FIGURE 14-8 Example of a PSA in the BBC WST campaign

weekly basis. Both programs were telecast in Hindi and dubbed into seven regional languages.

The cost of production and broadcast of the three campaigns from 2002 to 2007 was US$8.44 million.

EVALUATION

Nielsen's TAM data estimated the three campaigns to have cumulatively reached more than 200 million people in India from 2002 to 2007. During its final episodes from October 2006 to September 2007, *Jasoos Vijay* reached a cumulative audience of 70 million viewers, while *Haath Se Haath Mila* reached 50 million viewers; the PSAs reached 115 million viewers over 52 episodes. Because the Nielsen's panel does not cover towns with populations of less than 100,000 (where the majority of the Doordarshan's audiences live), the actual reach may have been significantly higher.

Jasoos Vijay climbed from 34th place at the start of the campaign to the 10th most popular TV program toward the end. Within the genre of action thriller programs, *Jasoos Vijay* continued to figure among the top three programs in India. *Haath Se Haath Mila* was very popular among the youth segment. The programs also won accolades and critical acclaim from many national and international organizations.

BBC WST conducted a baseline target audience survey in 2005 at the beginning of the last phase of the project and an endline survey in 2007 after the campaign went off air. The survey was conducted among 11,000 respondents (males and females aged 15 to 49 years) across 17 states in India. The sample represented 70 million semi-urban and rural viewers of Doordarshan.

The impact was measured by calculating changes in knowledge, attitude, and practice indicators between the baseline and the endline data of those exposed to BBC WST programs versus those not exposed to the programs. The impact was also assessed by analyzing the responses of 160 male viewers in 16 focus group discussions, 19 female viewers' in-depth interviews, and more than 23,000 letters and 4,000 e-mails received from audiences of the two programs.

The results revealed that the programs had the greatest impact on the knowledge, attitudes, and behavior of sexually active men. Data showed that a higher percentage of those exposed to BBC WST programs became aware of different routes of HIV transmission. Between the two programs, those exposed to *Haath Se Haath Mila* showed higher knowledge gains compared to those exposed to *Jasoos Vijay*, although *Jasoos Vijay* had a significantly higher reach than

Haath Se Haath Mila. While *Jasoos Vijay* had a wider family audience, *Haath Se Haath Mila* was popular among adolescents and younger audiences.

Further, exposure to the programs improved the knowledge of viewers about the methods of preventing HIV transmission from one person to another. Again, *Haath Se Haath Mila* viewers showed higher knowledge gains on methods of preventing HIV transmission compared to those exposed to *Jasoos Vijay.*

Qualitative group discussions indicated that viewers also attributed to the programs the improvement in their knowledge about voluntary counseling and testing centers (VCTCs) for HIV testing, the availability of condoms, the treatment of STIs and opportunistic infections like tuberculosis, and the availability of anti-retroviral drugs at government hospitals and health centers.

Data also showed that those exposed to BBC WST programs exhibited more positive and accepting attitudes toward people living with HIV/AIDS. After exposure to BBC WST programs, a significantly higher proportion said they would look after someone in their family who had HIV/AIDS. Similarly, a significantly higher proportion of those exposed to *Haath Se Haath Mila* disagreed with the statement that they would *not* like an HIV/AIDS infected person visiting their homes (see Figure 14-9).

Audiences narrated personal experiences through letters and e-mails about how their views on caring for and supporting people with HIV/AIDS changed after viewing the programs. Focus group discussions with a portion

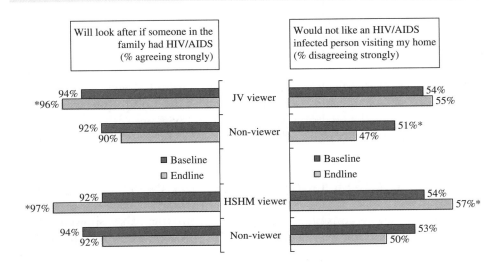

* Significant at $p < .05$

FIGURE 14-9 Change in attitudes toward people living with HIV/AIDS

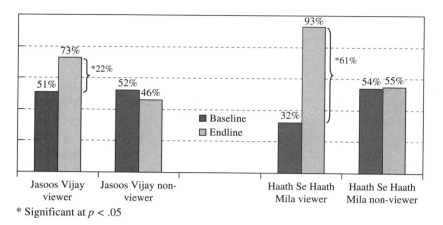

FIGURE 14-10   Consistent condom usage with commercial sex workers

of the audiences indicated that they had stopped feeling shy or embarrassed discussing sexual health problems, condoms, and HIV/AIDS with their partners, friends, and family members. Some audiences reported actions such as spreading accurate information about HIV/AIDS, STIs, and condoms within their communities and villages. There was clear evidence that the programs had initiated interpersonal and group communication on subjects that were traditionally considered taboo.

The biggest behavioral change was observed among those who reported having bought sex in the previous year. A significantly high percentage of those exposed to BBC WST programs reported consistent condom use with commercial sex workers every time they visited them (see Figure 14-10).

For a majority of the audiences who did not report multiple sexual partners or visits to commercial sex workers, there was clear evidence of program impact on the self- and collective efficacy levels of BBC WST programs.

LESSONS LEARNED FROM THE BBC WST CASE

Several factors were responsible for the success of the BBC WST programs. First, the educational entertainment ("edutainment") approach was thought to be more effective than a didactic and preachy approach for achieving the behavior change objectives of the communication campaign. The programs were created by experienced and qualified professionals, pretested, and produced in conformation with the production values and standards of BBC. The programs were shot on location using professional actors, properties, and technical equipment. *Jasoos Vijay* had all the ingredients of a Bollywood style thriller: helicopters, car chases, crime and suspense, songs, dances, and action sequences. *Haath Se Haath Mila* leveraged the appeal of movie stars and popular music to bond instantly with the youth.

Second, the portrayal of the detective hero, Vijay, as HIV-positive contributed greatly to dispelling myths and creating better awareness of HIV, its treatment, and its management. The stories and dramatic characters helped the programs achieve audience engagement, evidenced by thousands of letters and e-mails that arrived every month. The audiences identified with the characters, often looking at them as role models and forming para-social relationships with them. The programs pierced the cultural and social barriers in delivering messages related to sexual health and condoms—topics once considered taboo by Indian audiences.

Other factors responsible for the success of BBC WST's programs included choosing television as the main medium for reaching the masses, choosing the free-to-air national broadcaster Doordarshan, which provided a good reach; dubbing the program into seven regional languages; choosing the appropriate day and time for the telecasts and repeating the telecast of the programs; being consistent with the media consumption patterns and preferences of the target audiences; and continuously monitoring and pretesting as an intrinsic part of the creative development process, thus providing the creative team with feedback on program performance and audience feedback on the new story ideas under development.

SUMMARIZING THE TWO CASES

The two cases present diverse contraceptive social marketing efforts currently being undertaken to address the double burden of overpopulation and the high prevalence of HIV/AIDS in India.

PSI's EC campaign was regional in scope and targeted. It promoted EC pills (utilizing price, place, and promotion) in the poor segments of society through media and nonmedia options to address the population explosion.

BBC WST programs, on the other hand, were mass media–only edutainment vehicles that reached the general population in semi-urban and rural areas over a sustained period. BBC WST included the elements of drama as well as the celebrity value of Indian movie stars to spread information about HIV/AIDS and safe sex behaviors. These efforts were a good supplement to the targeted condom social marketing campaigns being carried out by the government of India and social marketing agencies.

Both case studies are excellent examples of the application of social marketing principles to important social problems reflected through clear strategy and implementation and robust research designs. Both applied the core components of marketing strategy—the 4Ps.

QUESTIONS FOR DISCUSSION

1. Because emergency contraception was a new technology with very few users, how would you identify the significant behavioral determinants differentiating "behaver" from "non-behaver" to overcome the barriers and triggers for adoption of the desired behavior?

2. List the advantages and disadvantages of the EC pill being an over-the-counter drug.

3. How can BBC WST extend the impact of the three TV campaigns? What other strategies would make the impact sustainable?

4. According to the BBC WST evaluation research, audiences developed para-social relationships with the program characters (e.g., *Jasoos Vijay*). Suggest ways of integrating this concept into impact monitoring models for behavioral change communications.

REFERENCES

Central Intelligence Agency (CIA). (2009). *The world factbook: India.* Retrieved July 28, 2009, from https://www.cia.gov/library/publications/the-world-factbook/geos/in.html

Ganatra, B., & Johnston, H. B. (2002). Reducing abortion-related mortality in South Asia: A review of constraints and a road map for change. *Journal of American Medical Women's Association, 57*(3), 159–164.

Goldman Sachs. (2003). *Global economics paper no. 99: Dreaming with BRICS: The path to 2050.* New York: The Goldman Sachs Group.

Harvey, P. D. (1999). *Let every child be wanted: How social marketing is revolutionizing contraceptive use around the world.* Westport, CT: Auburn House.

International Consortium for Emergency Contraception (ICEC). (2004). *Emergency contraceptive pills: Medical and service delivery guidelines,* 2nd ed. Washington, DC: Author.

International Institute of Population Sciences (IIPS) & Macro International. (2007). *National family health survey (NFHS-3), 2005–2006.* Mumbai: IIPS.

International Institute for Population Sciences (IIPS) & ORC Macro. (2001). *National Family Health Survey (NFHS-2), India, 1998–99: Rajasthan.* Mumbai: IIPS.

Mallik, R. (2003). *Beyond the magic bullet: Introduction of emergency contraceptive pills in India.* Takoma Park, MD: Center for Health and Gender Equity.

Ministry of Health and Family Welfare (MOHFW). (2005). *National rural health mission (2005–2012): Mission document.* Government of India. Retrieved July 28, 2009, from http://health.nic.in/NRHM/Documents/Mission_Document.pdf

Ministry of Health and Family Welfare (MOHFW). (n.d.). *National health policy 2002.* Government of India. Retrieved July 28, 2009, from http://mohfw.nic.in/np2002.htm

National Council of Applied Economic Research (NCAER). (2005). *The great Indian market: Results from the NCAER's market information survey of the households.* New Delhi: Author.

Ranjan, A. (2006). *Obstetric risk and obstetric care in central India.* New Delhi: Institute of Economic Growth, University of Delhi.

Singhal, A., & Rogers, E. M. (2002). A theoretical agenda for entertainment-education. *Communication Theory*, 14(2), 117–135.

Thapa, S., Prasad, C. V., Rao, P. H., Severy, L. J., & Rao, S. R. (1994). Social marketing of condoms in India. *Advances in Population: Psychosocial Perspectives 2*, 171–204.

UNICEF. (2007). *Progress for children report: A world fit for children, statistical review, number 6, December 2007.* New York: United Nations Children's Fund.

World Health Organization (WHO). (2006). *WHO country cooperation strategy: 2006–2011, India.* New Delhi: Country Office for India.

World Health Organization (WHO). (2007). *11 health questions about the 11 SEAR countries.* New Delhi: Regional Office for South-East Asia.

CHAPTER 15

Social Marketing Practices

Government and Private Partnerships in Controlling Diseases and Promoting a Healthy Lifestyle in Singapore

Kavita Karan

Social marketing involves applications of commercial marketing techniques, with the influence of voluntary behaviors as its core objective. In contemporary health-focused initiatives, the use of mass media and community-centered prevention strategies are a promising development, where empowerment of individuals and communities is attempted to achieve change at multiple levels (Andreasen, 2005; Lapinski & Witte, 1998). Although increasing global travel benefits most countries' economies, they also are believed to be responsible for the resurgence of vector-borne diseases such as SARS and dengue (Freimuth, Linnan, & Potter, 2002; Lee, Pong, & Karan, 2004). Singapore, like many other countries, needs to do more than just being vigilant about the spread of diseases; it also has to be competent in handling the challenges posed by the spreading of such infectious diseases (Fung, 2003).

Singapore has a reputation of being the land of campaigns. In the past two decades, noteworthy campaigns on the virtues of courtesy and family values have gone further to highlight risks associated with smoking, drugs, and alcohol consumption, as well as preventing diseases like SARS, bird flu, and dengue. Therefore, health communication and promotion campaigns are part and parcel of the Singaporeans' lifestyle; health authorities have launched a series of extensive public communications campaigns in relation to various social and health issues (Gauld, Ikegami, Barr, Chiang, Gould, et al., 2006). In addition, with the objective of building a nation of fit and healthy Singaporeans, the Ministry of Health (MOH) (2008) established the Health Promotion Board (HPB) (2009) in 2001 to drive its health promotion and disease prevention programs. As a holistic approach to healthy lifestyle advocacy, HPB's communication campaigns have focused, among others, on preventive measures to keep major diseases at bay and combat the outbreak of diseases. A specific department within the HPB, the Marketing and Communications Division, takes care of health promotion strategies within its organizational structure. The division has established important relationships with various communication and media outfits—both print and electronic—to disseminate information to the public. The department's Web site is a comprehensive source of information on healthy living, diseases, and health services. Besides educating citizens and identifying and controlling social and health problems, the public communications campaigns in Singapore also strengthen the government's agenda to encourage both locals and foreigners living in the country to treat Singapore as their "home" and tackle "our" problems in a collective manner.

Among the extensive campaigns the government has run, the SARS campaigns and the more recent dengue fever campaigns are fine examples of the success in having Singaporeans act collectively in response to the threat of diseases (Heng, Gh, How, & Chua, 1998; Lee et al., 2004). This chapter examines the social marketing efforts of two successful public health integrated marketing campaigns: one to combat dengue fever, which has threatened Singaporeans in the past few years, and an annual healthy lifestyle campaign that promotes greater awareness of health issues and motivates citizens to adopt preventive health practices to restrict the susceptibility to diseases.

SINGAPORE: A COUNTRY OVERVIEW

Located in Southeast Asia between Malaysia and Indonesia, Singapore is a tiny red dot in the world map with a total land area of 692.7 square kilometers. Founded as a British trading colony in 1819, it joined the Malaysian Federation in 1963 but became an independent nation in 1965. With a population of about 4.6 million in

2008, it has four major ethnic groups: Chinese (76.8%), Malay (13.9%), Indian (7.9%), and others (1.4%). Besides being a multiracial society, Singaporeans are also associated with many religions, including Buddhism (42.5%), Islam (14.9%), Taoism (8.5%), Hinduism (4%), Catholicism (4.8%), and other Christians and others (9.8%; Central Intelligence Agency [CIA], 2008).

The country has a parliamentary political system with the ruling People's Action Party (PAP) having won every election since its independence. Within the short span of four decades, Singapore has attained the status of a developed country in Asia with a free-market economy. It has an open, corruption-free environment and a stable economy, with its people enjoying one of the highest per capita incomes in the world (Singapore Department of Statistics, 2008). Fiscal stimulus, low interest rates, a surge in exports, and internal flexibility have led to a positive growth from 2004 to 2007 with an annual gross domestic product (GDP) growth averaging 7%. The economy depends heavily on exports, particularly in consumer electronics and information technology products (Singapore economic indicators, 2007).

Health Care: Government Initiatives and Private Support

The public health structure in Singapore is centralized under the care of the Ministry of Health (MOH), while the responsibility for food and the environment falls under the purview of the Ministry of Environment. The MOH is the nodal government agency on all health matters in Singapore. In 2001, the government established the HPB with the mission of *building a nation of fit and healthy Singaporeans*. Along with the HPB, other health organizations such as the Community Services (National University of Singapore), the Health Courses and Wellness Programs (Changi General Hospital), the Programs for the Elderly (MOH), and the Health@Work Program (National Healthcare Group) (2008) are actively geared toward promoting health care in Singapore. The MOH has identified the most common conditions that affect Singaporeans, and all programs are planned toward the prevention and control of such diseases. These include asthma, coronary heart disease, diabetes mellitus, hypertension, mental health, osteoporosis, pneumonia, stroke, and tuberculosis. The three principal causes of death in the country are cancer, heart disease, and pneumonia.

The healthcare system consists of both public and private sectors. The Singapore government believes that social welfare based on heavy taxes is not a viable option for the country because it will overburden public finance (Lim, 2004). Hence, the government is heavily involved in the health system, both in terms of regulation and implementation of policies, and it plays a key role in ensuring the right mix of policies to manage expenditure and service provision. Realizing the inflationary nature of healthcare costs, as well as the population's increasing demand for those services, the government tries to build a healthy population through preventive healthcare programs, complemented by the promotion of a healthy lifestyle.

The financing philosophy of the country's healthcare delivery system is based on individual responsibility and community support. According to its e-citizen Web site, the healthcare services in Singapore are provided by the government and private sectors in an 80:20 ratio. Patients are expected to co-pay part of their medical expenses, and government subsidies help keep basic health care affordable. The allocated budget of the MOH for the financial year 2008 was estimated to be at S$2.42 billion (US$1.65 billion), which is 17.4% higher than that of 2007. In 2006, the amount allocated was estimated to be around S$85 billion (US$59.4 billion). In 2005, the country spent about S$7.6 billion, or 3.8% of its total GDP, on health care, of which the government expended S$1.8 billion (Expenditure overview, 2007).

Primary health care in Singapore includes both preventive care and health education. The MOH places great emphasis on fitness and health and has been putting forth many workplace-based fitness programs and anti-smoking and healthy-eating campaigns. The National Environment Agency (NEA) (2005) works with agencies in both public and private sectors. The government believes that public communication campaigns serve as valuable tools to educate and influence the population. To achieve its mission, the HPB assumes the role of the main driver for national health promotion and disease prevention programs. Two of the major programs, the Anti-Dengue Campaign and the National Healthy Lifestyle Campaigns, are studied in detail.

CASE STUDY 1
The Anti-Dengue Campaign

BACKGROUND, PURPOSE, AND FOCUS

Dengue fever is an illness caused by infection through the transmission of a virus by the *Aedes* mosquito (Gubler, 1987) and is not new to Singapore. For almost 15 years the island country has been able to control the spread of the disease effectively. However, there has been resurgence in the last decade due to the combined factors of weaker immunity, transmission of the virus outside the home, an increase in the viability of the infection, and the adoption of a case-reactive approach in controlling the spread of infections (Ooi, Goh, & Gubler, 2006). In 2004, Singapore reported an outbreak of 9,259 dengue cases, which increased to 13,817 in 2005 (Burattini et al., 2008). To ensure the public's education and participation in preventing the spread of dengue, the NEA was identified as the lead agency in charge of the anti-dengue campaign to set up effective strategies to meet the challenge.

The main objective of this continuous campaign for the past few years has been to increase awareness among Singaporeans about the dangers of the disease and the importance of eradicating breeding sites. Campaigns are created by the NEA along with the MOH and the HPB. The mission of these agencies is to create awareness on the consequences of dengue fever, encourage the public to adopt preventive measures, and inculcate social and personal responsibilities in keeping the environment safe from the disease.

Prior research has shown that public involvement is crucial for the success of a vector control program (Chan, 1985). The two-pronged approach includes a national publicity strategy as well as a series of target group–specific initiatives. The dengue control program includes all the recommended control activities by the World Health Organization (WHO), namely, public health education and community participation, active breeding site detection, environmental management, reactive fogging of insecticides, and geo-referenced entomologic and clinical surveillance systems (Egger et al., 2008). The main thrusts of NEA's approach include

1. Preventive surveillance and control.
2. Public education and community involvement.
3. Enforcement.
4. Research.

Through mass and interpersonal forms, the campaign exposes the threats of dengue as a near-fatal disease and educates the masses on the methods of infection, consequences of infection, and measures to be taken to prevent the possible breeding of mosquitoes. It particularly focuses on methods of adopting regular cleaning practices in households. To involve the community, the country formed the Dengue Prevention Volunteer Groups (DPVG) in 1998, where members have been taking an active role in combating the deadly disease. At present, there are more than 6,000 DPVG members operating in 84 constituencies, including private and public housing communities.

TARGET MARKET PROFILE

From the beginning, the NEA recognized that engaging the public is the most crucial part in the island's fight to reduce mosquito breeding in households, which results in the spread of dengue. The target markets for the campaigns are the individual households in the country. Efforts are targeted at locations where breeding grounds for mosquitoes are rampant and where there is less access to fogging. The NEA's communications strategies target all Singaporeans and foreigners residing on the island. With Singapore's multiracial and multiethnic profile, it is imperative that innovative and multilingual communication strategies be developed.

One of the earliest nationwide campaigns on public education to control the spread of the dengue fever was the "Keep Singapore Clean and Mosquito Free" campaign in 1969, through which schoolchildren were educated to keep their surroundings clean and adopt preventive measures in their homes to control the breeding of mosquitoes. The impact of this campaign was tested through two surveys in 1992 and 1995, which showed that although the majority of Singaporeans were aware of the importance of dengue control, many did not believe that the mosquitoes were in their homes and were not motivated to prevent mosquito breeding (Heng et al., 1998).

In 2007, for example, in order to engage the youth, a parent–child dengue prevention activity was organized that included a digital photography competition entitled "Protect Yourself and Your Family." (See http://www.dengue.gov.sg/subject.asp?id=137 for more details on the process through which NEA engages the youth in Singapore in the fight against dengue.)

CAMPAIGN OBJECTIVES

The campaign is designed to meet the following specific objectives.

Behavior Objectives

Behavior objectives encourage individuals to take measures to deny the *Aedes* mosquitoes a place to breed. These include specific behaviors for source reduction and eliminate the further spread of the disease:

- Change water from flower vases every day.
- Throw away stagnant water from the bases of flower pots and other potted plants.

- Invert buckets and water containers after use to prevent stagnation of any stored water.
- Close pipes used for drying clothes to avoid accumulation of rain water.

Knowledge Objectives

Knowledge objectives encourage individuals to know and understand (1) the dangers of the disease, and (2) the facts about the spread of dengue through stagnant water, (3) the impact on health, and (4) the importance of eradication.

Belief Objectives

Belief objectives encourage individuals to know that eradicating the dengue virus is both a personal and social responsibility. They need to believe that their home is one of the primary breeding grounds of the disease and that they must make the effort to keep themselves and their families safe.

BARRIERS, MOTIVATORS (BENEFITS), AND COMPETITION

Despite prevention and control mechanisms and continued communication strategies, Singapore has seen a resurgence of the disease in the past decade because many residents in Singapore place full responsibility on the authorities with regard to controlling the spread of the disease. They also feel that their government's initiative in strengthening disease surveillance and control in the whole of Southeast Asia prevents the virus from reaching domestic shores (Ooi et al., 2006). However, inculcating responsible behavior among many Singapore residents remains a challenge—despite concerted efforts and constant reminders from the government.

Besides creating awareness, the nation needs to return to a vector control program based on the analysis of entomologic and epidemiologic data, where such data are collected from various sources and used to step up or plan new programs. The process of eradicating the potential breeding sites of the *Aedes* mosquitoes takes conscientious effort as well as time, and it must be perceived as a *personal responsibility* among the people. Because most of the potential breeding sites of the *Aedes* mosquitoes are within individuals' residences (such as flower pots, roof gutters, and gully traps), the inculcation of personal responsibilities and constant vigilance is one of the greatest challenges faced by the NEA. Another special concern is the movement of the disease from overseas, especially if Singaporeans travel without any prior medical precautionary checks before leaving the country. Besides private residences, there are public areas that are not within the immediate concern of individuals and that are left unchecked and undetected. These would include tree holes, roadside drains, and even discarded receptacles.

The expected result or benefit from the campaign is a clean and safe environment—free from the impending dangers of mosquito bites and fear of getting the disease and the resultant poor health. There is little competition as such, and the government is threatened by the fact that if the disease is not controlled, the spread could cause a major pandemic resulting in loss of life within the country and heavy economic losses as was the case during SARS in 2003.

POSITIONING STATEMENT

The NEA's objective is to encourage the agencies to create awareness, to call for active community participation in tackling the root of the problem of controlling the breeding of *Aedes* mosquitoes, and to educate people so they understand the near-fatal consequences and adopt preventive health practices to control the spread of the disease. The campaign is positioned to educate the target audience and influence them to participate in the prevention of the spread of the dengue fever.

CAMPAIGN STRATEGIES (4Ps) AND IMPLEMENTATION

The anti-dengue campaign is based on the data collected from reported cases. Efforts are made to educate the masses, provide incentives, and plan follow-up strategies for adopting practices. Frequent patrolling by the authorities and voluntary groups ensures that potential breeding sites are eradicated. The NEA works with various government agencies and private organizations, such as construction site owners as well as schools and town councils, to emphasize preventive messages and organize awareness events. A Web site (http://www.dengue.gov.sg) for dengue prevention and control is constantly updated to provide all the information needed by the people, even if they are not exposed to other media. (See http://www.dengue.gov.sg/subject.asp?id =51 for examples of communication posters by NEA.) The following sections present the marketing mix used to reach the segments of the target audience.

Product Strategy and Implementation

Core Product

The benefit promised and the expected outcome is that Singaporeans are warned about the dangers of dengue fever and the urgent need to adopt practices to control the disease.

Actual Product

The campaign's desire is to see residents use appropriate methods to reduce the breeding of mosquitoes in homes and surrounding areas and adopt personal care techniques.

Augmented Product

To facilitate this behavior, the NEA developed a Dengue Prevention Checklist that provides an overview of a series of preventive methods to be adopted at different times. The checklist is segmented into "time series" and includes tasks that need to be performed at "all times," "every other day," "once a week," and "once a month." With this checklist, the NEA wants to make sure that the public carries out the appropriate preventive actions to reduce the number of dengue cases. As part of the community involvement scheme, individuals are encouraged to sign up as volunteers in the Dengue Prevention Volunteer Group (DPVG) to help in patrolling to control the spread of diseases. In the area of patrolling and enforcement, dengue prevention officers generally issued "on-the-spot fines" for anyone who leaves water catchments unchecked and uncovered, especially during monsoon seasons when there is a greater possibility of the spread of disease. Because schools are also susceptible areas, they are required to send their operations managers for training in mosquito control and auditing pest control.

In addition, for those who are not familiar with the appropriate insecticides and other equipment needed to control and eradicate the breeding grounds, the NEA has compiled a list of vendors in Singapore that stock the appropriate insecticides and repellents. There is a dedicated Web site and a hotline to assist people when either making enquiries or reporting cases and to make the product even more accessible.

Price Strategy and Implementation

There is no formal price strategy for town councils to educate residents and implement the anti–dengue fever program. To encourage employers to take steps to protect their workers from dengue, the National Trades Union Congress (NTUC) *Fairprice*, a cooperative chain of stores, offers bulk discounts to unionized companies that purchase anti-mosquito products through their respective unions. As an incentive to individuals who sign up as volunteers in the DPVG, a reward system has been put in place, wherein members accumulate points that entitle them to enjoy special privileges at selected retail shops and food outlets. These little gestures give recognition to the volunteers, and the DPVG program owes its continued success to dedicated volunteers who share a deep-rooted and selfless concern for the safety of their community.

Place Strategy and Implementation

The potential breeding grounds for the *Aedes* mosquitoes can be found both inside and outside the home. Hence, the NEA has used a series of initiatives to ensure that appropriate preventive measures are in place. In 2006, NEA deployed approximately 500 officers for regular audits and inspections into the homes of Singaporeans. These officers were formed into teams and were in charge of specific sites around the island to identify any problematic areas and respond quickly to the problems. For areas outside the home, the NEA has partnerships with many agencies and organizations to administer a coordinated approach in combating the spread of diseases. For example, since 2001, an environmental control officer (ECO) scheme has been implemented at construction sites, where it is mandatory for an ECO to be engaged by the company. These ECOs are responsible for maintaining the pest and mosquito control works within the construction sites. The result has been a steep drop in the *Aedes* breeding areas. In 2008, breeding *Aedes* mosquitoes were found at only 6% of construction sites compared to 30% in 1999. The deployment of operations managers in schools to oversee the control measures has resulted in only 1% of the schools with mosquito-breeding sites, a figure down from 25% in 1999 (Tackling the dengue problem in Singapore, 2008).

Promotion Strategies and Implementation

Messages

The core messages of the campaign are to alert citizens about the breeding spots, educate them about the consequences, and control the spread of the disease. The campaign messages were "If they breed, you will bleed" and "Stop Breeding Danger." The messages are direct and hard-hitting to drive the citizens toward action, and the use of multimedia channels ensure that the messages reach most of the citizens.

Messages supporting the knowledge and belief objectives include:

- Stagnant water in pots, vases, buckets, and so on, can be a potential breeding place for mosquitoes. The water needs to be thrown out or changed daily, and buckets need to be inverted and kept without any water. The major breeding zones in the country were marked for people living in those areas to be more careful in adopting the practices.
- The symptoms of contracting dengue and the need to report were highlighted in the messages.
- Updates on people who contracted the disease in other countries were also communicated to the citizens. The number of cases and deaths reported and the fear of possible death were clear to inform the people to be careful.

Media Channels

The NEA ran the campaigns through advertising in various media including TV, radio, newspapers, magazines, posters, pamphlets, booklets, banners, mailers, videos, and a Web site that was regularly updated to provide all the information. Because Singapore is a multiethnic society, all communications materials are in the four official languages: English, Chinese, Malay, and Tamil. One of the most important features of the NEA's anti-dengue campaign was the support it received from the government in terms of resources, as well as the constant publicity in the media. The dengue situation in Singapore was reported on almost a daily basis, which helped keep the issue fresh in the minds of Singaporeans.

Print Media

The NEA regularly issued full- and half-page advertisements in all newspapers to remind readers of the dangers of dengue. The advertisements contained the precautionary methods required to control mosquito breeding. Posters and banners were also displayed on the streets and in the heartlands to constantly remind the public of the importance of preventive measures (examples of anti-dengue posters and mailers that are disseminated throughout Singapore are posted on http://www.dengue.gov.sg/subject.asp?id=51).

Broadcast Media

TV and radio commercials also promoted the preventive measures for controlling the breeding and spread of the disease. A hotline was set up to take calls about possible "hotspots" of mosquito breeding. The fact that Singaporeans are Internet savvy, a dedicated Web site (http://www.dengue.gov.sg) for dengue prevention and control is constantly updated for citizens even if they are not exposed to other media.

Grassroots Outreach and Public Events

Many public events allow residents to listen to the government and community workers. These events continue to be organized with high-level government representatives officiating (including the prime minister and other ministers) to show the government's full support and commitment to the fight against the disease. Campaigns were launched with fanfare at the national level and also in other districts of the country through smaller events. Some of these events included the launch of the "Keep Mozzies Away," "Fight against Dengue," and "Community Aedes Reduction Program" campaigns. These events allow members to interact with officials who reiterate the fears and consequences among the citizens. During such events, posters are displayed and demonstrations are held to further instill the sense of responsibility, believability, and the adoption of the stated practices. These events are well attended by the public and members of community and support groups and also receive extensive publicity through the media. (See http://www.dengue.gov.sg/subject.asp?id=31 for examples of awareness events organized by the NEA and its partners in Singapore.)

Budget

Most of the anti-dengue campaigns are generally funded by the government and the statutory boards in Singapore. The government has spared no effort or expense to ensure that the public is safe from the virus, at the same time remaining constantly vigilant about its possible resurgence. The annual budget has been increasing continuously for public health over the past few years to ensure that enough funds are available for the programs planned. For the 2007 fiscal year, the government set aside S$219 million (about US$153 million) for public health, including dengue prevention and control. This was about 11% more than the S$198 million budgeted for 2006. For 2008, S$271.1 million has been set aside, about 24% higher than the previous year (Expenditure overview, 2007).

CAMPAIGN EVALUATION

The efforts by the NEA and its partners, both in the public and private sectors, have paid off because the number of dengue cases has fallen rapidly since its last peak in 2007. During a three-day meeting of the core group on Asia-Pacific dengue partnership in Singapore in February 2007, the NEA's Director General for Public Health, Khoo Seow Poh, attributed Singapore's success in its fight against the spread of the dengue virus to the government's proactive rather than reactive approach. Only 3,100 dengue cases were reported in 2006, a significant decrease from 14,200 in 2005. This has been attributed to the dengue prevention campaign launched by the Singapore government (Experts call for Asia regional collaboration, 2007). In 2008, while the rest of the region saw an upswing in cases, Singapore bucked the trend, recording 7,032 case of dengue fever compared with 8,826 in 2007 (Jaganathan, 2009). This can be credited to the enhanced dengue control strategy put in place by the NEA, which costs a substantial amount a day (Khalik, 2008).

The efforts are ongoing as Singapore continues to live under the threat and impact of such a disease, particularly from the devastation brought by SARS in 2003 and the recurring threat of bird flu from neighboring and other countries. Therefore, Singapore's integrated dengue control program—which combines laboratory work and surveillance with aggressive vector control—worked to contain the disease last year and should continue to do so in the following years (Jaganathan, 2009). Its relentless effort in its fight against such contagious diseases has helped the island-state bring down the number of dengue cases.

CASE STUDY 2
National Healthy Lifestyle Program

BACKGROUND AND ENVIRONMENT

As a holistic approach to healthy lifestyle advocacy, the government's communication campaigns have focused not only on combating outbreaks of diseases, but also on promoting preventive measures and good health practices toward building a nation of fit and healthy Singaporeans. One of the longest-running campaigns in Singapore is the National Healthy Lifestyle Program that was launched in 1992 by former Prime Minister Goh Chok Tong and developed by the Ministry of Health (MOH). Over the years, the campaigns have been geared to raise awareness among Singaporeans of the importance of maintaining a healthy lifestyle and to equip them with the knowledge and skills to practice healthy eating, get regular exercise, and manage stress. In 1996, a civic committee on healthy lifestyles was set up to facilitate community involvement and participation in healthy lifestyle activities (Toh, Chew, & Tan, 2002).

Purpose and Focus

A National Healthy Lifestyle Campaign is being held annually to raise greater awareness and bring about behavioral changes in the people's eating and exercise habits in order to have a healthy lifestyle. A month-long *National Healthy Lifestyle Campaign* by the HPB is held annually to promote four components of a healthy lifestyle: regular exercise, healthy eating, no smoking, and stress management (Health Promotion Board, 2008). It endeavors to make the social and physical environment more supportive of healthy living in order to reduce morbidity and mortality in Singaporeans. With Singapore's multiracial and multiethnic population, programs are customized to cater to special ethnic groups, working populations, and senior citizens.

Strategy

Commercial marketing techniques are employed through aggressive advertising, sales promotion techniques, awards, and recognitions to motivate the general population. The messages highlight the importance of physical activities, healthy eating, and getting checked against diseases. It also involves mass participation and usually incorporates a mass physical activity like a group exercise or run. Most of the time, it is officiated by the prime minister or a senior minister of the cabinet, which is believed to add greater credibility and visibility to the campaign. Following the launch, the entire month is usually filled with planned activities to reach different sectors of the population through a mass media campaign with support from organizations involved in the campaigns. A key component of the program is the Healthy Lifestyle Ambassador Award. The award recognizes individuals who lead a healthy lifestyle and have made positive contributions to promoting such a lifestyle in their communities.

TARGET AUDIENCE PROFILE

Although the Healthy Lifestyle Program is intended to reach the general public, it adopts a multipronged approach to increase lifestyle practices to different segments of the population and in various settings like community centers and workplaces. It also features special programs for ethnic groups and senior citizens. The HPB collaborates with public, private, and community organizations to facilitate the adoption of healthy lifestyles.

CAMPAIGN OBJECTIVES AND PLANNED ACTIVITIES

The main objectives of the campaigns are to raise awareness among Singaporeans about the importance of a healthy lifestyle, to maintain a healthy body weight, and to equip them with the knowledge and skills to practice a healthy lifestyle. It also endeavors to make the social and physical environment more supportive of healthy living.

The marketing strategies were developed with the following objectives in focus:

- *Behavior objectives.* Influence the citizens to change their lifestyle to include good eating habits, regular exercise, and stress management techniques.
- *Knowledge objectives.* To create awareness and alert Singaporeans to the facts and consequences of common diseases and the need to prevent such diseases.
- *Belief objectives.* For people to believe that good health is of prime importance in life and that it is one's own responsibility to lead a good life through healthy diet and exercise.

BARRIERS, BENEFITS, AND COMPETITION

The major concern about the neglect of health is that Singapore is a fast-paced society, where the majority of the population is concerned with economic pursuits to create a better life for themselves and their children, which leaves little time to adopt healthy practices communicated by the government campaigns. Apart from time, the barriers for not pursuing a healthy lifestyle would include long working hours and not being able to rearrange their daily schedules to incorporate physical activities. This situation has resulted in a lifestyle that has physical activities at the bottom of an individual's priority list. Even when knowledge levels are high, there is still the need to induce people into taking concrete actions.

Another barrier to the success of the campaign is the multiracial and multicultural profile of Singapore, where the traditional dietary and lifestyle choices of the various ethnic groups vastly differ from each other. The HPB is faced with problems in developing different sets of persuasive messages and programs to suit the different target groups within the various ethnic segments of the population.

Competition comes from the country's well-organized expansive system of hotels, restaurants, food courts, and hawker centers that provide opportunities for citizens to experiment with a variety of food from these outlets. Many

Singaporeans tend to eat at these food courts near places of work and home; these temptations compete with the campaign messages and are likely to derail individuals' efforts in pursuing a healthy lifestyle.

Despite the problems, there is a high level of awareness of the disease among the citizens, with many adopting preventive measures, getting themselves checked against diseases, and also utilizing some form of health insurance. However, more still needs to be done not only to increase knowledge levels, but also to induce people into taking concrete actions. As the study by Karan (2007) has shown, there are great differences in terms of awareness of health issues and the adoption of healthy lifestyle practices.

POSITIONING

The positioning statement for the Healthy Lifestyle Program is "Healthy Life, Better Life," which exemplifies the importance, concern, and seriousness that the country shows toward the health of its citizens. The objective is to build a nation of healthy Singaporeans to adopt correct practices and make those practices part of their daily routine. To do this, the HPB uses various tactics and incentives and sometimes creates fear among the people to adopt good diet and exercise regimens and get medical checkups, or face the consequences of the simple flu or extreme health problems like cancer, stroke, and heart attacks.

CAMPAIGN STRATEGIES (4Ps) AND IMPLEMENTATION

To put its health communications message across to its target audience, the HPB has a dedicated in-house Marketing and Communications Division that leads the communication efforts in reaching out to the various segments of society.

Product Strategies and Implementation

Core Product

The program focuses on promoting the core product of a healthy lifestyle through the slogan, "Healthy Body and Healthy Mind." It gives the citizens an opportunity to lead a healthy lifestyle and describes the benefits of eating a balanced diet, getting regular exercise, and managing stress.

Actual Product

The desired behavior is for citizens to adopt the practices and reject the temptations to indulge in eating and avoiding exercise. (See the same section of the first case.) Efforts are made to plan strategies for the Chinese, Indians, and Malays. The HPB is constantly devising new ways to motivate and engage the public. One of its most recent developments is the renaming of the Healthy Lifestyle campaign to "Physical Activity." This allows the agency to be more focused and to plan initiatives that really get Singaporeans up on their feet and taking part in physical activities.

Augmented Product

The augmented product includes a variety of planned opportunities to motivate individuals to embark on the actual behavior of pursuing a healthy lifestyle. HPB has focused on messages and campaigns that are targeted at specific groups such as homemakers, health professionals, nutrition education facilitators, food industry professionals, food importers, wholesalers, retailers, manufacturers, caterers, and vendors to stress the benefits of a healthy lifestyle. For the Malays, HPB partners with the mosques and other Malay/Muslim organizations to develop innovative ways to educate and engage the Malay community. These have included quizzes, cooking and exercise sessions, telematches, and interactive exhibitions. For example, in 2004, exercise routines with a local twist were introduced to the Malay community. Sheikarobics is a 30-minute workout that incorporates *silat*, a form of martial arts, with aerobics. It is suitable for both males and females—with the benefits of improving cardiovascular fitness and strengthening and toning body muscles. As for the Malay women, customized exercises specially tailored for women wearing kebayas—Kebayarobics—were also developed.

To encourage workplace health, the Fitness@Work program is targeted at the working population. Furthermore, the HEALTH (Helping Employees Achieve Life-Time Health) Award was introduced in 1998 to give national recognition to workplaces with commendable workplace health promotion programs. In partnership between the HPB and the California Fitness Centre, the program encourages the working population to incorporate a regular exercise schedule into their daily lives. To achieve this goal, weekly exercise sessions are planned near workplaces. PowerWalk is another initiative that encourages brisk walking at the parks and nature reserves in Singapore. The objective is to inject low-intensity exercising into the lives of all age groups, especially those who lead sedentary lifestyles.

Price Strategies and Implementation

To encourage Singaporeans to adopt a healthy lifestyle and to take responsibility for their health, HPB provides incentives as well as low-cost health checkups in organizations. For example, under the agency's Workplace Health Promotion initiative, employees whose company is part of the Health PRO program will automatically enjoy a 50% subsidy for healthy lifestyles–related activities with selected providers of the agency. Other programs such as the Check Your Health community health-screening program was targeted at the elderly aged 50 years and older. Priced at a highly subsidized fee of S$5 (US$3), this screening program is easily accessible to lower- and middle-income groups.

To adopt healthy eating practices, innovative schemes are developed for different target groups. Club Foodies is a forum set up by HPB is to encourage diners to share their healthier food experiences. One of the HPB's programs was the Healthier Chinese Cuisine Program and Healthier Restaurant Program, which motivated people to use selected restaurants that were serving healthier food. These restaurants were committed to reducing the use of oil, salt, and sugar in their food preparation, while adding more fruits or vegetables to the menu. Individuals were awarded with shopping vouchers if they chose to dine at HPB-recommended restaurants.

To ensure that good eating habits start early in age, the HPB has programs such as Fruitie Veggie Bites (FVB), which was specially designed for primary school students. Students were given a card to facilitate their purchases of fruits and vegetables at school. Classes with the highest fruit and vegetable intake and extensive involvement in physical activities won a prize. Another major incentive named after the program was the Healthy Lifestyle Ambassador Award to recognize individuals who live healthy lifestyles and serve as models for others.

Place Strategies and Implementation

To ensure that the targeted audiences have more opportunities to adopt the desired behavior by participating in more physical activities, HPB's strategies included mass activities that allow for maximum participation and socialization among the participants—for example, the month-long National Healthy Lifestyle Campaign generally involves mass activities like the grand Healthy Lifestyle Carnival in 2004, a three-day fitness expo in 2005, a Healthy Lifestyle Showcase and Food Bazaar in 2006, and a theme party at Singapore's Botanic Garden in 2007. To keep the campaign's momentum going, the entire month is usually filled with many activities to reach different sectors of the population. During the other months of the year, there is a wide range of healthy lifestyle activities for the public to choose from. These activities are largely held jointly with HPB's partners from both the public and private sectors. These partnerships generally include collaboration with the Community Development Councils (CDCs) for the Central Singapore On the Move (CSOTM) initiative—a program launched in June 2004 to motivate individuals to take brisk walks regularly.

The HPB keeps evolving new ideas and themes into the annual campaigns with diverse activities. Some of the wide-ranging events include the following: Great Singapore Workout, Mental Health Education Program, National Smoking Control Campaign, AIDS Campaign, Family Run, Supermarket Program, "Ask For" Program, Restaurant Program, National Floor Ball Carnival, Soccermania, Dance-a-thon, National Fitness Fiesta, Healthier Food Exhibition, Sheares Bridge Run & Army Half Marathon, the 2+2 Innovation Exhibition, FunFITT aerobic workout, and "Vote for Your Most Helpful Stall" Contest.

Promotion Strategies and Implementation

Messages

The main messages and promotional strategies are devised to motivate and persuade citizens to adopt healthy lifestyle practices and participate in the various activities planned by the HPB. The style and tone are sometimes hard-hitting for prevention of diseases (like the anti-dengue campaign) and sometimes toned down—especially when the objective is to change long-term behaviors of people toward healthy eating by incorporating fruits and vegetables and also exercising regularly.

Messages supporting knowledge and belief objectives include:

- The promotion of the four components of a healthy lifestyle: regular exercise, healthy eating, no smoking, and managing stress.
- The need to include two fruits and vegetables in the diet, ask for less gravy and oil, and also eat at restaurants that have been identified by the HPB for serving healthier food.
- The facts and figures of the most common general and lifestyle diseases affecting Singaporeans, and the ways to control them through diet, exercise, and medical checkups.

Messengers

The messengers are many—from the prime minister and other members of the cabinet to the citizens themselves, who actively participate and support the annual campaign.

Budget

In 2007, the MOH allocated SG$86 million toward promoting good health to Singaporeans, including the National Healthy Lifestyle Program, the National Smoking Control Program, and the Workplace Health Promotion Program. This amount went up to SG$93 million in 2008 (Expenditure overview, 2008).

Channels and Grassroots Outreach

The HPB works closely with various media outlets in Singapore to disseminate useful and important information to promote health-related programs to the public. Health education materials such as articles for newspapers and magazines, as well as pamphlets, booklets, posters, exhibition panels, and scripts for slide-tape presentations, video programs, and radio talks, are widely produced and distributed.

Most media organizations have reporters specializing in reporting health news. Advertisements for various programs are extensively placed in the local English, Malay, and Tamil newspapers. Promotional materials are distributed through community centers, polyclinics, and hospitals. Like any other government agency, a well-organized Web site provides comprehensive information on healthy living, disease prevention, and health services.

The HPB also maintains a Health Information Center (HIC), HealthLine, and HealthZone. HIC is a specialized resource library of books, journals, and audiovisual materials on health education, health promotion, and disease prevention. HealthLine is a toll-free telephone information service on health issues that provides personalized counseling services, where trained nurses answer questions on various aspects of health and disease prevention and there is a 24-hour, prerecorded health information service. Health Zone is a theme exhibition on healthy lifestyles covering nine topics: exercise, nutrition, substance abuse, dental care, eye care, growth and development, health for the elderly, mental health, and lifestyle diseases.

Web and Interactive Elements

New media technologies are used to reach a highly techno-savvy population, and the HPB has been at the forefront of using channels such as computer games, screen savers, e-cards, and podcasts. Allowing users to download audio files from the Internet, podcasting offers users the convenience of listening to health programs at their convenience, even when they are on the go. The first podcast featured 13 episodes of *Health Talk with Nancy Sit*, a talk show with the popular Hong Kong celebrity that covered female-related illnesses such as cervical cancer and breast cancer and other general health topics like nutrition, osteoporosis, and depression. In 2006, it jointly commissioned a Malay drama series with the Media Development Authority (MDA), *Erlin Montel*, an eight-episode series on the Suria (Malay) channel, highlighting the importance of eating right, regular physical activities, and staying or becoming smoke-free. The light-hearted drama series relates the story of an overweight lady, who tries to lose weight, and her relationship with a smoker, who tries to quit smoking. The drama unfolds their trials and temptations/tribulations as well as their successful efforts in achieving a healthy and balanced lifestyle. Finally, the storyline ends on a positive note with their marriage. Currently, the information available via HPB podcasts covers a wide range of topics, including the type of sports, red wine and health, packing a healthy lunch to work, and ways to inculcate healthy eating habits in children.

CAMPAIGN EVALUATIONS AND LESSONS LEARNED

Singapore provides ample opportunities for people to take part in their own health development and adopt better health practices through its philosophy of education and persuasion. Continuous and sustained efforts by the MOH and the HPB in Singapore have led to an increased level of knowledge among Singaporeans on health issues, lifestyle diseases, and adoption of healthy practices. A study found that Singaporeans obtain health-related information largely from the print media, followed by outdoor media, electronic media, the Internet, medical institutions, and word-of-mouth (Karan, 2007).

An important issue that is particularly important in this country is the role of government as it spearheads the national campaigns through the ministries and the statutory boards. The partnerships with community organizations and involvement of volunteers from the community are a good measure of individual as well as collective responsibility in health promotion and preventive measures. The nation's health and the need to combat diseases are the primary concerns of the government, unlike other countries, where most of the health awareness programs are carried out to a large extent by nongovernmental organizations. In Singapore, the system of incentives in forms of awards, cash incentives, and other rewards that are offered to citizens who adopt healthy practices have a definite impact on citizens—as evident from the successful strategies used in both the antidengue and healthy lifestyle campaigns. A system of fines and legal measures for noncompliance of rules and regulations is a good method of keeping checks and balances for implementing the programs.

The HPB's Workplace Health Program has been able to achieve significant results since 2004. Employees who exercise more than three times a week increased from 38.1% in 2004 to 46.2% in 2007; employees with hypertension reduced from 20.1% to 9.5%; employees with diabetes reduced from 8.2% to 2.5%; medical cost per employee went down from S$660 to S$467 (Achieving workplace health, 2008).

Singapore's short- and long-term strategies in building a nation of healthy people have gained considerable success. Although there are continuous efforts (like annual healthy lifestyle campaigns) as well as ongoing shorter campaigns for combating diseases and preventive measures, a lot has yet to be achieved in the years to follow.

One of the pressing concerns with regard to the continuity of the healthy lifestyle initiatives is the overwhelming number of campaigns that Singaporeans are inundated with on a daily basis. As Karan's (2008) study shows, the messages from the various campaigns could have been lost within the clutter of the many campaigns in Singapore. Another concern is the stagnation of the campaign message. These methods of social engineering and restrictive practices may have a negative impact on the citizens. In the fast-paced lifestyle of many Singaporeans, it has become an excuse for many to take the easy way out by not exercising, but visiting slimming centers to maintain a visually trim and toned physique—thus hiding, perhaps, a poor cardiac self. Despite the limitations, the government and all supporting organizations are continuously making efforts not only to educate and motivate people toward better health practices, but also to provide the necessary infrastructure and facilities for exercising and by recommending restaurants for healthy eating and offering programs for managing stress. Incentives for regular medical checkups for screening and control of diseases for Singaporeans have had a good response, and the majority of Singaporeans are covered by health insurance.

Although the efforts are noteworthy, a more organized system of a few messages at a time is needed, rather than the many different messages currently presented, which can lead citizens to be indifferent to the campaigns with limited attention paid—unless the situation is life-threatening, like SARS and the possibly fatal bird flu and dengue fever. However, the lessons from the outbreak of SARS and threats of bird flu and dengue fever have kept the country's health and environmental agencies well prepared and on the alert in dealing with such crisis situations. It remains to be seen how the NEA, the HPB, the supporting government and private organizations, and grassroots workers can continuously come up with fresh and innovative ideas to engage the different age and ethnic groups in Singapore to persuade them of the importance and merits of physical activities to attain their overall objective of controlling diseases and improving the lifestyle of Singaporeans in terms of physical, social, and mental well-being.

QUESTIONS FOR DISCUSSION

1. What strategies and tactics has the Singapore government used in preventing the spread of dengue fever across the country? Suggest two other techniques that would enable the citizens, particularly the youth, to act fast and adopt the preventive techniques.
2. What is the importance of using new media technologies in health communication? Taking examples from Singapore and two other countries, evaluate the strategies used in health communication. Do you think these initiatives are sustainable in reaching different audiences?
3. What impact do cultural factors have on the success of a campaign? Because most countries today are multicultural societies like Singapore, what are some of the problems faced by communicators in planning multiple strategies for various segments of the population?

NOTES

1. Medisave, introduced in 1984, is a national medical savings scheme that helps individuals place part of their income into a Medisave account to meet their future personal or immediate family's hospitalization, day surgery, and certain outpatient expenses.
2. MediShield is a low-cost catastrophic illness insurance scheme. Introduced in 1990, the government designed MediShield to help members meet medical expenses from major or prolonged illnesses, which could not be sufficiently covered by their Medisave balance.
3. ElderShield is an affordable severe disability insurance scheme that provides basic financial protection to those who need long-term care, especially during old age. It provides a monthly cash payout to help pay out-of-pocket expenses for the care of a severely disabled person.

REFERENCES

Achieving workplace health the BP way. (2008). Retrieved July 28, 2009, from http://creative.asiaone.com/2008/IA/hpb_IA080404/Issue3/spotlight.html

Andreasen, A. R. (2005). *Social marketing in the 21st century.* Thousand Oaks, CA: Sage Publications.

Burattini, M. N., Chen, M., Chow, A., Couthinho, F. A. B., Goh, K. T., Lopez, L. F., et al. (2008). Modelling the control strategies against dengue in Singapore. *Epidemiology and infection*, 136(3), 309–319.

Central Intelligence Agency (CIA). (2008). *The world factbook.* Singapore. Retrieved July 28, 2009, from https://www.cia.gov/library/publications/the-world-factbook/geos/sn.html#People

Chan, K. L. (1985). *Singapore's dengue hemorrhagic fever control programme: A case study on the successful control of Aedes aegypti and Aedes albopictus using mainly environmental measures as part integrated vector control.* Singapore: Ministry of Health of Singapore.

Egger, J. R., Ooi, E. E., Kelly, D. W., Woolhouse, M. E., Daviesa, C. R., & Colemana, P. G. (2008). Reconstructing historical changes in the force of infection of dengue fever in Singapore: Implications for surveillance and control. *Bulletin of the World Health Organization 2008,* 86(3), 187–196.

Expenditure overview. (2007). Retrieved July 28, 2009, from http://www.mof.gov.sg/budget_2008/expenditure_overview/social_dev.html

Expenditure overview. (2008). Retrieved July 28, 2009, from http://www.mof.gov.sg/budget_2008/expenditure_overview/social_dev.html

Experts call for Asia regional collaboration to tackle dengue. (2007). Retrieved July 28, 2009, from http://english.people.com.cn/200702/09/eng20070209_348681.html

Freimuth, V., Linnan, H. W., & Potter, P. (2002). *Emerging Infectious Diseases,* 6(4), 11, 337.

Fung, A. (2003, April 9). SARS: How Singapore outmanaged the others. *Asia Times Online.* Retrieved July 28, 2009, from http://www.atimes.com/atimes/China/ED09Ad03.html

Gauld, R., Ikegami, N., Barr, M. D., Chiang, T. L., Gould, D., & Kwon, S. (2006). Advanced Asia's health systems in comparison. *Health Policy,* 79, no. 2–3: 325–336.

Gubler, D. J. (1987). Current research on dengue. In H. K. F. Harris (Ed.), *Current topics in vector research.* New York: Springer Verlag.

Health Promotion Board. (2000). Singapore Youth Tobacco Survey 2000. Retrieved July 28, 2009, from http://www.hpb.gov.sg/hpb/default.asp?pg_id=1288

Health Promotion Board. (2008). Retrieved July 28, 2009, from www.hpb.gov.sg

Heng, B. H., Goh, K. T., How, S. T., & Chua, L. T. (1998). Knowledge, attitude, belief and practice on dengue and *Aedes* mosquito. In K. T. Goh (Ed.), *Dengue in Singapore* (pp. 167–183). Singapore: Institute of Environmental Epidemiology, Ministry of the Environment.

Jaganathan, J. (2009, January 30). NEA monitoring recent dengue spike. *The Straits Times* (Daily Newspaper) Singapore.

Karan, K. (2007). *Prevention is better than cure: Health communication campaigns and health behaviors in Singapore.* Paper presented at American Academy of Advertising's Fourth Asia-Pacific Conference, Seoul, Korea.

Karan, K. (2008). Impact of health communication campaigns on health behaviors in Singapore. *Social Marketing Quarterly,* 14(3), 85–108.

Khalik, S. (2008, December 23). Dengue cases down but chikungunya up. *The Straits Times* (Daily Newspaper) Singapore.

Lapinski, M. K., & Witte, K. (1998). *Health communication campaigns, health communication research: A guide to developments and directions.* Westport, CT: Greenwood Press.

Lee, A., Pong, E., & Karan, K. (2004). *SARS in Singapore: Moving and nation to be socially responsible.* Paper presented at the International Intercultural Conference, Taipei, Taiwan.

Lim, M. K. (2004). Shifting the burden of health care finance: A case study of public–private partnership in Singapore. *Health Policy,* 69(1), 82–93.

Ministry of Health. (2008). Retrieved July 28, 2009, from www.moh.gov.sg

National Environment Agency (NEA), National Trades Union Congress (NTUC) and companies team up to help our workers combat dengue. (2005). Retrieved July 28, 2009, from http://app.nea.gov.sg/cms/htdocs/article.asp?pid=2599

National Healthcare Group. (2008). Retrieved July 28, 2009, from www.nhg.com.sg

Ooi, E.-E., Goh, K.-T., & Gubler, D. J. (2006). Dengue prevention and 35 years of vector control in Singapore. *Emerging Infectious Diseases*, 12(6), 887–893.

Singapore Department of Statistics. (2008). *Ministry of Finance.* Retrieved July 28, 2009, from www.mof.gov.sg

Singapore economic indicators. (2007). Retrieved July 28, 2009, from http://asiabusinessadvisory.com/eco-sing.html

Tackling the dengue problem in Singapore. (2008). *Ministry of Health.* Retrieved July 28, 2009, from www.moh.gov.sg

Toh, C. M., Chew, S. K., & Tan, C. C. (2002). Prevention and control of non-communicable disease in Singapore: A review of national health promotion programs. *Singapore Medical Journal*, 43(7), 333–339.

CHAPTER 16

Reducing Drink Driving Road Deaths

Integrating Communication and Social Policy Enforcement in Australia

Samantha Snitow and Linda Brennan

In 1989, 776 people were killed on the roads in Victoria, Australia. In 1994, the number had been slashed to 378, a reduction in the road toll of 51%. In this short period, Victorian roads became "the safest roads of anywhere in the world" (Black, 1995, p. 8). This chapter examines the initiatives implemented and the strategies utilized in Victoria, which led to this achievement in public health behavior and attitude change.

AUSTRALIA: A COUNTRY OVERVIEW

Australia is the sixth largest country in the world in geographic area, with a relatively small population size of just over 21 million people (Australian Bureau of Statistics, 2009a). Located between the Pacific and Indian oceans, 71% of the population lives in urban areas along the narrow eastern coastline. The narrow strip of coastline between the Great Dividing Range and the sea is often the only place where sufficient rainfall and water supply are to be found to enable a significant population to exist. The heart of Australia is mainly desert and is very sparsely populated. The Indigenous peoples of Australia are often to be found in these isolated desert regions. Australian Indigenous peoples are said to be the oldest continuous culture on earth, with cultural traditions dating back more than 40,000 years. Settled by Britain in 1788, Australia is now a multicultural country with many waves of settlement from across Europe, Asia, the Middle East, and, more recently, Africa (Australian Bureau of Statistics, 2009b).

Australia is a constitutional monarchy and a member of the Commonwealth of Nations. Australia's government is structured in three main levels: federal, state, and local. There are six states and two territories in the Australian federal system. The states are relatively self-governing. Although federation of the six colonies occurred in 1901, the states and territories often compete for funding, resources, and access to international markets.

While Australia is a very healthy country from the perspective of the World Health Organization (WHO), Indigenous Australians are among the least healthy in the world. They have a life expectancy nearly 20 years less than the non-Indigenous population of Australia and have significantly higher rates of many diseases compared with non-Indigenous Australians. Common health issues found among this population generally relate to diseases caused by the Western lifestyle. The prevalence of many burdens of disease such as cancers, diseases of the circulatory system, diabetes, kidney disease, and respiratory conditions are significantly higher in the Indigenous population, due to the higher rates of risk behaviors, including tobacco smoking, alcohol and substance abuse, and obesity. As a consequence, the Australian national health priorities (NHPs) largely relate to the aging population, Westernized diet, and lifestyle issues. The priorities are arthritis and musculoskeletal conditions, cancer control, cardiovascular health, diabetes, injury prevention and control, mental health, and asthma. These priority areas were developed by the Australian government as a response to WHO's global strategy, Health For All, by 2000. The national health priority areas account for approximately 80% of all diseases and injuries in Australia. These are issues that have the potential to reduce their impact on the health of Australians through changes in policy and the development of health promotional initiatives.

While these public health priorities occupy the majority of government effort and funding, other risk factors for the population abound. For example, alcohol, illicit drugs, and poverty among certain groups are also major issues facing public health services. Alcohol-related crashes are responsible for more than 4,000 deaths annually and more than 47,000 hospitalizations (Commonwealth of Australia, 2006). A particular facet of alcohol-related health is trauma due to drink driving.

This case study is an example of how one state government (Victoria) is addressing the problem.

The Problem of Drink Driving in Australia

In Australia, the term "drink driving" refers to a motorist who is driving after the consumption of alcohol and is impaired to some degree. Unlike in the United States, the term "drunk driving" is rarely used in Australia, and when it is, it is used mainly to refer to someone suffering from the effects of alcohol, such as a slurring of words or stumbling. This distinction may be due to the fact that in Australia, the general belief of the community is that one does not need to be visibly drunk to be impaired and dangerous behind the wheel; hence, the wide-scale problem is *drink driving*, and thus the term *drunk driving* is too narrow and misleading.

Road fatalities became an increasingly serious issue in the 1970s and 1980s in Australia. According to the Australian Transport Safety Bureau (ATSB), there were 3,798 road fatalities in 1970, representing 30.4 deaths per 100,000 persons, or 8 per 10,000 registered vehicles. The number of deaths fluctuated within the 3,000 to 4,000 range throughout the 1970s and mid-1980s. Early efforts by government agencies did help bring attention to the issue within the community but had little or no effect on driving behaviors.

In 2001, on average in Australia, road accidents resulted in one death each day, one severe brain injury occurred every four days, a paraplegic or a quadriplegic was produced every 17 days, someone was admitted to the hospital every three hours, and there was a person injured every 30 minutes (Transport Accident Commission [TAC], 2002). On roads only within the state of Victoria, 330 people died, 6,642 people were seriously injured, and 16,274 people suffered minor injuries. Across the whole of Australia, road accidents cost the country AU$17 billion (approximately US$12.5 billion) in 2003, more than the annual defense budget. These statistics portrayed a very grim reality, especially considering that they described one of the safest jurisdictions in the world in terms of road accidents at the time. In 2000, Australia was rated the 11th safest nation out of all OECD nations[1] in regard to the road toll

---

[1]The Organization for Economic Co-operation and Development (OECD) is a group of 30 countries whose work covers economic and social issues. The OECD is a measure often used by Australia for international comparisons covering a range of issues. The OECD is comprised of the following countries: Australia, Austria, Belgium, Canada, Czech Republic, Denmark, Finland, France, Germany, Greece, Hungary, Iceland, Ireland, Italy, Japan, Korea, Luxembourg, Mexico, Netherlands, New Zealand, Norway, Poland, Portugal, Slovak Republic, Spain, Sweden, Switzerland, Turkey, United Kingdom, and United States.

per 100,000 population and the 8th safest for the number of deaths per 10,000 registered vehicles (Australian Transport Safety Bureau, 2002).

Statistics like those mentioned provide an explanation as to why the WHO recently reported its prediction that road traffic injuries would be "the third leading contributor to the global burden of disease and injury" by 2020 if appropriate action is not taken (World Health Organization [WHO], 2004, p. 1). According to WHO, an estimated 1.2 million people are killed worldwide every year in road crashes, while an additional 50 million are injured.

Reducing Drink Driving: Past Efforts and Major Milestones

VicRoads is a government organization that focuses on the roads themselves, vehicles, traffic management, driver licenses, and regulation. VicRoads launched smaller public education campaigns throughout the 1980s in Victoria, which also had little or no effect on the community's attitudes and behaviors. It was in 1986 that the first all-encompassing step was taken to combat the road toll. Under the Victorian Transport Accident Act of 1986, the Transport Accident Commission (TAC) was established.

The TAC is a third-party government insurance agency whose mission is to "ensure that road accident victims received adequate compensation and the cost of road accidents to the community was reduced" (TAC, n.d.). The TAC is responsible for paying the compensation and early rehabilitation costs for people injured in transport accidents and also for minimizing the cost and occurrence of transport accidents. With regard to its responsibility of minimizing the cost and occurrence of transport accidents, the TAC implemented a variety of initiatives, from a graphic advertising campaign to the execution of stationary random breath testing. It is this advertising campaign that is examined in this chapter's case study.

CASE STUDY
Anti–Drink Driving Campaign

CAMPAIGN BACKGROUND, PURPOSE, AND FOCUS

In late 1989 the Transport Accident Commission of Victoria hired GREY Advertising Melbourne to develop an advertising campaign that would bring road safety to the forefront of the community's social agenda. The goal of the campaign was to make motorists, regardless of age or gender, reconsider their attitudes and behaviors with regard to drink driving and speeding. Moreover, advertisements were needed to promote two new initiatives, random breath-testing (RBT) "booze buses" and speed cameras. The resulting drink driving campaign was a theme that would remain unchanged and in use from December 1989 to November 2003. Under the banner, "If you drink, then drive, you're a bloody idiot," 20 television advertisements were produced between 1989 and 2000 (see Figure 16-1). These ads, along with the legislation and enforcement that supported them, were considered to play an important role in the minimization of deaths on the road resulting from drink driving.

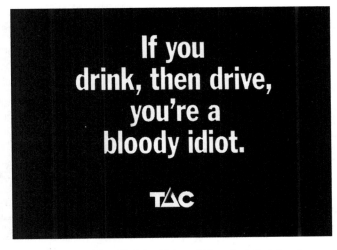

FIGURE 16-1   The Drink, Drive, Bloody Idiot tagline
Courtesy of the Transport Accident Commission and GREY Advertising Melbourne, Australia

This initiative was successful due to the integration of three major campaign elements, which can be summarized by the tripartite model for behavioral compliance: a legislation element, an enforcement element, and an advertising element. This model is illustrated in Figure 16-2. Because space does not allow all three elements to be examined in-depth in this chapter, here is a brief synopsis.

Legislation

Over the course of four decades, 11 regulations and pieces of legislation were introduced in Victoria that were directly related to efforts to minimize drink driving. They ranged from setting the BAC, or blood alcohol concentration, limit at 0.05 to dictating penalties and broadening enforcement circumstances.

Of all the legislation implemented in Victoria, there are three major pieces that had notable influences on changing drink driving behaviors: the legal BAC limit, the legality of random breath testing, and the immediate suspension of licenses for drink driving offenders.

Blood alcohol concentration is a measurement of the amount of alcohol in the body. In Victoria,

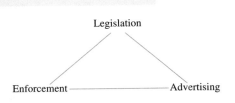

FIGURE 16-2   The tripartite model of behavioral compliance for effective social marketing campaigns

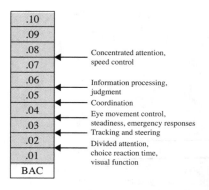

FIGURE 16-3   BAC levels and impairment

NHTSA, as cited on MADD's web site: http://www.madd.org/stats/0,1056,1182,00.html (accessed on 07/06/04)

and all of Australia, the legal BAC allowed for fully licensed drivers is 0.05 (which means motorists may not have more than 50 milligrams of alcohol per 100 milliliters of blood in their bodies). This level has been the law since 1966, well before drink driving became a societal issue. Therefore, the BAC level has not been an issue of vocal debate among Victorians—it is mostly accepted that the legislators who created this law did the research to ensure that 0.05 was an appropriate level. This has since been confirmed by an array of research studies that have shown that impairment from alcohol can begin at levels as low as 0.02 (Burns & Fiorentino, 2001; Moskowitz, 2001; Preusser, 2002). Figure 16-3 illustrates varying levels of impairment based on BAC levels.

The legality of random breath testing, implemented in 1976, is another key piece of Victorian legislation. The Victoria Police are allowed to breath test any driver in any vehicle anywhere in the state. Also, any motorist over the age of 15 who is taken to a hospital after an accident must allow a blood sample to be taken and analyzed.[2] It is important to note that a major reason this legislation was accepted by the community is the Australian concept of "mateship": that Victorians put the community good before the rights of the individual.

The third important piece of legislation is the legal penalties for driving with a BAC over the 0.05 limit. The BAC level at arrest plays a large role in determining the severity of punishments for drink driving. Therefore, less discretion is involved in assigning the punishments, and those who have acted grossly irresponsibly (driving with an extremely high BAC) are penalized differently than those whose actions may not be viewed as equally irresponsible (driving with a BAC slightly over the legal limit.) The majority of illegal BACs result in an immediate, on-the-spot suspension of license, ranging in length from six months to two years. Monetary fines of varying degrees are also imposed on offenders.

Enforcement

In terms of enforcement, Victoria found a "silver bullet"—a solution to a problem that, when implemented properly, had a relatively immediate and profound effect on the issue at which it was aimed. Random breath testing, as noted earlier,

---

[2]This rule does not apply if the first doctor responsible for the patient's care or treatment believes the taking of a blood sample would be prejudicial to the individual's proper treatment or care.

is the ability for police to test drivers for an illegal BAC without any suspicion of impairment. This is done in two ways in Victoria: stationary and mobile RBT. Stationary RBT is when police set up booze buses (mobile, RV-like police units with evidentiary breath-testing units on board) along streets and the highways, and test drivers randomly selected as they approach a booze bus (see Figure 16-4). Mobile RBT is when police officers pull drivers over for another offense (such as speeding) and additionally test their BAC. In both cases, motorists are given a breath test that takes 30 seconds—if their BAC is 0.049 or

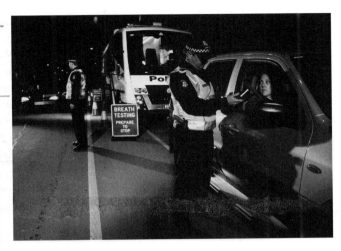

FIGURE 16-4   A Victoria police mobile breath testing stop
Courtesy of the Transport Accident Commission and GREY Advertising Melbourne, Australia

below, they simply roll up the window and drive on. If they fail the preliminary BAC test, they then must take a test on an evidentiary machine. If they fail this test, dependent upon the BAC level, their licenses are immediately suspended or they are issued a fine on the spot. Victorian RBT policies utilize deterrence theory when executing their random breath testing—*deterrence* is a method of gaining control through the use of fear (of being caught). Legislation created in Victoria now dictates that "every police car is a booze bus," meaning that every traffic stop in the state may result in a breath test.

Advertising

As will be discussed in more detail later, Victoria utilized a combination of high-fear, emotional threat advertising and low-fear, informational advertising to educate Victorians about drink driving legislation and enforcement and to alter community attitudes regarding the acceptability of drink driving. The campaign was part of integrated marketing campaign (IMC), which promoted the same message throughout multiple media outlets and through sponsorship of high-profile Victorian events. The drink driving campaign had a theme that remained unchanged and in use from December 1989 to November 2003. This allowed for a clear and consistent message to be delivered over time to many people. A majority of these advertisements contained emotive, graphic, shock-style threat appeals. Some of the ads were enforcement-related, utilizing an informative style. One was humorous, specifically related to the TAC's sponsorship of a sporting team. A majority of the ads remained on air for three to five years, rotated between enforcement and emotive styles and alternated with other road safety messages (e.g., speed, fatigue, and seat belt use).

The purpose of the campaign was twofold: (1) to reduce the negative health behavior of drinking and driving, and (2) to change the attitude of the Australian community that drink driving was an acceptable behavior.

TARGET AUDIENCES

At the broadest level, the entire Victorian community was the target audience of this campaign, because a major goal of the campaign was to make drink driving a socially unacceptable behavior. Therefore, the attitudes of the entire community—both those who drove and those who were passengers—had to be addressed and (ideally) altered. The overall target audience for the campaign was "Australian motorists" because the state borders are permeable and it is not possible to constrain a campaign within state boundaries. However, segmentation of the audience is a critical aspect of social marketing. The "bloody idiot" campaign contained advertisements targeted at families, at younger drivers, and at rural drivers. While the "drink, drive, bloody idiot" slogan was targeted at the entire Victorian community, individual advertisements were themed to segments of that greater audience. Older drivers and younger drivers had different viewpoints on drink drivers and drink driving and thus needed different advertisements targeting their concerns (e.g., taking care of their family versus peer acceptance). Understanding target groups was a key program strategy for the TAC. Each of these segments could have responded to different cues in advertisements they felt were relevant to their lives. To this end, the TAC commissioned Sweeney Research to conduct market research before and after each advertisement was run to ensure an understanding of what was relevant to each group. This allowed the TAC to design various advertisements specifically geared toward each of the various segments of their target audience.

CAMPAIGN OBJECTIVES

The campaign comprised three different types of objectives in terms of behavior, knowledge, and belief.

Behavior Objectives

The primary behavior objective of this campaign was to decrease the amount of drink driving through the increase of the adoption of alternate behaviors (including designating a driver, walking, utilizing public transport, and taking a cab). It was believed this would result in a decrease in alcohol-related crashes and, therefore, injuries and death. Research demonstrated that a decrease in crashes of at least 13% could be expected (Elder et al., 2004) as a result of mass media campaigns. Advertising, legislation, and enforcement would be a powerful combination.

Each phase of the campaign was built on promoting a different desirable behavior. In the early stages of the campaign, the focus was on changing attitudes and promoting safer alternatives. Later phases built in the appearance of social norms relating to drink driving and providing skills to support behavioral change. In addition to their messages about the effects of drink driving (with images of death, injury, and grief), the TAC advertisements also advocated the alternative, desirable behaviors noted earlier.

Knowledge Objectives

The TAC wanted to develop an awareness of the consequences of drink driving. Utilizing informational, low-fear threat advertisements throughout the "bloody idiot" campaign, they simultaneously served two different purposes. This style of advertising increased the target audiences' awareness of the repercussions of getting caught perpetrating the undesirable behavior, in addition to increasing their fear that they would actually be caught. In this case, the repercussions included fines, an immediate loss of license, and condemnation from family and friends. The informational advertisements were also used to highlight and reinforce the message that community members would be caught if they performed this behavior, due to random breath testing and the fact that every police stop, regardless of the offense (such as a broken taillight), resulted in a breath test. The objective was to ingrain the knowledge in all Victorians of the risks and the consequences of committing the undesirable behavior.

Belief Objectives

Changing people's beliefs about drink driving represented the major challenge for the TAC campaigns. First, drinking has always been embedded in Australia culture, with most social functions being "lubricated" by alcohol. Second, there was an established culture of car ownership that saw a car as defining the self (Solomon, 2002). This made it very difficult to go out to a social occasion without the cherished car, leaving some to feel that they had no choice but to drink and drive. Thus, a major longer-term objective was to shift some of the entrenched beliefs about what it meant to be a social Australian who did not drink and drive.

In contrast to the informational, low-threat ads, the TAC used the high-fear, emotive advertising to show the damaging effects of drink driving. The creation of the societal attitude that drink driving was considered unacceptable was a way to convince community members that it was instead acceptable to drink less and drive your car, or to drink the same amount but leave the car at home.

Attitude change influences behavioral change, and vice versa. It can be difficult to change one if the other remains stationary. However, in regard to the issue of attitude and behavior change related to advertising goals, there is sufficient evidence that indicates that forced behavior change often leads to long-term changes in attitude (Donovan, Henley, Jalleh, & Slater, 1995). In addition to attempts to change community attitudes through high-fear, threatening advertising, forced behavior was simultaneously changed through booze bus enforcement and the application of deterrence theory. The change in behavior in turn led to changes in attitude.

BARRIERS, MOTIVATORS (BENEFITS), AND COMPETITION

Barriers to Performing the Behavior

There were many barriers the campaign had to contend with when trying to get Australians to reduce and ultimately cease the undesirable behavior of drink driving. The most prominent of these barriers were the social culture of drinking in Australia, individuals' inability/difficulties in gauging their BAC levels, the remoteness in the rural areas of Australia, intentions versus actions, and the perception of a difference between drink driving and drunk driving.

- *The social culture in Australia is a major barrier to change.* Alcohol plays a major role in the larger Australian social society, and it is understood that beer consumption is an Australian pastime (Pettigrew, 2002). Its function is versatile, illustrated by the clichéd image of "mates having a few drinks 'round the barbie," the prevalence of alcohol at sporting events, and the almost iconic status of the major beer brands. Australians were the ninth largest per capita consumers of beer in the world as of 1999 (Commonwealth of Australia, 2001). In a country in which alcohol is ingrained to such a degree in the culture, some of the negative consequences of alcohol consumption (e.g., drink driving) are bound to occur.

• *Gauging BAC is a problem.* One of the major problems discovered during this case study was the lack of knowledge regarding BAC that exists in the community. People simply cannot tell if they are over the limit or not. The direct consequence of this is "guesstimating" BAC levels and taking a risk by driving without certainty. Because BAC can be influenced by an individual's metabolism, their levels of sleep and recent food consumption, the pace at which they are drinking, and the size of their drinks (not all drinks served are one standard drink), there is no absolute guide to determining one's BAC. Potential solutions, including coin-operated breathalyzers and handheld breathalyzers, that were available were not reliably accurate or consistently maintained.

• *The bush telegraph is used in rural areas.* While random breath testing through the use of booze buses was demonstrated to be one of the most effective road safety tools for metropolitan Melbourne, it was also demonstrated to be quite counterproductive in rural Victoria. Through research conducted by the Monash University Accident Research Centre (Cameron, Diamantopoulou, Mullan, Dyte, & Gantzer, 1997), it was uncovered that booze buses were actually increasing the level of deaths in alcohol-related accidents on minor roads in small country towns. When booze buses were implemented in these small towns, the "bush telegraph" was put into use. *Bush telegraph* is a term used to describe when people in a small community contact each other to notify them of where the breath testing is occurring so that they can drive alternate routes. The outcome of this was that motorists were still drinking and driving, but they were taking back roads that were poorly lit, poorly maintained, and less familiar to them. These factors, enhanced by the effects of alcohol, resulted in an increase in deaths along those back roads.

• *My intentions were good (but my actions were a problem).* One issue that warrants attention is that regardless of how good an individual's intentions were when they were sober, plans changed once they were intoxicated. A motorist may have driven to a pub with the intention of taking a cab or getting a ride home, but if she or he drank enough, her or his behavior often subsequently contradicted those intentions. This highlights the fact that advertising in itself is of little assistance once a motorist is drunk and still in a position to drive (i.e., has access to a car). Therefore, it was important to promote alternative desirable behaviors that involved leaving the car at home.

• *I'm not drunk; I've only had a few.* Victorian community members were shown to draw a distinction between "drink driving" and "drunk driving," which then led to some attitudinal difficulties. Although the gray area between the two varied by community member, a strong distinction was drawn. *Drink driving* was perceived to occur after someone had an amount of alcohol that did not necessarily appear to impair him or her—they were not slurring their words or falling over. Conversely, all community members identified *drunk driving* as driving when an individual was critically affected by alcohol—through visible behaviors such as the slurring of words or stumbling when trying to walk. This distinction between drink driving and drunk driving led to the growth of several undesirable attitudes: that driving a little bit over the legal limit was not a problem, that driving short distances was an acceptable behavior, and that there was not any harm driving at BAC levels below the legal limit.

Motivators and Perceived Benefits

While there were many barriers to convincing Australians to avoid drinking and driving, there were many motivations and perceived benefits highlighted throughout the campaign: motivating drivers to avoid the risk of losing their license on the spot, of having to pay a fine, or of losing points on their license. A motivating factor was also the conviction that avoiding drinking and driving was the socially correct thing to do; this was best exemplified through a focus on the Australian culture of "mateship"—taking care of others and being concerned and acting in their best interests. The benefits of drinking and driving should not outweigh the perceived costs.

Competition

The TAC campaign had sufficient resources to overcome much of the competition for "mind space." However, the competition for the hearts and minds of drink drivers still took a generation to succeed. For example, the alcohol industry still advertises nationally at more than AU$125 million (US$112 million) per year (Cornelius, 2008). While currently the industry is constrained by legislation to advertise drinking responsibly, most drinkers believe that they *are* drinking responsibly. Further, the advertising industry is strongly lobbying for less legislation around alcohol advertising under the banner of freedom of speech.

Perhaps the strongest competition for these campaigns is the aforementioned culture of drinking prevalent in Australia. Overcoming this culture will take generational change. To this end, the TAC is partially funding organizations such as Drinkwise, an evidence-based organization focused on promoting change toward a more responsible drinking culture in Australia. Drinkwise is aimed at parents to help inform them about how their drinking may influence their children's choices about drinking in the future.

Further competition for the TAC message comes from the large amount of advertising and clutter that exists in Australia (with more than AU$9 billion, about US$8 billion, spent annually; Cornelius, 2008). This has generated stronger and stronger messages in an effort to cut through the clutter.

POSITIONING

One of the major goals of the TAC's "bloody idiot" campaign was to position drink driving as a socially unacceptable and dangerous behavior. Alternate behaviors—including designating a driver, taking public transport, and leaving the car at home—were positioned as replacements that could be used to eliminate the undesirable behavior.

CAMPAIGN STRATEGIES (4Ps), IMPLEMENTATION, AND EVALUATION

Product Strategies

The core benefits of the campaign were that decreasing alcohol intake would lead to a "safer" existence. That is, if you kept your intake at a moderate level (less than 0.05), then you would be able to drive home safely, you would not hurt others, and you would not be fined (or lose your license). The practice of drinking moderately (keeping one's BAC under 0.05) was the actual product. The augmented products were the random breath tests and police "presence," speed cameras, Web site information, bumper stickers, stubby holders (beer can coolers), and so on. Just about anything drinking related can be found with a TAC logo. However, while there is a great deal of merchandise available, not all items are officially endorsed. Notwithstanding the lack of official support, these additional items provide tangible reminders of the implicit threat of being caught drink driving.

Pricing Strategies

One of the largest costs to the audience is having to give up the social and emotional value of drinking—in addition to having to give up driving after drinking. Australia's culture highly values both drinking and driving (often over long distances). Hence, the cost of not drinking and driving was originally seen as being very high. In Australia, people who do not drink are sometimes ostracized, and people who do not drive after drinking lose their autonomy. The TAC, therefore, had to develop a value for the product that decreased the perceived cost of not drinking and increased the perceived risk of getting caught. Some of the costs presented were fines (financial) and/or loss of license if caught (time and financial cost of alternative transport), physically hurting friends and/or family (emotional), loss of income (financial), loss of "face" or embarrassment at getting caught (psychological), and loss of autonomy (psychological). Some of the benefits presented were increases in individual actions being socially responsible, or mateship appeal (emotional); the ability to still have fun as a designated driver (social and emotional); and increased well-being from drinking in moderation (financial and physical).

Place Strategies

Drink driving takes place in both urban and rural areas, although it is more prevalent in rural districts. This is partially due to the lack of available alternatives (such as public transportation) and a stronger drinking culture in rural Australia. For the campaign to be effective, the combination of placement of enforcement techniques, advertising, and education strategies was highly scientific. Algorithms for where the enforcement would be placed were developed in conjunction with the police and the proposed advertising campaign (including timing and location). This was to ensure that the highly localized and targeted techniques had maximum impact. The elements of a particular campaign would be combined. For example, billboard advertising would be present with a snapshot from a TV ad, because both were a curiosity builder (before the TV campaign) and a reminder (during and after the TV campaign). New media were also used to distribute the messages. For example, "Go Melbourne" was an online program created to encourage community members to plan how they were going to get home before they went out drinking. A downloadable guide was developed and posted on a TAC Web site, which included all of the licensed (alcohol-serving) premises in metropolitan Melbourne and all of the train, tram, and bus locations, as well as taxi stands. Also utilizing the Internet, a Web site was created for young drivers who have their learner's permits to educate them about the rules and risks associated with drinking and driving.

Promotion Strategies

The TAC "bloody idiot" campaign was an integrated campaign that combined mass media with relevant new media. Mass communication was a driving feature of the campaign, illustrated by the 70% use of the budget on television advertising (GREY Advertising Melbourne, 1995). This was aided by a large-scale IMC campaign. Multiple mass communication channels were used for this campaign, as was recommended by Wallack and Dorfman (2001), in order to ensure that the message reached the audience and directed them to the behaviors they were supposed to undertake. Press, radio, outdoor, Sky Channel, and cinema advertising were all used, as was the Internet in the latter stages of the campaign. Expanding from the main media, promotional products were distributed ranging from T-shirts to bike lights. These media and promotional tools were used to promote TAC's position as a road safety organization committed to the Victorian community.

Market research conducted prior to the campaign recommended that the key messages had to be "acceptable" to the target audiences; the advertising style had to be "attention-grabbing" and confronting; the ads should be localized to the communities to increase their salience; and the campaign should be resourced to a high degree, which ensured that key target groups received high levels of the campaign messages (Healy & Forsyth, 1996). To this end, the TAC spent millions of dollars on both advertisement development and media buy to place the advertisements (Cameron & Newstead, 1996).

Because the target audience was so broad, the decision was made to segment the audience according to the type of appeals that would be most effective in each subgroup. Emotional appeals focused on images and feelings, while informational/rational appeals emphasized deductive logic, objective informational content, and cognitive processing. Informational appeals gave the consumer target audience details about what was being advertised. For consumer products, informational appeals provided details about the benefits and qualities of the product (Belch & Belch, 2009). In public health campaigns, informational advertisements gave details about new legislation, enforcement efforts, or options for help (e.g., a hotline to call). Emotional appeals tried to elicit feelings and emotions in relation to a product or a brand. The emotional appeals used by the TAC leveraged fear, guilt, and shame to help break through advertising clutter and to make the issue personal to individual Australians.

Each of the phases of the campaign was built around a different type of cost or price. Some advertisements focused on the immediate grief experienced by those directly affected by a drink driving death. Others illustrated the long-term effects of a crash, ranging from a lifetime of rehabilitation to lost productivity from physical impairment or the lack of a job due to not being able to get to work without a license. Two specific examples are outlined here:

- In *Bush Telegraph*, a father has a last beer, pushed into his hand by his friends as "one for the road," before he heads off with his young son.

After remarking to his son, "maybe I should have passed on that last beer," they drive off; after driving through a stop sign, their car is demolished by a tanker truck (see Figure 16-5). The implication of death is without question, and the scene ends with the same friends who started the ad by literally saying, "Go on, take it, one more beer won't kill you" receiving a call that their friend and his young son are dead. The feeling of guilt is palpable as the "drink, drive, bloody idiot" slogan fades off the screen. The cost of living a lifetime with guilt was enhanced by the knowledge that not only could they have stopped the death of a friend, but indirectly they were responsible for it.

- *Glasses* was an advertisement that utilized both informational and emotive approaches. The ad began with a car driving on a highway, looking out at the road from the driver's point of view. A pint glass comes on the screen, in the driver's line of vision. Four pint glasses are brought into the field of view sequentially, with each one increasing the blurriness of the scene ahead. This was educational in showing the visual impairments that result from increasing levels of alcohol in the blood (see Figure 16-6). With the pint glasses blurring the road ahead, it is jarring when the car slams into a parked truck. The advertisement shifts into the emotive phase as it continues, with police delivering the news to the deceased's wife. She crumples into hysterics, as a young daughter starts crying and keeps asking, "What's wrong mummy? What's wrong?" The heartbreaking emotion the mother experiences emphasizes the cost to those who are left behind after a drink driving death.

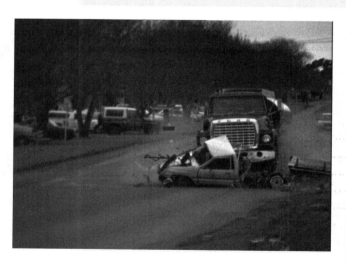

FIGURE 16-5   A screen shot from *Bush Telegraph*, an example of the highly graphic, high-fear advertisements utilized by the TAC

Courtesy of the Transport Accident Commission and GREY Advertising Melbourne, Australia

In conjunction with these hard-hitting ads, there were also ads that presented more subtle costs such as the loss of "face" due to being unable to drive to work and the potential loss of income for those who need to drive to work. Each advertisement had a clear indication of the cost of noncompliance. Each ad was designed to demonstrate this cost to a different emotional appeal segment.

In addition to the shock of the content of the advertisements, which featured realistic crashes, bodies, and the emotional aftermath, there was some shock around the slogan theme itself. In the late 1980s, the use of the word "bloody" was akin to swearing. The use of such a word in primetime television, on large billboards, and on radio was compounded by the fact that the proponent of the slogan was a government agency. The direct outcome of this was intense publicity and media scrutiny.

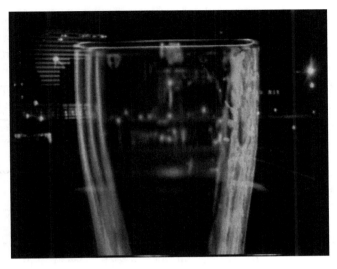

FIGURE 16-6   A screen shot from *Glasses*, which illustrates the visual effects of alcohol impairment from behind the wheel

Courtesy of the Transport Accident Commission and GREY Advertising Melbourne, Australia

CAMPAIGN BUDGET AND TIME FRAME

One of the major contentions about the TAC advertising campaign was its cost. The TAC spent millions of dollars annually (approximately AU$16 million, about US$9 million) both on producing the television advertisements and on media spend to place them (TAC, 2004a), in addition to the creation and placement of radio advertisements, billboards, and the other aspects of their IMC campaign. Critics of the TAC's advertising campaigns argue that the massive advertising spending and highly dramatic tactics may not have been necessary to secure similar results, if the amount of enforcement and media spending were equal to that which was spent in Victoria (e.g., Donovan, Jalleh, & Henley, 1999). Although the TAC advertising was successful in the reduction of casualty crashes, the use of less costly and perhaps less dramatic advertisements could be more cost beneficial.

Research has documented that persistence and a long time frame are essential aspects of a successful social marketing campaign (Chapman Walsh, Rudd, Moeykens, & Moloney, 1993). The "If you drink, then drive, you're a bloody idiot" slogan ran unchanged from December 1989 to October 2003 in Victoria and was present in any aspect of the TAC ads related to drink driving. The campaign lasted 14 years, which is a long time in advertising terms. Therefore, a long time frame and persistence were both achieved.

Although outside the scope of this chapter, the TAC's "drink, drive, bloody idiot" campaign is in place to this day. The theme has been slightly changed to reflect the changing attitudes and behaviors of the community members. The new slogan is, "Only a little bit over? You bloody idiot."

CAMPAIGN OUTCOMES

Behavioral

The tripartite approach is the platform for success in this campaign. In the case of Victoria, all three aspects were present and integrated. Legislation was implemented, enforced, and advertised. Enforcement was also advertised. Advertising turned drink driving into a socially unacceptable behavior. Accordingly, the number of driver deaths on Victorian roads related to alcohol dropped from more than 100 in 1989 at the start of the campaign to approximately 50 in 2000 (TAC, 2004). While the numbers have fluctuated slightly since the end of the period examined in this case study, to date the numbers are still more than 50% lower than they were at the start of the campaign.

Interviews with community members indicated that behaviors have distinctly changed over the past 15 years in the state. While 15 years ago many Victorians would drink and drive, regardless of the distance they had to travel, who was in the car with them, or how close they were to the legal limit, today these behaviors have, for the most part, been abandoned by the greater Victorian community. Instead, more desirable behaviors have been adopted. The younger community members tend to leave their cars at home, designate drivers, and generally try to plan their transportation ahead of time. The older respondents take taxis a majority of the time and walk or take public transport at other times. If they drink, they have their partners (the designated drivers) drive home. Those interviews also indicated that the use of personal breathalyzers and BAC calculations based on body weight and number of drinks are new behaviors adopted by some community members to avoid driving with an illegal BAC.

Community members have also changed their behaviors in relation to the drinking and driving of others. Hesitations over trying to stop a family member or close friend from drinking and driving seem nonexistent today, whereas 15 years ago stopping someone from drink driving was not a consideration. In addition to discouraging others from drink driving, there is a general sense of reluctance for sober individuals to get into a car with a drink driver.

Some undesirable behaviors have not yet been eradicated. There are still some drivers who have minimized their drink driving but will drive when they feel they are only slightly over the limit or when they are only driving short distances. There are also those who drink drive intentionally when they are well over the legal limit; these recidivists (repeat offenders) represent a very small percentage of the community but a large percentage of the drink driving offenders.

Knowledge

It has been documented through a decline in the road toll and quantitative studies that Victorian attitudes regarding drink driving have changed over the past two decades. In 1989, drivers did not think about "drink driving"; it was a nonissue. If you went out and drank, you drove home. If the police stopped you, they would generally give you a warning and let you go. No one condemned the behavior, so no one gave it much thought. Drinking and driving was simply the "norm." Now, attitudes have shifted on two different levels. Drinking and driving is considered a socially unacceptable thing to do—those who do drink and drive are often condemned by their family members and peers. Most community members will not drink and drive because they believe the behavior is wrong. The other new attitude is that the consequences of drink driving are not worth the risk.

Belief

Although the attitude of the majority in the Victorian community toward drink driving has changed, a minority of the population still believes that drink driving is not wrong under any circumstances or that drink driving is acceptable under certain conditions. Some interviewees said they would be more likely to chastise others for being "stupid enough to get caught," which indicates that some community members believe that driving a bit over the limit is not a serious offense. This belief is representative of a new barrier to anti–drink driving campaigns—the community needs to be fully convinced and constantly reminded that drinking even a bit over the limit is dangerous and is, therefore, an undesirable behavior.

SUMMARY

The TAC advertising campaign has followed the principles of social marketing, utilizing many strategies recommended by Chapman Walsh and others (1993):

1. Persistence and a long time frame are essential.
2. Segmentation of the audience is critical.
3. Understanding target groups is a key program strategy.
4. Teaching consumers skills supports behavior change.
5. The integration of feedback improves program effectiveness.

The success of the TAC campaign has shown the importance of using social marketing theory to guide the development and implementation of social marketing campaigns. By adopting time-tested techniques successful for commercial advertisers, the TAC was able to make its road safety messages pertinent to the Victorian community and, therefore, gain the audience's attention. It has been illustrated that none of the tripartite model components was strong enough on its own to change behaviors. It was only through the support of the other elements that change could be achieved and maintained. Although 0.05 legislation was in place in Victoria as early as 1966, this legislation was not strictly enforced until 1990. The RBT by itself would not have been accepted as quickly and easily as it was, had it not been for the advertising that positioned drink driving as a social threat and socially unacceptable act, triggering a community desire for reducing this threat.

The advertising itself, while bringing the drink driving issue to the forefront of community concern and even affecting the attitudes of some, was not strong enough by itself to motivate a large number of community members to alter their behavior. It was only when the legislation was enforced and the issue was made a public concern that behaviors, as well as attitudes, were changed. Throughout Victoria's drink driving campaign, all three aspects were present and integrated. Legislation was implemented, enforced, and advertised. Enforcement was also advertised. Advertising positioned drink driving as a socially unacceptable act. Hence, the number of deaths on Victorian roads related to alcohol dropped significantly.

QUESTIONS FOR DISCUSSION

1. Which elements of the TAC's "bloody idiot" campaign do you think would be transferable to other efforts to change undesirable health behaviors?

2. Which components of the campaign do you believe were the most successful in altering community attitudes and behaviors?

3. If you were planning a social marketing campaign but had a more limited budget than the TAC, which elements would you decrease reliance on?

ACKNOWLEDGMENT

The authors would like to thank Caitlin Brennan for her research assistance in the preparation of this case study.

REFERENCES

Australian Bureau of Statistics. (2009a). *Population clock*. Retrieved July 28, 2009, from http://www.abs.gov.au/ausstats/abs%40.nsf/94713ad445ff1425ca25682000192af2/1647509ef7e25faaca2568a900154b63

Australian Bureau of Statistics. (2009b). *Australian social trends*. Retrieved July 28, 2009, from http://www.abs.gov.au/AUSSTATS/abs@.nsf/mf/4102.0?opendocument?utm_id=LN

Australian Transport Safety Bureau. (2002). *International road safety comparisons: The 2000 report*. Civic Square, Canberra ACT: Author.

Belch, G. E., & Belch, M. A. (2009). *Advertising and promotion: An integrated marketing communications perspective* (8th ed.). Boston: McGraw-Hill Irwin.

Black, A. (1995, January 1). It's official: Vic roads worlds safest. *Sunday Herald Sun*, pp. 8–9.

Burns, M. M., & Fiorentino, D. (2001). *The effects of low BACs on driving performance*. Washington DC: Transportation Research E-Circular.

Cameron, M., Diamantopoulou, K., Mullan, N., Dyte, D., & Gantzer, S. (1997). *Evaluation of the country random breath testing and publicity program in Victoria, 1993–1994* (No. CR 126). Clayton: MUARC.

Cameron, M., & Newstead, S. (1996). *Mass media publicity supporting police enforcement and its economic value*. Paper presented at the Public Health Association of Australia 28th Annual Conference.

Chapman Walsh, D., Rudd, R. E., Moeykens, B. A., & Moloney, T. W. (1993). Social marketing for public health. *Health Affairs*, 104–119.

Commonwealth of Australia. (2001). *Alcohol in Australia: Issues and strategies*. Canberra: Commonwealth Department of Health and Aged Care.

Commonwealth of Australia. (2006). *National alcohol strategy: Towards safer drinking cultures*. Retrieved July 28, 2009, from http://www.alcohol.gov.au/internet/alcohol/publishing.nsf/Content/B83AD1F91AA632ADCA25718E0081F1C3/$File/nas-06-09.pdf

Cornelius, P. (2008). *Australia's top advertisers* (Special report). Melbourne, Australia: Nielsen Media Research Pacific.

Donovan, R., Henley, N., Jalleh, G., & Slater, C. (1995). *Road safety advertising: An empirical study and literature review*. Canberra: Donovan Research for Federal Office of Road Safety.

Donovan, R., Jalleh, G., & Henley, N. (1999). Executing effective road safety advertising: Are big production budgets necessary? *Accident Analysis and Prevention*, 31, 243–252.

Elder, R. W., Shults, R. A., Sleet, D. A., Nichols, J. L., Thompson, R. S., & Rajab, W. (2004). Effectiveness of mass media campaigns for reducing drinking and driving and alcohol-involved crashes: A systematic review. *American Journal of Preventive Medicine*, 27(1), 57–65.

GREY Advertising Melbourne. (1995). An entry into the 1995 AFA Effectiveness Awards by GREY Advertising Melbourne (Category: Social Advertising).

Healy, D., & Forsyth, I. (1996, September 30). *Road safety mass media advertising in Victoria*. Paper presented at the Symposium on Mass Media Campaigns in Road Safety, Scarborough Beach, WA.

Moskowitz, H. (2001). *Laboratory studies of the effects of low BACs on performance*. Washington, DC: Transportation Research E-Circular.

Pettigrew, S. (2002). A grounded theory of beer consumption. *Qualitative Market Research*, 5(2), 112–122.

Preusser, D. F. (2002). *BAC and fatal crash risk*. Paper presented at the 16th International Conference on Alcohol, Drugs and Traffic Safety, Montreal, Canada.

Solomon, K. (2002). *My car, my space, my life: Young people's attitudes to driving*. Unpublished Honours Thesis, Monash University, Clayton, Victoria, Australia.

Transport Accident Commission (TAC). (2002). *2002 TAC Annual Report*. Melbourne: Transport Accident Commission.

Transport Accident Commission (TAC). (2004). *Drink driving statistics*. Retrieved July 28, 2009, from http://www.tacsafety.com.au/jsp/content/NavigationController.do?areaID=12&tierID=1&navID=A9348A54&navLink=null&pageID=164

Transport Accident Commission (TAC). (2007). *BAC statistics*. Retrieved July 28, 2009, from http://www.tacsafety.com.au/jsp/content/NavigationController.do?areaID=12&tierID=1&navID=A9348A54&navLink=null&pageID=164

Transport Accident Commission (TAC). (n.d.). *VCE Legal Studies Resource*. Melbourne: Author.

Wallack, L., & Dorfman, L. (2001). Putting policy into health communication. In R. E. Rice & C. K. Atkin (Eds.), *Public communication campaigns* (3rd ed., pp. 389–399). Thousand Oaks, CA: Sage Publications.

World Health Organization (WHO). (2004). *World report on road traffic injury prevention* (abstract only). Geneva: Author.

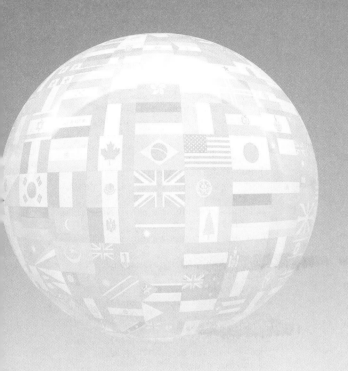

Index